SO-EJV-432

STATUS OF THE CURABILITY OF CHILDHOOD CANCERS

The University of Texas System Cancer Center
M. D. Anderson Hospital and Tumor Institute
24th Annual Clinical Conference on Cancer

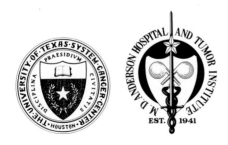

Published for
The University of Texas System Cancer Center
M. D. Anderson Hospital and Tumor Institute
Houston, Texas, by Raven Press, New York

The University of Texas System Cancer Center
M. D. Anderson Hospital and Tumor Institute
24th Annual Clinical Conference on Cancer

Status of the Curability of Childhood Cancers

Edited by

Jan van Eys, Ph.D., M.D.
and
Margaret P. Sullivan, M.D.

Department of Pediatrics
The University of Texas System Cancer Center
M. D. Anderson Hospital and Tumor Institute
Houston, Texas

RC 261
A 2
C 641c
1979

Raven Press ▪ New York

367564

Raven Press, 1140 Avenue of the Americas, New York, New York 10036

© 1980 by Raven Press Books, Ltd. All rights reserved. This book is protected by copyright. No part of it may be reproduced, stored in a retrieval system, or transmitted, in any form or by any means, electronic, mechanical, photocopying, recording, or otherwise, without the prior written permission of the publisher.

Made in the United States of America

Library of Congress Cataloging in Publication Data

Clinical Conference on Cancer, 24th, Anderson Hospital
    and Tumor Institute, 1979.
    Status of the curability of childhood cancers.

    Includes indexes.
    1. Tumors in children–Congresses. 2. Prognosis–
Congresses. I. Van Eys, Jan. II. Sullivan,
Margaret P. III. Anderson Hospital and Tumor
Institute, Houston, Tex. IV. Title. (DNLM:
1. Neoplasms–In infancy and childhood–Congresses.
2. Neoplasms–Therapy–Congresses. QZ266 S797 1979)
RC281 . C4C54 1979   618.92'994075   79-5469
ISBN 0-89004-478-3

This volume is a compilation of the proceedings of The University of Texas System Cancer Center M. D. Anderson Hospital and Tumor Institute 24th Annual Clinical Conference on Cancer, held November 8 and 9, 1979, in Houston, Texas.

The material contained in this volume was submitted as previously unpublished material, except in the instances in which credit has been given to the source from which some of the illustrative material was derived.

Great care has been taken to maintain the accuracy of the information contained in the volume. However, the Editorial Staff and The University of Texas System Cancer Center cannot be held responsible for errors or for any consequences arising from the use of the information contained herein.

Preface

Childhood cancer is a small part of the overall morbidity of cancer. However, pediatric oncology has become the benchmark for achievements in clinical cancer research and treatment development. Indefinite, continuous, complete, unmaintained remissions are commonplace for children with cancer. It is therefore rational to talk about cures in childhood cancer. Cure does not mean that children with cancer have survived 5 years; rather, it means that children will not die of their cancer within the period of a normal life-span. It is hard to face cure as a concept; it is easier to assume that the disease is always there, just controlled. But that is a self-serving protection for physicians. The "almost cure" allows continued control of the patient; it allows the view that the medical status of the child is always transient and never an end point. Yet it is clear we do cure the cancers, and that permanent late effects are the price for that cure. Therefore, there is need for a conference that examines the status of the curability of childhood cancers, to meet the challenge of the concept of cure, to define cure so that we can learn from the consequences of our methods of cure. In that way we may begin to learn about the process of cancer—what makes children who get it different from those who don't.

With a cure rate of approximately 50%, care and cure of cancer in children are decades ahead of care and cure of cancer in adults. It is true that childhood cancers are quantitatively and often qualitatively different from cancers in adults. It is true that children are not just small adults. They do tolerate chemotherapy significantly better than do adults, but that is not the whole story. In fact, focusing on such differences between childhood and adult oncology obscures the significant and real advances made in childhood cancer care. There is not one obvious breakthrough that can be identified as the singular point of departure for this progress. If there has been a breakthrough, it has been the willingness of all concerned with the care of the child with cancer to work together. Real multimodal approaches with surgery, radiotherapy, chemotherapy, immunotherapy, and pharmacological monitoring are accepted as the norm in pediatric oncology. Cooperative trials with agreed end point reporting and statistical control began in pediatrics. Supportive therapy has made chemotherapy feasible. Care of the whole child is a generally accepted concern. Long-term follow-up is understood as a major need. A real attempt at laboratory approaches to pediatric cancer is reemerging. It is from those steps that amazing progress, from the introduction of antifolates and actinomycin D by Sidney Farber to the 50% cure mark, was realized in the short span of 30 years. Even a decade ago, cure was only a realistic hope and not an accepted achievement.

This conference should be a celebration. But cure has its consequences. Cure comes at the price of late effects, not only the obvious consequences of ablative surgery, but also late effects of radiotherapy and chemotherapy. There are psychological and social consequences. Children who have had cancer are not the same as children who never contracted the disease. Children who survive cancer are not the same children they were before the disease. But the cure rate is so high that having had cancer as a child will become epidemic in the population. The late effects of therapy will be with us for many years. The need to learn how to minimize the physical and psychological costs is of the highest priority.

One of the most dreaded of the late effects is the development of second malignancies. Since our success spans only a few decades at most, the full magnitude of that problem is not known. It teaches us the sobering lesson again that no disease is ever conquered by cure. But the phenomenon of second malignancies has given us the unique opportunity to observe the development of cancer in a well-defined population prospectively. Lessons in the epidemiology of cancer are beginning to emerge. We are beginning to talk about prevention. We are beginning to discuss tailoring our therapy to the patient, identifying those patients at especially high risk of second malignancies. The view of cancer as an acquired or inherited genetic disease is compelling.

One theme of this conference was well summarized by Dr. Hartmann, who observed that "in pediatric cancer we slew a dragon maybe only to have awakened a new one." While this is an up-to-date summary of the status of childhood cancer care, these proceedings contain little retrospective description: there is no resting on laurels. Instead of crushed laurels, the reader will find the future. The future is still uncertain, but filled with renewed hope.

Many who attended this conference were present at the previous conference on childhood cancer held at M. D. Anderson Hospital in 1969. The promise of cure, voiced so carefully then, is now at least partially realized. There is now promise of an understanding of etiology and a realization of prevention. It is hoped that this volume will be used as a basis for designing epidemiological, therapeutic, psychological, and laboratory studies to conquer cancer once and for all. A decade hence, a new conference may document major further progress.

The Editors

Acknowledgments

We would like to thank all those who helped make this 24th Annual Clinical Conference possible, especially the National Cancer Institute, the American Cancer Society, Texas Division, Inc., and the *National Enquirer.*

We are grateful to the members of the Program Committee, Jan van Eys and Margaret P. Sullivan, cochairpersons, Alberto G. Ayala, Robert D. Lindberg, Ellen R. Richie, Marvin M. Romsdahl, and W. W. Sutow, for organizing the conference.

Finally, we would like to extend our appreciation once again to the Department of Scientific Publications, M. D. Anderson Hospital and Tumor Institute, and especially to Diane L. Culhane, Editor, for compiling and editing this monograph.

Contents

Status of the Curability of Hemopoietic Malignant Diseases

The Future Beyond Cure

Contributors

Alberto G. Ayala
Department of Pathology
The University of Texas System Cancer
  Center
M. D. Anderson Hospital and Tumor
  Institute
Houston, Texas 77030

Jean B. Belasco
Children's Cancer Research Center
The Children's Hospital of Philadelphia
Philadelphia, Pennsylvania 19104

Robert Benjamin
Department of Developmental
  Therapeutics
The University of Texas System Cancer
  Center
M. D. Anderson Hospital and Tumor
  Institute
Houston, Texas 77030

J. M. V. Burgers
Werkgroep Kindertumoren Emma
  Kinderziekenhuis
Antoni van Leeuwenhoek Ziekenhuis
The Netherlands Cancer Institute
Amsterdam, The Netherlands

James J. Butler
Department of Pathology
The University of Texas System Cancer
  Center
M. D. Anderson Hospital and Tumor
  Institute
Houston, Texas 77030

Ayten Cangir
Department of Pediatrics
The University of Texas System Cancer
  Center
M. D. Anderson Hospital and Tumor
  Institute
Houston, Texas 77030

Patricia Carter
Department of Nutrition and Food Service
The University of Texas System Cancer
  Center
M. D. Anderson Hospital and Tumor
  Institute
Houston, Texas 77030

Rafael C. Chan
Division of Radiotherapy
The University of Texas Health Science
  Center at Dallas
Dallas, Texas 75235

Betsy Cohen-Teitell
Department of Nursing
The University of Texas System Cancer
  Center
M. D. Anderson Hospital and Tumor
  Institute
Houston, Texas 77030

Edward M. Copeland
Department of Surgery
The University of Texas System Cancer
  Center
M. D. Anderson Hospital and Tumor
  Institute
Houston, Texas 77030

Giulio J. D'Angio
Children's Cancer Research Center
The Children's Hospital of Philadelphia
Philadelphia, Pennsylvania 19104

J. de Kraker
Werkgroep Kindertumoren Emma
  Kinderziekenhuis
Antoni van Leeuwenhoek Ziekenhuis
The Netherlands Cancer Institute
Amsterdam, The Netherlands

J. F. M. Delemarre
Werkgroep Kindertumoren Emma
  Kinderziekenhuis
Antoni van Leeuwenhoek Ziekenhuis
The Netherlands Cancer Institute
Amsterdam, The Netherlands

Sarah S. Donaldson
Department of Radiology
Division of Radiation Therapy
Stanford University School of Medicine
Stanford, California 94305

G. J. Draper
Childhood Cancer Research Group
Department of Paediatrics
University of Oxford
Oxford, England

Philip R. Exelby
Department of Surgery
Memorial Sloan-Kettering Cancer Center
New York, New York 10021

Lawrence S. Frankel
Department of Pediatrics
The University of Texas System Cancer
  Center
M. D. Anderson Hospital and Tumor
  Institute
Houston, Texas 77030

Antonio Frias
Dwight D. Eisenhower Army Medical
  Center
Fort Gordon, Georgia 30905

Stephen L. George
Biostatistics Section
St. Jude Children's Research Hospital
Memphis, Tennessee 38101

John R. Hartmann
Division of Hematology/Oncology
The Children's Orthopedic Hospital and
  Medical Center
Seattle, Washington 98105

Robert C. Hickey
Executive Vice President
The University of Texas System Cancer
  Center
Director
M. D. Anderson Hospital and Tumor
  Institute
Houston, Texas 77030

Norman Jaffe
Department of Pediatrics
The University of Texas System Cancer
  Center
M. D. Anderson Hospital and Tumor
  Institute
Houston, Texas 77030

F. Leonard Johnson
Division of Hematology/Oncology
The Children's Orthopedic Hospital and
  Medical Center
Seattle, Washington 98105

Alfred G. Knudson, Jr.
The Institute for Cancer Research
The Fox Chase Cancer Center
Philadelphia, Pennsylvania 19111

Nancy L. Krejmas
Children's Cancer Research Center
The Children's Hospital of Philadelphia
Philadelphia, Pennsylvania 19104

Charles A. LeMaistre
President
The University of Texas System Cancer
  Center
M. D. Anderson Hospital and Tumor
  Institute
Houston, Texas 77030

Brigid G. Leventhal
The Johns Hopkins Oncology Center
The Johns Hopkins University School of
  Medicine
Baltimore, Maryland 21205

Bruce Mackay
Department of Pathology
The University of Texas System Cancer
  Center
M. D. Anderson Hospital and Tumor
  Institute
Houston, Texas 77030

Anna T. Meadows
Children's Cancer Research Center
The Children's Hospital of Philadelphia
Philadelphia, Pennsylvania 19104

Robert W. Miller
Clinical Epidemiology Branch
National Cancer Institute
Bethesda, Maryland 20205

John A. Murray
Department of Surgery
The University of Texas System Cancer
  Center
M. D. Anderson Hospital and Tumor
  Institute
Houston, Texas 77030

Chris O. Ortiz
Department of Nursing
The University of Texas System Cancer
  Center
M. D. Anderson Hospital and Tumor
  Institute
Houston, Texas 77030

Betty Pfefferbaum
Department of Pediatrics
The University of Texas System Cancer
  Center
M. D. Anderson Hospital and Tumor
  Institute
Houston, Texas 77030

Donald Pinkel
Division of Pediatrics
Familian Children's Hospital
City of Hope National Medical Center
Duarte, California 91010

Irma Ramirez
Department of Pediatrics
The University of Texas System Cancer
  Center
M. D. Anderson Hospital and Tumor
  Institute
Houston, Texas 77030

Ellen R. Richie
Department of Pediatrics
The University of Texas System Cancer
  Center
M. D. Anderson Hospital and Tumor
  Institute
Houston, Texas 77030

Marvin M. Romsdahl
Department of Surgery
The University of Texas System Cancer
  Center
M. D. Anderson Hospital and Tumor
  Institute
Houston, Texas 77030

Margaret P. Sullivan
Department of Pediatrics
The University of Texas System Cancer
  Center
M. D. Anderson Hospital and Tumor
  Institute
Houston, Texas 77030

W. W. Sutow
Department of Pediatrics
The University of Texas System Cancer
  Center
M. D. Anderson Hospital and Tumor
  Institute
Houston, Texas 77030

H. Grant Taylor
Department of Pediatrics
The University of Texas System Cancer
  Center
M. D. Anderson Hospital and Tumor
  Institute
Houston, Texas 77030

O. A. van Dobbenburgh
Werkgroep Kindertumoren Emma
  Kinderziekenhuis
Antoni van Leeuwenhoek Ziekenhuis
The Netherlands Cancer Institute
Amsterdam, The Netherlands

Jan van Eys
Department of Pediatrics
The University of Texas System Cancer
  Center
M. D. Anderson Hospital and Tumor
  Institute
Houston, Texas 77030

A. Vos
Werkgroep Kindertumoren Emma
  Kinderziekenhuis
Antoni van Leeuwenhoek Ziekenhuis
The Netherlands Cancer Institute
Amsterdam, The Netherlands

P. A. Voûte
Werkgroep Kindertumoren Emma
  Kinderziekenhuis
Antoni van Leeuwenhoek Ziekenhuis
The Netherlands Cancer Institute
Amsterdam, The Netherlands

William J. Zwartjes
Department of Oncology and Hematology
The Children's Hospital
Denver, Colorado 80218

Introduction

Charles A. LeMaistre, M.D.

President, The University of Texas System Cancer Center

I am pleased to welcome you to the 24th Annual Clinical Conference. Each fall The University of Texas System Cancer Center sponsors this forum to allow practicing physicians to share current information on cancer therapy and discuss mutual problems in the hope that a sounder knowledge of a particular type of cancer will result.

Over the years, the key to the success of M. D. Anderson's clinical conferences has been the timely choice of topics, each selected to represent an area of intense clinical investigation in which rapid changes made sharing of new information imperative. This year's conference is no exception. "The Status of the Curability of Childhood Cancers" comes at a time when more pediatric cancer patients than ever before are being cured, and when measures are being taken to ensure that the future lives of those patients are as full as possible.

There is another reason the timing of this conference is opportune. As I am sure you are all aware, 1979 has been designated the International Year of the Child. The year has been dedicated to the improvement of the lives of children throughout the world. Certainly the area of children's health is one that bears scrutiny during this year. We are pleased to dedicate this conference to improving the health of children with cancer, and to honor those of you who have devoted not only this year but every year to helping children.

The accomplishments in the area of cancer in children are readily apparent to anyone who studies the control and cure rates achievable in many types of pediatric cancer today and compares them to the rates of just a few years ago. By reviewing the results published in the monograph from M. D. Anderson's last clinical conference on childhood cancers, *Neoplasia in Childhood,* we can see how far pediatric cancer management has advanced in the last decade or so.

In his opening remarks at that 1967 conference, Dr. R. Lee Clark observed that "all of us are especially hopeful, even optimistic, that we can attain success in curing or controlling cancer in these children." I know many of you here today attended that conference and some of you presented papers. It must give you a great sense of accomplishment to know that those hopes have been realized for more than half of all childhood cancer patients.

During that conference, much attention was focused on the treatment of

Wilms' tumor, then as now the second most common solid malignant tumor in children. Encouraging progress was then beginning to be made with a multimodal approach that included chemotherapy. The addition of dactinomycin and vincristine sulfate marked a turning point in the management of Wilms' tumor. The 2-year survival rate was about 49% in 1967. Today the cure rate is more than 90% for patients with localized tumors, and the overall survival rate, even in those with spread of disease, is 80%. The management of Wilms' tumor has progressed to the point where patients today can be treated with equal success by their own physicians and at major cancer centers.

Osteosarcoma was another solid tumor that was regarded in 1967 as carrying a hopeless prognosis in almost all patients. The 5-year survival rate had remained unchanged for decades, ranging from 5% to 20%, regardless of treatment. With the addition of adjuvant multidrug chemotherapy to surgery in the mid-1970s, more than half of such patients are now free of disease after 3 years or more.

A third solid tumor discussed in detail in 1967 was rhabdomyosarcoma, which had a 5-year overall survival rate of about 35%. In one paper presented at that conference, Dr. Wataru Sutow described a course of treatment called VAC, a combination of vincristine, actinomycin D, and cyclophosphamide. That treatment has since proved to be extremely successful in the management of rhabdomyosarcoma, especially when used with other agents. By full use of the multimodal approach, rhabdomyosarcoma is now controllable in 90% of patients, and 80% are surviving free of disease for longer than 5 years.

Additionally, some of the hematopoetic malignancies have shown encouraging results, aided by the delineation of distinguishing characteristics and better staging procedures. Probably the greatest success has occurred in acute lymphocytic leukemia. Some time ago the addition of chemotherapy to existing treatment forms enabled physicians to obtain remission rates of 80–90%, but median survival was only 3 years. Now, through the use of maintenance chemotherapy, central nervous system prophylaxis, and supportive measures, therapy can be discontinued after 3 years, with only a 20% subsequent relapse rate, in children with good prognoses. Good remissions are now achievable in acute granulocytic leukemia patients who can tolerate the maximum amount of therapy. The favorable progress in the treatment of Hodgkin's disease has meant that minimal treatments can be outlined for patients with favorable presentations to minimize late effects of therapy.

The gratifying upswing in the outlook for childhood cancer patients has brought pediatric oncologists to the point of encountering new problems. Attention is now being given to questions about how the therapy children receive now will affect their later lives, both physically and mentally. Consideration is being given to normalizing the lives of childhood cancer patients while they are receiving treatment to ensure they will not be handicapped mentally and emotionally when they rejoin their peers. The last session of this conference is devoted to exploring these all-important points.

I would like to express my thanks to the National Cancer Institute and the Texas Division of the American Cancer Society for their assistance in co-sponsoring this conference. In addition, I would like to extend a special note of appreciation to the *National Enquirer* for its significant contribution toward the support of this conference.

HEATH MEMORIAL AWARD LECTURE

Status of the Curability of Childhood Cancers,
edited by J. van Eys and M. P. Sullivan.
Raven Press, New York © 1980.

Introduction of Heath Memorial Award Recipient

Robert C. Hickey, M.D.

Executive Vice President, The University of Texas System Cancer Center, and Director,
M. D. Anderson Hospital and Tumor Institute

The Heath Memorial Award recipient this year, Dr. Giulio J. D'Angio, is a distinguished academician and radiotherapist who graduated from Columbia University in 1943 and Harvard Medical School in 1946. He is currently Professor of Radiation Therapy and Pediatric Oncology at the University of Pennsylvania School of Medicine in Philadelphia.

Dr. D'Angio's training in pediatric pathology and radiology has been exemplary. From 1953 to 1964 he held radiation therapy posts of increasing responsibility at the Boston Children's Hospital, the Massachusetts General Hospital, and other institutions. In 1964 he became director of the Division of Radiation Therapy at the University of Minnesota, and in 1968, chairman of the Department of Radiation Therapy at Memorial Hospital for Cancer and Allied Diseases, as well as chief of the Division of Radiotherapy Research at Sloan-Kettering Institute. Dr. D'Angio assumed his present position at the University of Pennsylvania in 1976.

He has received much peer recognition as a radiotherapist, but Dr. D'Angio deserves a special accolade for his work in pediatric oncology. He is well known for his efforts to ensure that the treatment pediatric cancer patients receive will have as few harmful effects as possible. He was among the first to call attention to the late effects of radiation in children, and is the former chairman of a 13-institution study group that analyzed these late effects. He also organized the National Wilms' Tumor Study, which has served as the prototype for similar study groups.

Dr. D'Angio is currently chairman of the National Wilms' Tumor Study Committee, a Fellow of the American Academy of Pediatrics, and a member of numerous societies, including the American Association for Cancer Research, American College of Radiology, American Society of Therapeutic Radiologists, Royal Society of Medicine, and International Society of Pediatric Oncology. For his works, he has received a number of awards, including the American Cancer Society Annual National Award in 1978.

The Heath Memorial Award commemorates Guy H., Dan C., and Gilford

3

G. Heath, brothers of the late Judge William Heath, former chairman of the Board of Regents of The University of Texas System. It is presented annually to individuals who have made, in the words inscribed on the back of the medallion, "outstanding contributions to the care of the patient with cancer." Dr. Giulio J. D'Angio is a most fitting recipient.

Status of the Curability of Childhood Cancers,
edited by J. van Eys and M. P. Sullivan.
Raven Press, New York © 1980.

It Ain't Necessarily So

Giulio J. D'Angio, M.D.

*Department of Radiation Therapy, University of Pennsylvania, and
Children's Cancer Research Center, Children's Hospital of Philadelphia,
Philadelphia, Pennsylvania*

Sporting Life, one of the characters in the operetta *Porgy and Bess,* sings at one point, "The things that you're liable to read in the Bible—it ain't necessarily so."

I'm not here today to engage in a theological debate with religious fundamentalists. Insert "medical" before "Bible" and my topic will be clearer—or, to be even more precise, the line might read, "The things one may read or hear as current medical dogma—it ain't necessarily so."

What does this have to do with the status of the curability of childhood cancers, which is the focus of this conference? Let me explain. Certainly we can rejoice that better cure rates are being recorded in pediatric oncology. These can no doubt be attributed to the more widespread employment of modern, aggressive, multimodal therapy, but the very success of these proven methods has created its own perhaps predictable problems. It has, for example, led to the use of these often vigorous and therefore toxic therapies in blanket, indiscriminate attacks against any and all of a variety of malignant diseases at any stage; survival, when it follows, is cited as documentation of the efficacy of the specific treatments employed. Ladies and gentlemen—it ain't necessarily so, nor are cause and effect always clear even when simpler therapies are employed.

Childhood cancer is a complex of diseases, and diseases within diseases, that have their own special and sometimes seemingly contradictory natural histories. It is rather like a picture done as a mosaic. One can see the whole composition and can distinguish the individual components represented, but truly to understand the work, one must appreciate that the whole is made up of individual bits, each with its own shape, shading, and hue. Pediatric oncology is like that. It is no longer appropriate, for example, to ask, "How does one treat leukemia, or Wilms' tumor, or neuroblastoma, or rhabdomyosarcoma?" We now have knowledge, imperfect though it may yet be, of prognostic variables for these entities—the shapes, shades, and hues, if you will, of the disease mosaic. The question posed a moment ago should be answered by another set of questions, "What age is the child?" "What stage is the tumor?" "What was the initial white blood cell count?" Then therapy can be fitted to the threat to life and well-being, and—important for this and similar conferences—the efficacy of any treatment can be evaluated with better accuracy.

Let me try to be more specific, and to do so largely by recalling personal observations made over the years with the collaboration of numerous colleagues to whom I remain eternally grateful. Let us first consider a benign condition, the hemangioma. It is well recognized that hemangiomas may grow for a period, but that the vast majority undergo spontaneous resolution. In short, simple observation is all that is usually required.

There are exceptions, however. Laryngeal lesions and cavernous hemangiomas involving the parotid regions provide examples (Figure 1). These tumors tend to involve more of the nearby tissues as they grow. Laryngeal obstruction can result and kill the patient. The parotid hemangioma, if left untreated, sometimes enlarges to involve adjacent structures, or it may ulcerate. The consequent scarring or the engrossment of contiguous parts can produce irremediable deformities, as shown in the baby in Figure 1. The tracheostomy tube needed to prevent asphyxia can be seen, as can the progression of the lesion over the passage of some weeks to affect the pinna of the ear extensively. There also is ulceration of the central portion of the lesion.

Radiation therapy was given to this child. Tangent fields were used to avoid the underlying developing mandible and tooth buds. The deeper portions of the lesion were thus left untreated, but this was all right. What was needed was a reminder for Mother Nature to speed her work—there is no need in such cases to be aggressive and to use large fields or high doses. Modest doses of a few hundred rad each were delivered to selected portions of the lesion, without any attempt to include the entire tumor. Figure 1 *(right bottom)* shows the results several years later. The tumefaction is gone, but there is residual deformity because of the ulceration, and there is elephantiasis of the pinna. Thus, several years later there is little trace of the severe deformities present in infancy. The patient is a very normal-looking girl, with her hair combed

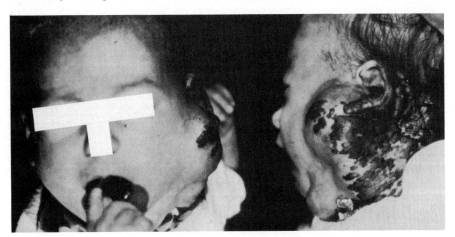

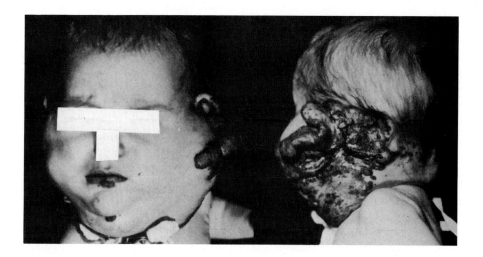

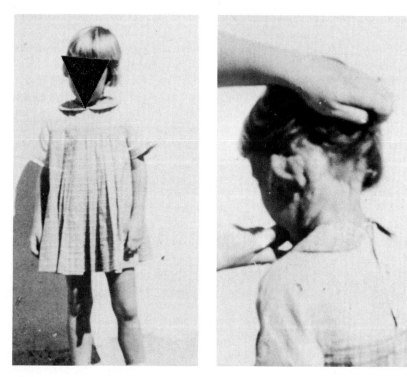

Figure 1. Left, Infant girl with capillary and cavernous hemangioma involving lip, face, larynx, and left side of face and parotid. Top, Enlargement and spread of lesions a few weeks later. Bottom, Appearance several years later.

down on the left, and there is nothing to remind us of the grotesque deformity of the face that was present many years before.

Several points can be made in reviewing this case. First, hemangiomas can enlarge with time. Second, they undergo spontaneous resolution, as did the untreated lesions in the case just described. Let me pause here for a moment. Anyone giving routine treatment to children with strawberry hemangiomas, regardless of whether the therapy involves high doses of vitamins, the spreading of salves, or the twiddling of dials, would be able to claim great success for his methods. But we could all sing in unison, "It ain't necessarily so," couldn't we? The third point I would like to make is that treatment is nonetheless sometimes needed. The case just reviewed illustrates some of the indications. The Kasabach-Merritt syndrome, or so-called platelet-trapping hemangioma, provides another because of the associated coagulopathy, which can be life threatening in some patients. Fourth and fifth, if radiation therapy is used, modest doses to part of the lesion suffice to initiate resolution, which can then be left to proceed on its own. The therapist thus can exclude the more sensitive structures from even the low treatment doses that are administered in such circumstances.

Let us now consider another lesion, histiocytosis X. This is not a monolithic entity, it is now generally agreed. Eosinophilic granuloma of bone is rarely lethal, but it can lead to deformity and local problems. One problem is the so-called wafer vertebral body. Recommendations regarding management have included the administration of a few hundred to a few thousand rad of radiation therapy, the use of anticancer chemotherapeutic agents or antibiotics, and various other measures. How successful are these treatments? A retrospective study undertaken at the University of Minnesota some years ago can be cited in this regard (Nesbit et al. 1969). The method used in the analysis was based on follow-up X-ray films taken of the same child over a period of years. The growth capacity of the collapsed bone was assessed by measuring its subsequent increase in vertical height, if any, with time, and by comparing the dimensions with those of a normal vertebral body immediately above or below the diseased one. The heights of the two vertebral bodies were then plotted according to time. One of the vertebral bodies that was totally collapsed and was given radiation therapy retained its capacity for growth. The growth curve paralleled that of its normal neighbor. It might readily be concluded that radiation therapy is a very effective means of dealing with the problem.

It ain't necessarily so.

Another untreated collapsed vertebral body in the same child showed good residual growth capacity, and its growth rate also paralleled that of its normal neighbor. Other cases studied showed the same thing. It is thus clear that the results are the same, regardless of whether or not treatment is given. As with hemangioma, however, there are indications for radiation therapy, and again like hemangioma, the therapy is designed more to prevent or alleviate problems than to secure a given end result. Treatments can therefore be gentle and carefully attuned to solving a specific, usually transient difficulty. The investigators at the University of Minnesota, for example, concluded that irradiation should be used if there is local pain or only early collapse (Nesbit et al. 1969). Then it seems reasonable to avoid further loss of height by irradiating the part to arrest the process and to promote healing. What about the dose for eosinophilic granuloma of bone? Good results have been reported after 2,000 to 3,000 rad or more, and such doses, it might be concluded, should be used in these cases. The Minnesota group looked into this matter, also, and concluded that the response rate was not improved when doses in excess of 600 rad or so were used in various clinical settings (Smith et al. 1973).

This is not to say that all elements of the complex of diseases grouped together under the single term "histiocytosis X" can be treated in a similar fashion. There is no doubt that patients with widespread involvement of soft tissues are at pronounced risk. Rather, the conclusions can be drawn that eosinophilic granuloma of bone can be a self-limited process, that treatment is not mandatory immediately, that well-defined criteria should be met before treatment is given, and that relatively modest doses of radiation can produce the desired effect.

Why discuss benign and paramalignant conditions in a cancer conference? Because the principles elaborated in the discussion up until now have their counterparts in the natural histories of some of the malignant diseases that afflict children, and these, in turn, have obvious implications regarding both treatment and the accurate assessment of the results of that treatment. Certainly the general and specific, relatively straightforward methods that apply to cancer in adults are not always germane to those cancers that are found in younger patients. There are subsets of children within each tumor type whose clinical courses vary greatly. Some of these patients develop widespread metastases early, and currently available treatments are of little avail. Others with what seems to be the same tumor type have a clinical course that is remarkably benign. It is therefore essential that the clinician-investigator have a thorough grasp of the many nuances of pediatric oncology before he either prescribes treatment or judges its result in an individual child or a group of children with the same nominal diagnosis.

Neuroblastoma can be taken as an example. Surely neuroblastoma, being such a very malignant lesion, should be treated aggressively in all children if disaster is to be avoided. Not long ago it was almost universally accepted that a child with neuroblastoma required surgical removal of the primary lesion if at all possible, and that postoperative radiation therapy and chemotherapy should be given.

It ain't necessarily so.

Evidence, including a randomized clinical trial conducted by the Children's Cancer Study Group, now makes it clear that neither postoperative radiation therapy nor chemotherapy adds significantly to survival in children with stage I disease, that is, with tumors confined to the organ or structure of origin (Evans et al. 1976). That is not to say that every child with stage I disease will survive, although almost all will do so after simple surgery. In fact, all 22 stage I children in the Children's Cancer Study Group trial are living. Fourteen of them received no chemotherapy, and nine of these received no radiation therapy (Evans et al. 1976). Thus, it would appear that neither of the two therapeutic measures mentioned can be expected to make an appreciable difference in outcome. More remarkable, of course, are children with stage IV-S disease. As is well known, these include patients who have widespread involvement of the liver, the skin, the bone marrow, or any combination of those sites, but no roentgenographic evidence of osseous metastases (D'Angio et al. 1971). The striking fact is that the tumor cells in these patients continue to proliferate for a while and then disappear spontaneously. Some patients will show an enlarging nodule in one site while the disease is regressing in another. In short, the tumor cells in most of these patients go away with little if any therapy. A review of 31 IV-S children under 13 months of age by Evans and co-workers (1978) shows that 87% are surviving at 2 years, in sharp contrast with the 31 children with stage IV disease. The 2-year survival of the latter is 42%, and the curve has not plateaued yet (Figure 2).

Anyone who treats stage IV-S patients with vigorous chemotherapy, radiation therapy, or both, must keep these results with minimal treatment in mind before attributing to the treatments employed what will surely be a gratifyingly good survival rate. Indeed, this factor appears to have misled Bodian years ago when he reported excellent results in neuroblastoma children given vitamin B12

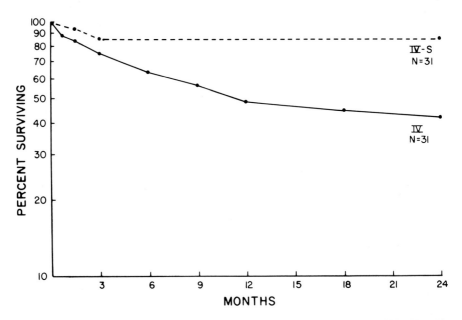

Figure 2. Survival of patients with metastatic neuroblastoma in the 1st year of life; life-table analysis by stage.

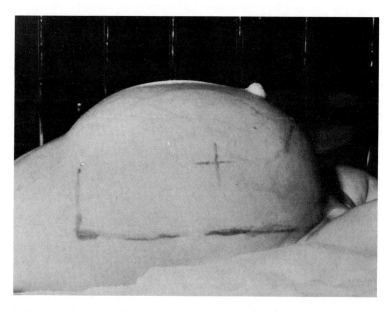

Figure 3. Patient with stage IV-S neuroblastoma, with massive liver enlargement. Skin marks indicate transverse table lateral portal used for radiation therapy.

(Bodian 1959). Many of his successes were achieved in what we now know were stage IV-S children. It is well, also, to recall the fact that infection secondary to immunosuppression following aggressive chemotherapy caused the only two deaths in another group of 20 stage IV-S children under 12 months of age reviewed a few years ago (Evans et al. 1971). Too vigorous therapy of these infants—and most stage IV-S patients are under 12 months of age—in inexperienced hands might well lead to worse, not better, results than those obtained with no treatment at all.

The major problem in these children arises from the site and size of the tumor, rather than from any propensity of the tumor to metastasize widely in the manner characteristic of cancer. The liver causes the chief difficulty. It can sometimes become enormous, completely filling the abdomen, as was true in the child shown in Figure 3. Under those circumstances, local compression of the renal vasculature, elevation of the diaphram, or both, can threaten survival by producing renal or pulmonary compromise. In other situations the disease in the liver can lead to an associated coagulopathy, which in turn can be lethal (Evans et al. 1980).

Does this sound like what was said when the lowly hemangioma was under discussion? If so, is it such a wrench to accept here what our own eyes see when we were comfortable with the same kinds of observations there? I do not wish to press the similarities too hard, but certain harmonies, at least, can be heard. The threat to life is again one of tumor site and size, rather than the inexorable course usually associated with the word "cancer".

Under these circumstances, the principles discussed for the management of the child with hemangioma can be applied to the patient with stage IV-S neuroblastoma. The aim of therapy should be to reduce bulk as might be needed, and this can usually be accomplished by gentle chemotherapy or by irradiation of the liver using opposing lateral fields directed upward about 5 or 10 degrees, the posterior edge of the beam being placed at the level of the anterior margin of the vertebral body so as to avoid the underlying kidneys and, in girls, the ovaries. Quite modest doses are then delivered. At the Children's Hospital of Philadelphia, 150 rad given on each of three successive days seem to have sufficed in some (Evans et al. 1980). In others an additional 450 rad have been necessary because regression of the liver was not sufficiently prompt. As with the child with hemangioma, then, a period of watchful waiting before any treatment is given is not unreasonable. When treatment is thought necessary, low doses to a portion of the tumor-bearing volume suffice to achieve the desired result.

These approaches to what is generally a most malignant tumor of childhood may at first glance seem bizarre, major departures from what is accepted as proper care for a cancer patient. But we are not dealing with cancer in the classic sense. Some of the neuroblastoma constellations, especially the one just described, behave in a fashion that makes one think of aberrations of embryological development and maturation, rather than cancer (D'Angio et al. 1971). The so-called in situ neuroblastoma described by Beckwith and Perrin (1963) fits this description, too. Indeed, it has been suggested that stage IV-S neuroblastoma can best be understood if one views the disease as a type of neurocristopathy with multifocal primary tumors, rather than metastatic involvement (Schimke 1980). I subscribe to that view. This is not to say that any one of the nodules may not have or develop full "malignant" properties, or that no child with stage IV-S will ever develop classical, progressive, stage IV neuroblastoma. That certainly can happen in an occasional child, and Knudson (1980) has suggested a mechanism to explain this seemingly contradictory behavior. Then the disease behaves as it does with neuroblastoma patients in general and cure may be difficult (Evans et al. 1971).

Examples of differences in clinical evolution that are associated with certain clinicopathologic patterns can also be cited for Wilms' tumor (Breslow et al. 1978). Several factors of prognostic importance in this disease were identified in the first National Wilms' Tumor Study (NWTS-1). First, one can no longer be satisfied with the simple diagnosis Wilms' tumor. Rather, one must specify whether the lesion is of the so-called favorable histologic (FH) type or falls into one of the categories grouped under the term unfavorable histology (UH). That this makes an enormous difference is shown by the fact that only 53 of 268, or 20%, of the NWTS-1 patients with FH relapsed, compared with 24 of 34, or 71%, of those with UH. Moreover, younger children with FH tumor have an excellent prognosis; fewer than 10% relapse and most of those can be retrieved, so the survival rate is extremely high. On the other side of the fence, patients with UH lesions and positive lymph nodes have a very poor prognosis; all 13 children in NWTS-1 with that combination of findings relapsed, and most died. These and the several other subsets of Wilms' tumor patients with different clinical courses who are being identified must be kept in mind whenever treatment regimens are being designed or their results evaluated.

Acute lymphatic and undifferentiated leukemias present similar echelons of aggressive behavior. Children with high initial white blood cell counts fare less well than those with counts under 20,000, for instance. There are other important facets of the disease that are only now becoming better understood—the role of central nervous system so-called prophylaxis, for example, and its impact on bone marrow relapse and survival rates.

The Children's Cancer Study Group undertook two randomized clinical trials to examine these questions. Patients were randomized among four treatment groups in one trial, CCG-101 (Nesbit et al. 1977). The first group received 2,400 rad to the craniospinal axis and 1,200 rad to the infradiaphragmatic organs, the thymus, and the testis in the boys. The second group received 2,400 rad craniospinal irradiation, the third received cranial irradiation with 2,400 rad plus intrathecal methotrexate (IT/MTX), and the fourth received only IT/MTX in doses that subsequent events made clear were insufficient. In a later study, CCG-143, patients were randomized between craniospinal radiation therapy and cranial radiation therapy plus IT/MTX, as in CCG-101, but the radiation therapy doses were reduced to 1,800 rad (Nesbit et al. 1979).

The various outcomes are shown in Table 1, where the CCG-143 patients are labeled 5 or 6 according to whether they were given axial or cranial irradiation, respectively. As can be seen, the results 4 years after randomization were similar in all the irradiated groups (Littman et al. 1979). Equal protection of the central nervous system was obtained, and the bone marrow relapse and survival rates are very much the same. Of great interest and importance, however, are the results in Regimen 4 patients, who were not irradiated and received only IT/MTX. Their CNS relapse rate is much higher, 38%, yet their bone marrow and survival rates are the same as those in the irradiated groups. These data can be interpreted to indicate that CNS relapse does not inevitably and

Table 1. *Percentages of Children Relapsing or Dying, by Intensification Regimen, 48 Months After Therapy for Leukemia*

Endpoint	CNS Intensification Regimen					
	1	2	3	4	5	6
Death	32	27	29	29	28	22
Bone marrow relapse	28	26	30	29	31	22
CNS relapse	5	8	9	38	3	14

inexorably lead to bone marrow relapse and death in children who are receiving good, modern, multiple-agent chemotherapy in competent hands.

This conclusion seems to run counter to the personal experience of many pediatric oncologists. They recall that patients who develop CNS disease almost inevitably go on to bone marrow relapse and death. But that sequence today applies chiefly to patients who have already had some good form of CNS protection and who then develop meningeal leukemia in spite of intrathecal medication, radiation therapy, or both.

It has seemed logical to assume, as a result of these kinds of observations, that the bone marrow is "reseeded" from the "sanctuary" site, but it ain't necessarily so. Another interpretation of the data and the observations cited is that there is a hard core of patients who have an especially aggressive, progressive form of leukemia, and for whom our current therapies are inefficient. Central nervous system disease after adequate protection is, in these patients, not a leading cause of worse to come, but rather an announcement that active disease is present and that bone marrow relapse and death can be predicted. For children not given effective CNS prophylaxis, meningeal disease has less ominous connotations, although the hard core is obviously going to be present in this subset, too. That seems the best explanation for the results in CCG-101; otherwise, why with such a high CNS relapse rate are the eventual bone marrow relapse and survival rates in Regimen 4 patients similar to those in patients given better CNS protection?

In summary, these results seem to mean that CNS prophylaxis does not have a major impact on bone marrow relapse and survival rates. Let it be made clear that there is every reason to provide "prophylaxis" of the CNS in poor prognosis patients at least, so that recurrent bouts of meningeal involvement with their disturbing side effects and potentially lethal outcomes can be avoided. Given this shift in focus, however, the elucidation of CNS problems in leukemia can proceed more deliberately, with the identification of CNS high-risk factors and devising of means of avoiding the undesirable and sometimes fatal secondary effects of some prophylactic methods currently in use. The CCG-143 results with 1,800 rad, for instance, encourage one to test low-dose radiotherapy regimens in suitable circumstances and not to be fixed on a "magic number" approach.

Still other examples can be adduced. In a major pediatric hospital, it was the practice to give postoperative irradiation to the ipsilateral iliac and para-aortic lymph nodes in boys with embryonal cell carcinoma of the testis. The results were excellent; all the children survived. Two observers at the same institution surveyed the results. One concluded that proper treatment included routine postoperative irradiation of the sites described; the other, a skeptic, concluded that if the results were uniformly good, treatment probably had little to do with the outcome, and recommended that no postoperative irradiation be given—a recommendation that now appears generally accepted.

It is the willingness of pediatric oncologists to entertain the null hypothesis in selected clinical situations that has led and will lead to a better understanding of the childhood cancers and the therapies that are appropriate and necessary for each condition. This is important because all treatments have their side effects, and the late deleterious consequences of cancer treatment are becoming factors of major concern as survival rates climb (D'Angio 1976). These delayed effects can take any of the following forms:

1. Disruption of function
   a. Impaired growth and development
   b. Damage to the central nervous system—psychologic, neurologic and intellectual
   c. Gonadal aberrations—reproductive, hormonal, genetic and teratogenic
   d. Disturbances of function in other organs and structures such as the liver, kidney and lung
2. Oncogenesis
   a. Benign
   b. Malignant

Surely, then, the aim of therapy must be to achieve maximum benefit at minimum price. A willingness to sing along with our friend from *Porgy and Bess,* therefore, is not being radical; it may well prove conservative in the truest sense, or preservative, if you will. Refining therapy to its bare, critical essentials has everything to recommend it when the tender tissues of children are under consideration.

Looking backward for a moment, we can see we have come a long way toward curing childhood cancer. Advances have been made largely through observations and treatments developed by individuals or groups in single institutions, and then confirmed in well-designed cooperative clinical trials. This one-two sequence has been extremely rewarding, and there is not only plenty of room for both types of investigation, but also a real need. Failure to follow that pattern can lead to such unfortunate situations as the current uncertainty regarding the role of high-dose methotrexate as adjuvant chemotherapy for osteogenic sarcoma.

Both individual institutions and cooperative groups have contributions to make to an understanding of the natural histories of childhood tumors—the one through sustained personal study, the other through modern statistical and computer methods that can be used to sort the myriad data accumulated in group data centers.

It is time to summarize. I could go back to *Porgy and Bess* and echo, "I'm preaching this sermon to show it ain't necessarily so." Let me take another tack, however, and do it quickly: childhood cancer is a labyrinth. It is easy for the unwary traveler to follow the mistaken path of *ad hoc* reasoning. This must be avoided like the plague, because, walking the wrong way, we not only lose time, but also are likely to fall into a trap, to the injury of the children we carry on our shoulders.

Now on to the conference, with this envoi, paraphrased from another well-known song from a different famous operetta—changed a little in wording, and much in intent:

> Our object, so sublime,
> We shall achieve in time:
> To let the therapy fit the threat,
> The therapy fit the threat.

ACKNOWLEDGMENT

This investigation was supported in part by grants CA-11722, CA-11796, and CA-14489, awarded by the National Cancer Institute, Department of Health, Education and Welfare.

REFERENCES

Beckwith, J. B., and E. V. Perrin. 1963. In situ neuroblastomas: A contribution to the natural history of neural crest tumors. Am. J. Pathol. 43:1089–1100.

Bodian, M. 1959. Neuroblastoma. Pediatr. Clin. North Am. 6:449.

Breslow, N. E., N. F. Palmer, L. R. Hill, J. Buring, and G. J. D'Angio. 1978. Wilms' tumor: Prognostic factors for patients without metastases at diagnosis. Results of the National Wilms' Tumor Study. Cancer 41:1577–1589.

D'Angio, G. J., ed. 1976. Proceedings of the National Cancer Institute Conference on the Delayed Consequences of Cancer Therapy: Proven and potential. Cancer 37(suppl.):999–1236.

D'Angio, G. J., A. E. Evans, and C. E. Koop. 1971. Special pattern of widespread neuroblastoma with a favorable prognosis. Lancet 1:1046–1049.

D'Angio, G. J., K. M. Lyser, and G. Urunay. 1971. Radiation Therapy Grand Rounds. Neuroblastoma, stage IVS: A special entity? Clin. Bull. 1:61–65.

Evans, A. E., V. Albo, G. J. D'Angio, J. Z. Finklestein, S. Leikin, T. Santulli, J. Weiner, and G. D. Hammond. 1976. Cyclophosphamide treatment of patients with localized and regional neuroblastoma: A randomized study. Cancer 38:655–660.

Evans, A. E., G. J. D'Angio, and J. Randolph. 1971. A proposed staging for children with neuroblastoma: Children's Cancer Study Group A. Cancer 27:374–378.

Evans, A., R. Chard, and E. Baum. 1978. Do children with IV-S neuroblastoma need treatment? Proc. Am. Soc. Clin. Oncol. 19:367.

Evans, A. E., J. Chatten, G. J. D'Angio, J. M. Gerson, J. Robinson, and L. Schnaufer. 1980. A review of 17 IV-S neuroblastoma patients at the Children's Hospital of Philadelphia. Cancer, in press.

Knudson, A. G., Jr. 1980. Why the genetics of neuroblastoma? *in* Advances in Neuroblastoma Research, A. Evans, ed. Raven Press, New York, in press.

Littman, P., G. J. D'Angio, M. Nesbit, H. Sather, J. Ortega, M. Donaldson, and D. Hammond. 1979. Radiation therapy (RT) factors in prophylactic central nervous system (CNS) irradiation for childhood leukemia: A report from Children's Cancer Study Group (CCSG) (Abstract). Int. J. Radiat. Oncol. Biol. Phys. 5(suppl.):99.

Nesbit, M., M. Donaldson, J. Ortega, R. Hittle, D. Hammond, J. Weiner, and H. Sather. 1977. Influence of an isolated central nervous system (CNS) relapse on subsequent marrow relapse in childhood lymphoblastic leukemia (ALL) (Abstract). Proc. Am. Assoc. Cancer Res. 18:143.

Nesbit, M. E., S. Kieffer, and G. J. D'Angio. 1969. Reconstitution of vertebral height in histiocytosis X: A long-term follow-up. J. Bone Joint Surg. 51A:1360–1368.

Nesbit, M. E., H. N. Sather, L. L. Robison, G. J. D'Angio, P. Littman, M. Donaldson, and G. D. Hammond. 1979. Presymptomatic CNS treatment in childhood acute lymphoblastic leukemia (ALL): Comparison between 1800 and 2400 rad (Abstract). Proc. Am. Soc. Clin. Oncol. 20:343.

Schimke, R. N. 1980. The neurocristopathies, fiction or fact, *in* Advances in Neuroblastoma Research, A. Evans, ed. Raven Press, New York, in press.

Smith, D. G., M. E. Nesbit, G. J. D'Angio, and S. H. Levitt. 1973. Histiocytosis X: Role of radiation therapy in management with special reference to dose levels employed. Radiology 106:419–422.

DEFINITIONS AND SCOPE

Status of the Curability of Childhood Cancers,
edited by J. van Eys and M. P. Sullivan.
Raven Press, New York © 1980.

Definitions and Scope

W. W. Sutow, M.D.

Department of Pediatrics, The University of Texas System Cancer Center M. D. Anderson Hospital and Tumor Institute, Houston, Texas

Twelve years ago at this conference, Dr. Sidney Farber (1969) cautiously charted the course for pediatric oncology. He identified the goals, and pointed out the landmarks in the slow progress to that point. Dr. Giulio D'Angio (1980) reviewed today the solid gains that have been made since that time. He told a remarkable success story.

Table 1 outlines the positive achievements that have been conceived, developed, field tested, and established by many who were here in 1967 and are in the audience again today. The principles and strategies demonstrate significant advances in the management of children with cancer.

In 1967 Dr. Farber stressed the "total care" concept. Since then we have learned, progressed, matured. At this conference today we are examining what might be termed the "total cure" concept—cure of the whole child. If total cure is our goal, then we need a good understanding of what constitutes total cure.

The first segment of this clinical conference will address that subject—first, by defining, from various viewpoints, the criteria for the cure of childhood cancer and, second, by identifying the scope of that goal.

Table 1. *Major Achievements in the Treatment of Childhood Cancers Since 1967*

Multidrug chemotherapy	Total care concept
Adjuvant chemotherapy	Recognition of late effects
Multidisciplinary cancer therapy	Genetic implications
"Sanctuary" therapy	Refinement of therapy
Cure of metastatic disease	Preoperative chemotherapy
Identification of prognostic factors	"Second look" operations

REFERENCES

D'Angio, G. J. 1980. It ain't necessarily so, *in* Status of the Curability of Childhood Cancers, J. van Eys and M. P. Sullivan, eds. Raven Press, New York, pp. 5–16.

Farber, S. 1969. The control of cancer in children, *in* Neoplasia in Childhood (The University of Texas System Cancer Center Twelfth Annual Clinical Conference on Cancer 1967). Year Book Medical Publishers, Inc., Chicago, Ill., pp. 321–327.

Status of the Curability of Childhood Cancers,
edited by J. van Eys and M. P. Sullivan.
Raven Press, New York © 1980.

Criteria for Biological Cure of Cancer

Donald Pinkel, M.D.

Division of Pediatrics, Familian Children's Hospital, City of Hope National Medical Center, Duarte, California

Biological cure of cancer means freedom from the disease without risk of relapse or need for further treatment. The patient biologically cured of cancer lives out his life without experiencing the cancer again and ultimately dies of some other disorder.

MEASURING THE BIOLOGICAL CURE RATE

In the patient biologically cured of a cancer, all cancer cells are eliminated or no longer behave like cancer cells. It is impossible to determine this clinically, so one must continue to follow these patients. Cured patients remain free of cancer after cessation of treatment and demonstrate little or no risk of relapse, recurrence, or metastases (Frei and Gehan 1971).

To determine whether patients are cured, they must be followed throughout their lifetimes for evidence of recurrence. If their cancers persist, a steady, possibly slow relapse rate should be expected. If the cancers do not persist, a plateau in cancer-free survival time should be observed, reflecting the absence of the cancer cell activity that would result in relapse. Graphs of cancer-free survival are the primary tools, then, for determining whether cancers are curable and in what proportions of patients. These graphs must be based on actual observations, rather than actuarial projections from preliminary data. In addition, semi-logarithmic scales are used to distinguish between apparent and real changes in relapse rates (Pinkel 1979b).

Cancer is a heterogeneous group of diseases with various natural histories and responses to treatment. The cure rate should be ascertained for each type of cancer in accordance with its clinical course. For example, medulloblastoma patients continue to relapse many years after initial therapy (Harisiadis and Chang 1977), while children with Wilms' tumors are usually free of the risk of recurrence if they remain continuously free of tumor for 2 years (Lemerle et al. 1976). Two-year disease-free survival suggests cure for children with Wilms' tumor, but not for those with medulloblastoma.

The age of the patient can be a variable in assessing cure. Infants with neuroblastoma have a higher cure rate than older children, independent of disease stage.

Infants who remain free of neuroblastoma for 1 year are usually cured, but older children can experience recurrences many years after initial treatment (Jaffe 1976, Pinkel et al. 1968). Again, with medulloblastoma, older children tend to relapse later than younger children (Harisiadis and Chang 1977). For this reason one must be more cautious in pronouncing cures of these tumors in older children.

Treatment is a major factor in curability. Children with acute lymphocytic leukemia treated by multiple drugs and preventive meningeal therapy have a higher cure rate than those treated by single drugs and no preventive meningeal therapy. However, treatment that results in longer remission and survival does not always lead to a higher cure rate (Pinkel 1979b).

Finally, as in all scientific assessments, reproducibility of data is important. A cure rate reported by one group of physicians needs to be confirmed by other groups who use comparable methods of diagnosis and treatment with comparable clinical skill.

In summary, the biological cure rate is measured by determining the plateau of continuous complete remission or cancer-free survival for a given type of cancer, taking into consideration patient age and treatment. Once this measurement is ascertained, one can predict the chance for cure of a given cancer patient on the basis of the patient's type of cancer, age, treatment, and duration of continuous freedom from evidence of cancer. If the patient's cancer-free survival time is well out on the plateau, the patient can be considered cured.

ESTABLISHING CURE RATES

Scant information is available about cure rates for childhood cancers treated by modern therapy. This is due in part to the relatively brief time since these methods were generally adopted, and in part to emphasis on such parameters as remission rate, median duration of remission, median survival, and 3 or 5-year survival. These parameters indicate advances in clinical control of cancer that may lead to better cure rates, but are not themselves measures of cure.

The present experience with acute lymphocytic leukemia in children illustrates the establishment of a cure rate for a form of cancer. In 1967–70, 76 children who developed complete remissions at one institution were treated with preventive meningeal irradiation and multiple-drug chemotherapy (Pinkel 1979a). Their initial continuous complete remission durations are illustrated in Figure 1. Approximately one half of the patients have remained in initial continuous complete remission for 9–11 years and have been off therapy for 6–9 years. Only one patient relapsed after 4 years of leukemia-free survival, and none relapsed after 5½ years. The patients currently surviving continuously free of leukemia demonstrate no risk of relapse and are presumptively cured.

The reproducibility of this cure rate is suggested by the results at another institution that used the same principles but different methods of therapy (Haghbin et al. 1980). Between 1969 and 1973, 70 children with acute lymphocytic

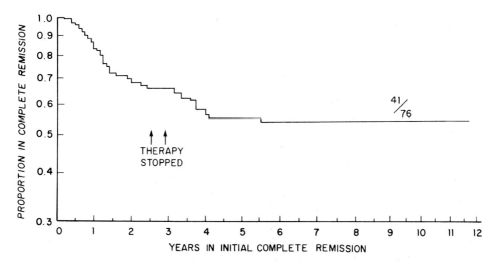

Figure 1. Semilogarithmic graph illustrating initial continuous complete remissions in children with acute lymphocytic leukemia who received preventive meningeal irradiation and combination chemotherapy in 1967–70 at St. Jude Children's Research Hospital.

leukemia developed complete remissions and subsequently received multiple-drug continuation chemotherapy and preventive meningeal treatment. Forty of the children have remained in continuous complete remission for 6–10 years and have been off therapy for 3–6 years (Figure 2). One child relapsed in the 3rd year after cessation of therapy and one in the 4th year, but none in the

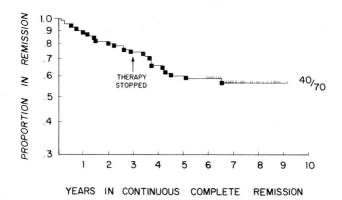

YEARS IN CONTINUOUS COMPLETE REMISSION

Figure 2. Semilogarithmic graph illustrating initial continuous complete remissions in children with acute lymphocytic leukemia treated with preventive meningeal therapy and combination chemotherapy at Memorial Hospital in 1969–73. The risk of relapse in survivors has diminished and a plateau of continuous complete remissions is being achieved. The configuration of the curve resembles that in the St. Jude study, suggesting that the cure rate for acute lympho-cytic leukemia is reproducible. (Reproduced with permission from Haghbin, M., et al., Cancer, in press.)

5th or 6th years. The results suggest that the children presently surviving free of leukemia are at little or no risk of relapse and are probably cured.

THE PROBLEM OF SECOND CANCERS

Children whose cancers have been removed or destroyed are at some risk of second cancers. Several mechanisms appear to be involved in causing these second cancers.

Some children's cancers are genetically determined. Second cancers that are phenotypically similar may develop in these children simultaneously with the first cancer or following its removal. In retinoblastoma and Wilms' tumor, for example, bilateral neoplasms often occur simultaneously or sequentially. The second cancers develop because of the vulnerability of a specific tissue to a specific genetic determinant. Less frequently, children with a genetic predisposition to cancer develop second cancers that are phenotypically different from the first. For example, osteogenic sarcoma sometimes develops in the limbs of children who have recovered from bilateral retinoblastoma (Aherne 1974). In this instance more than one tissue is susceptible to the genetic determinant for cancer. Finally, the term "second cancer" might be applied to cancers that occur in the offspring of patients cured of genetically determined cancers. The best current example is the development of retinoblastoma in children of patients cured of retinoblastoma. This may be related to the fact that retinoblastoma has long had a high cure rate, allowing children with this tumor to grow up and reproduce. As cure rates for other childhood cancers increase, the problem of second cancers in children of survivors may also increase.

Other second cancers in children have no apparent genetic basis. Of recent interest is the occurrence of second leukemias or lymphomas in children who are being or have recently been treated for one of these forms of cancer. Children with acute lymphocytic leukemia can develop malignant histiocytosis, Hodgkin's disease, or acute myelocytic leukemia, and leukemia can occur in patients with Hodgkin's disease (Karcher et al. 1978, Woodruff et al. 1977, Ravindranath et al. 1978, Coleman et al. 1977). The relatively early onset of these second cancers, often during treatment for the first, and the biological relationship between the cancers suggest that some leukemia and lymphomas involve several types of leukocytes and that selective pressures of cancer therapy result in the emergence of a cancer that was present but not recognizable initially. Another possibility is that the second cancer represents an early response to the cancer-producing effects of radiation and chemotherapy in highly susceptible immuno-suppressed persons.

Some nongenetic second cancers in children are clearly caused by cancer therapy. Second cancers different in histology from the first can occur many years later in therapeutic radiation portals (Li 1977).

We can define biological cure only with respect to the presenting cancer. Criteria for biological cure must be applied independently to second cancers.

SUMMARY

The criteria for biological cure of cancer can be summarized as follows:

1. Completion of all cancer treatment;
2. Continuous freedom from clinical and laboratory evidence of cancer;
3. Minimal or no risk of relapse, as indicated by actual cancer-free survival experience for the particular tumor, its treatment, and the age of the patient, as plotted on a semilogarithmic graph, and as determined independently in two or more cancer centers.

Children with cancer are at risk of second cancers that may be genetically determined, possibly related to the first cancer and selected by therapy, or the result of cancer therapy. Biological criteria for cure need to be applied separately and independently to these second cancers.

REFERENCES

Aherne, G. 1974. Retinoblastoma associated with other primary malignant tumours. Trans. Ophthalmol. Soc. U.K. 94:938–944.

Coleman, N., C. J. Williams, A. Flint, E. J. Glatstein, S. A. Rosenberg, and H. S. Kaplan. 1977. Hematologic neoplasia in patients treated for Hodgkin's disease. N. Engl. J. Med. 297:1249–1252.

Frei, E., III, and E. A. Gehan. 1971. Definition of cure for Hodgkin's disease. Cancer Res. 31:1828–1833.

Haghbin, M., M. L. Murphy, C. Tan, B. Clarkson, H. Thaler, S. Passe, and J. Burchenal. 1979. A long-term clinical follow-up of children with acute lymphoblastic leukemia treated with intensive chemotherapy regimens. Cancer, in press.

Harisiadis, L., and C. H. Chang. 1977. Medulloblastoma in children: A correlation between staging and results of treatment. Int. J. Radiat. Oncol. Biol. Phys. 2:833–841.

Jaffe, N. 1976. Neuroblastoma: Review of the literature and an examination of factors contributing to its enigmatic character. Cancer Treat. Rev. 3:61–82.

Karcher, D. S., D. R. Head, and J. D. Mull. 1978. Malignant histiocytosis occurring with acute lymphocytic leukemia. Cancer 41:1967–1973.

Lemerle, J., M. F. Tournade, R. G. Marchant, R. Flamant, D. Sarrazin, F. Flamant, M. Lemerle, S. Jundt, J. M. Zucker, and O. Schweisguth. 1976. Wilms' tumor: Natural history and prognostic factors. Cancer 37:2557–2566.

Li, F. P. 1977. Second malignant tumors after cancer in childhood. Cancer 40:1899–1902.

Pinkel, D. 1979a. The Ninth Annual David Karnofsky Lecture: Treatment of acute lymphocytic leukemia. Cancer 43:1128–1137.

Pinkel, D. 1979b. Cure of the child with cancer: Definition and prospective, in Care of the Child with Cancer. American Cancer Society, New York, pp. 191–200.

Pinkel, D., C. Pratt, C. Holton, D. James, Jr., E. Wrenn, Jr., and H. O. Hustu. 1968. Survival of children with neuroblastoma treated with combination chemotherapy. J. Pediatr. 73:928–931.

Ravindranath, Y., S. Inoue, B. Considine, J. Lusher, and W. W. Zuelzer. 1978. New leukemia in the course of therapy of acute lymphoblastic leukemia. Am. J. Hematol. 5:211–223.

Woodruff, R. K., R. J. Brearley, J. M. A. Whitehouse, T. A. Lister, A. G. Stansfeld, J. S. Malpas, S. B. Sutcliff, E. I. Thompson, and R. J. A. Aur. 1977. Hodgkin's disease occurring during acute leukaemia in remission. Lancet 2:900–903.

Status of the Curability of Childhood Cancers,
edited by J. van Eys and M. P. Sullivan.
Raven Press, New York © 1980.

Criteria for Functional Cure of Cancer

Betty Pfefferbaum, M.D.

*Department of Psychiatry, The University of Texas Medical School, Department
of Pediatrics, The University of Texas System Cancer Center M. D. Anderson
Hospital and Tumor Institute, Houston, Texas*

With the cure rate for childhood cancer approaching 50%, it behooves us
to determine the nature and consequences of these apparent cures. Perhaps
the best way to examine the criteria for functional cure of childhood cancer
is to determine the reactions of children to the illness, review the sequelae of
treatment, examine current behavioral and psychological symptoms associated
with cancer cure, and, finally, delineate the criteria by which functional cure
may be identified.

Of course, different children react differently to the crisis of an illness. Some
are more vulnerable than others. Some seem to have a remarkable ability to
withstand the stresses imposed by illness. The child's preillness strengths and
weaknesses help determine his emotional and behavioral status at cure. While
reactions to illness vary with the child, family, and situation, there are some
common denominators. Variables that need to be routinely examined when
assessing a child's reaction to illness include the child's emotional and cognitive
development, the nature and severity of the illness, the parent-child relationship,
and the reaction of adults, particularly the parents, to the illness.

During the diagnostic and treatment phases, the child may develop new symptoms, lose previously developed functions, or even become nonfunctional. He
may seek reassurance, withdraw, or become aggressive. The stresses and reactions
during the early phases of the illness may predispose him to later difficulties
in various areas. Any number of sequelae may follow maladaptation to the early
stresses of the illness or to reaction to these stresses. Psychological sequelae
may include disturbances in relationships, behavior disorders, neurotic disorders,
and school problems.

In an attempt to assure functional cure, current theory advocates "normalization" of the child during the treatment years. Normalization means that the
child is encouraged to participate and function in an essentially "normal" atmo-
sphere throughout treatment and up to the cure itself. This is likely to be difficult
for the child and his family, who may experience the need for normalization
as an additional burden to that created by the illness itself. However, the normalization process is beneficial to the child's overall development. It forces the

27

child, from the earliest stages of his illness, to live with his handicap in the real world. The child is not shielded from rudeness, criticism, or ostracism imposed by others, but is forced to live with and adapt to them. He is encouraged, sometimes even pushed, to participate in activities that may at the time seem beyond him. His adaptive skills, including physical, emotional, social, and educational skills, are developed and maintained.

The crisis of an illness such as cancer is similar in many ways to other crises. As in any crisis, several outcomes are possible. The individual may return to his preillness level of functioning, he may grow as a result of the crisis, or he may develop psychological or behavioral problems. Since the child is a developing organism who must continue to develop despite the tragedy of the illness, the first possibility, that of returning to the preillness level of functioning, is a negative outcome, as is the development of psychological and behavioral problems. To achieve functional cure at some point, normal psychological growth and development must not be precluded.

In many ways, an illness such as cancer might better be viewed as a series of crises (Pfefferbaum 1979). The child's status as he enters the cure phase depends in large measure on what he has experienced previously and on how he has emerged from each of the numerous crises of his illness. The child confronted with cancer and its treatment experiences repeated attacks. Each successive assault may increase the threat to his ego integrity or provide increased strength. The result determines the child's emotional status and degree of function at cure.

Before delineating the criteria for functional cure, let me first review a few studies that have attempted to assess the nature and extent of problems in long-term cancer survivors. At least three kinds of reactions may result in symptoms. First, a problem during an acute phase of the illness may cause immediate disturbances of function that continue and result in chronic symptoms. For example, an adolescent patient might become depressed during the treatment years and turn to drug abuse as a means of escape. If such a patient continues to abuse drugs after the crisis, he will have developed a chronic problem and long-term psychological maladaptation. Second, the problems encountered during the early phases of the illness may have psychological sequelae. For instance, the fact of having had cancer, even with biologic cure, may lead some individuals to be denied employment, military entry, and health and life insurance. These social consequences can have great influence on an individual's psychological status. His inability to succeed in certain endeavors may also be taken as a reflection of his psychological functioning. Finally, long-term or late sequelae of the cancer illness or treatment may cause disturbances in functioning after the cure. For example, the treatment of cancer may result in sterility, which will not cause difficulty until the patient tries to reproduce, at which time he may experience a psychological disturbance.

Reports on the cognitive, psychological, social, and educational status of cured cancer patients are contradictory.

Neurological examinations, psychometric instruments, and school perfor-mance have been used to investigate long-term effects on cognitive functioning. Soni et al. (1975) reported a retrospective and prospective study of leukemia patients receiving craniospinal irradiation or cranial irradiation with intrathecal methotrexate. They found no neurological or psychological impairment at 18 months or 4 years after irradiation, but they noted that the lack of impairment did not rule out undetected or future declines in functioning. Verzosa et al. (1976) concluded that there were no significant long-term neuropsychological problems in children 5 years after central nervous system irradiation and intrathe-cal methotrexate. In this study, schoolteachers reported that children with cancer were average or above average on several academic dimensions, but graded about one third of the children below average in energy level, motivation, atten-tion span, and concrete-abstract thinking. Further follow-up on these patients has revealed problems not previously detected, especially in mathematical and recall ability (G. Marten, unpublished observation). Two other studies have identified neurological and cognitive problems in long-term survivors of child-hood cancer. McIntosh et al. (1976) found learning disabilities, abnormalities in motor, perceptual, behavioral, and language development, and neurological symptoms, including seizures, in almost half the patients studied. Eiser and Lansdown (1977) found that younger children (mean age 6.3 years) treated with cranial irradiation and chemotherapy differed from those in the matched control groups on tests measuring quantitative, memory, and motor skills.

Studies of psychosocial adjustments also offer conflicting conclusions about the long-term effects of childhood cancer. In a descriptive study of a small sample of cancer survivors, Obetz and co-workers (unpublished observation) found good overall adaptation in cancer survivors. Holmes and Holmes (1975) found that over 70% of those in their sample reported that cancer had had no particular effect on their present life. One fourth described themselves as having moderate to marked disability related to the cancer. While the authors admitted that "disability" was difficult to quantify, their overall impression of the patients' psychosocial status was favorable. Li and Stone (1976) found dis-abling psychiatric illness uncommon in long-term survivors, but they pointed out the need for more intensive investigation.

A series of scientific reports from long-term follow-up studies at the Sidney Farber Cancer Center (unpublished observation) describe some of the psychoso-cial problems that may accompany childhood cancer. These reports cite emo-tional turmoil in patients and families and highlight discrimination experienced by patients seeking employment and insurance. While some of the data are still being analyzed, preliminary findings show that, on psychiatric examination, approximately one fifth of survivors had psychiatric problems (J. O'Malley, unpublished observation). Other measures have revealed that 59% of these survi-vors of childhood cancer had psychosocial adjustment problems, although half were only mildly impaired. Those patients showing good adjustment were younger at the time of diagnosis and were socially more mature. The time since diagnosis was significant, with better adjustment in patients who were further from diagnosis. Psychological adjustment was related to estimated verbal IQ, depression, manifest anxiety, and self-esteem (G. Koocher et al., unpublished observation). Twenty-eight percent of the survivors felt cancer had had "much effect" on their current or future occupation, and almost 70% reported it had had "some" or "a major" impact on their life, either positively or negatively (J. O'Malley, unpublished observation).

Although few studies of long-term survivors have been completed and those reported have contradictory findings, it remains difficult to imagine that cancer does not dramatically affect the life of an individual both at the time of illness and treatment and after the pronouncement of cure.

How, then, do we assess functional cure, once biologic cure has been achieved? What areas should we look at to determine whether or not the patient has progressed adequately to functional cure? First, of course, is the patient's emotional state. Is he depressed, exceedingly anxious, excessively defensive, or psychotic? Second, we should look at interpersonal relationships, for these shed light not only on the patient's functional adaptation, but on his intrapsychic status as well. It is important to examine the patient's relationships with his relatives, peers, and authorities, either school personnel, military personnel, or employers. Third, the patient's educational status, including both academic and social standing, needs to be examined, as it reflects his adaptation to the occupational and social expectations of society. The patient's ability to function appropriately at school or on the job is a crucial indicator of functional cure. Finally, the patient's plans for his future and his overall outlook are important variables in assessing functional cure.

In discussing the child's adaptation after the illness, treatment, and cure, I would like to cite the Group for the Advancement of Psychiatry's report on the classification of childhood psychopathologic disorders: "Although the criteria for the assessment of healthy responses are still somewhat subjective and impressionistic, a positive assessment can be made, at least in terms of part functions and their relation to total functioning, allowing for developmental level" (1966, p. 220). The GAP classification includes assessments of intellectual, social, emotional, and personal and adaptive functioning. Intellectual functioning involves "adequate use of capacity, intact memory, reality-testing ability, age-appropriate thought processes, some degree of inquisitiveness, alertness and imagination." Social functioning includes "an adequate balance between the dependent and independent strivings, reasonable comfort and appropriate love in relationships with other children and adults, . . . and age-appropriate capacities to share and empathize with peer group representatives." Emotional functioning involves "general mood quality, some degree of stability of emotional responses, some capacity for self-perspective, some degree of frustration tolerance, sublimation potential, and some capacity to master anxiety and to deal with conflicting emotions." Personal and adaptive functioning involve "a degree of flexibility, drive toward mastery, coping capacities, and adaptive or integrative capacity, the latter making possible the balanced use of defenses, some degree of self-awareness, the existence of self-concept, the capacity to use fantasy in play in constructive fashion, and other criteria" (p. 220).

Precise requirements for functional cure are difficult to delineate. The child should move from the illness to the cure, maintaining the usual array of emotional capacities that exist in the "normal" child. The child's relationships with his family, peers, and community should be no more disturbed than those of the "normal" child. He should maintain hope for and experience the same variety of interpersonal relationships that most individuals do. His performance at school and later on the job should be age and situation appropriate.

What is difficult in assessing these aspects of living is finding some means of measuring them. This is difficult in the general population as well, and assessment tools are not basically different for childhood cancer patients. The child's adaptation must be considered in the context of his having been made aware of his vulnerability through a life-threatening illness. On the other hand, assessment of his status should include the recognition that the illness was only one part of his development and that other factors contributed to his psychological and functional adaptation.

In a society with apparently increasing chaos, with large numbers of children presenting with behavior disorders, neurotic symptoms, and other psychopathologic syndromes, with an increasing incidence of family disruption, with more and more children experiencing academic failure, with the insecurity associated with continued inflation and serious unemployment, and with increasing numbers of alternative life-styles, it becomes more and more difficult to measure the direct effects of the cancer episode. One is led to the conclusion that for the child with cancer to be pronounced functionally cured, he must meet the same standards for healthy adaptation that would be applied to any child of his age and stage of development. Certainly the child with cancer has a different "real world" from that of many of his peers, and his "normal" may be different from theirs. What is required, then, for functional cure is an emotional sense and a behavioral expression of "normal" in the child, what one mother called "not normal like it used to be, but a new normal" (Pfefferbaum 1979).

REFERENCES

Eiser, C., and R. Lansdown. 1977. Retrospective study of intellectual development in children treated for acute lymphoblastic leukemia. Arch. Dis. Child. 52:525–529.

Group for the Advancement of Psychiatry. 1966. Psychopathological Disorders in Childhood: Theoretical Considerations and a Proposed Classification. Vol. VI, Report No. 62. Group for the Advancement of Psychiatry, New York.

Holmes, H. A., and F. F. Holmes. 1975. After ten years, what are the handicaps and lifestyles of children treated for cancer? Clin. Pediatr. (Phila.) 14:819–823.

Li, F. P., and R. Stone. 1976. Survivors of cancer in childhood. Ann. Intern. Med. 84:551–553.

McIntosh, S., E. H. Klatskin, R. T. O'Brien, G. T. Aspnes, B. I. Kammerer, C. Snead, S. M. Kalavsky, and H. A. Pearson. 1976. Chronic neurologic disturbance in childhood leukemia. Cancer 37:853–857.

Pfefferbaum, B. 1979. Reacting to a crisis, *in* The Normally Sick Child, J. van Eys, ed. University Park Press, Baltimore, pp. 99–110.

Soni, S. S., G. W. Marten, S. E. Pitner, D. A. Duenas, and M. Powazek. 1975. Effects of central-nervous-system irradiation on neuropsychologic functioning of children with acute lymphocytic leukemia. N. Engl. J. Med. 293:113–118.

Verzosa, M. S., J. A. Rhomes, J. V. Simone, H. O. Hustu, and D. P. Pinkel. 1976. Five years after central nervous system irradiation of children with leukemia. Int. J. Radiat. Oncol. Biol. Phys. 1:209–215.

Status of the Curability of Childhood Cancers,
edited by J. van Eys and M. P. Sullivan.
Raven Press, New York © 1980.

Supportive Therapy with Curative Intent

Jan van Eys, Ph.D., M.D., Edward M. Copeland, M.D.,* H. Grant Taylor, M.D., Ayten Cangir, M.D., Patricia Carter, R.D.,† Betsy Cohen-Teitell, R.N., M.A.,‡ and Chris O. Ortiz, R.N.‡

*Departments of Pediatrics, *Surgery, †Nutrition and Food Service, and ‡Nursing, The University of Texas System Cancer Center M. D. Anderson Hospital and Tumor Institute, Houston, Texas*

The outcome of medical treatment has always been determined as much by the ability to support the patient until the disease is overcome as by the disease-specific therapy. In pediatric oncology this is more obvious than in many other disease areas. Our present consideration of cure would not have been possible without the ability to deliver supportive therapy. Much of modern blood component therapy has grown out of leukemia therapy. Infection control has made possible intensive chemotherapy.

The need for supportive therapy is greatly determined by the primary treatment. Many of our current concepts of supportive care were derived from experience at a time when primary therapy was primitive and usually palliative. As primary therapy research progressed, supportive therapy research was pursued apace. It follows, then, that when primary therapy becomes curative in intent, supportive therapy must do so also. Unfortunately, supportive therapy is often still viewed as a mode of countering iatrogenic disease.

Supportive therapy with curative intent should support the patient, not the doctor. This paper will attempt to highlight that distinction, using as a paradigm nutritional support, though concepts will first be illustrated with examples from other modes of supportive treatment.

THE MODALITIES OF SUPPORTIVE CARE IN PEDIATRIC ONCOLOGY

Certain specific modalities of supportive care are generally recognized. All nursing care is supportive care, vital to the ultimate successful outcome of the therapy, but specific modes of supportive therapy care are usually singled out as separate areas of management and research, including blood component therapy, infection control, treatment, and prevention, autologous bone marrow transplantation, nutritional support, and psychosocial support. The last area will not be dealt with here, as it is discussed extensively elsewhere in this book.

However, the distinction between amelioration of iatrogenesis and independent patient support with curative intent is clearest in the area of psychosocial support. The former is represented by the death-and-dying movement, which effects psychological euthanasia to prepare for the possible failure to achieve cure. The latter includes support of normal child development to produce a truly cured child, which is parallel with, not subservient to, medical care (van Eys 1977a, 1979a).

The degree to which more biological modalities of support were specifically adapted to oncology varies. Antibiotics were not designed for oncology, but antibiotic researchers enthusiastically use cancer patients as the test arena. However, protected environments are almost exclusively the domain of adult cancer research. Closer ties to cancer research can be found in the area of blood component therapy; but a great spur to blood component technology came also from hemophilia research. Workers in infectious disease and blood banking have had mutually beneficial relationships with oncology, but they are not wholly dependent on each other. Autologous bone marrow transplantation is almost exclusively related to oncological management, while nutritional support has only recently gained a place in cancer care (Copeland et al. 1976).

THE HISTORY OF SUPPORTIVE CARE IN PEDIATRIC ONCOLOGY

There are many reviews of the use of supportive care in pediatric oncology. What we are concerned with here is the *conceptual* history of supportive care, which is best illustrated by a brief review of the use of platelets in pediatric leukemia treatment. First, it must be remembered that all modern cancer care originated in pediatrics. Many of our early chemotherapeutic attempts were directed against childhood leukemia. Many early drugs tested were spectacularly effective, yet patients died. They rarely died from organ malfunction through tumor invasion, but rather from infection and hemorrhage. Infection was attributed to granulocytopenia, and bleeding to thrombocytopenia. Susceptibility to infection is far more complicated than granulocytopenia, as will be touched upon later, but bleeding and thrombocytopenia are related. In a landmark paper, Gaydos et al. (1962) reported that patients with platelet counts below 20,000/ mm^3 were very prone to bleeding (Figure 1), and that the danger of bleeding was proportional to the number of circulating platelets. That paper was published when cancer chemotherapy was very primitive. Table 1 shows the chronological relationship between the development of platelets as supportive care and milestones in leukemia treatment.

The ability to use platelets for transfusion was demonstrated shortly after the report by Gaydos and co-workers. By 1966 the effectiveness of platelet transfusion had been proven (Alvarado et al. 1965, Freireich 1966). Prophylaxis was demonstrated to be feasible in 1963 (Freireich et al. 1963), but not proven effective until the early 1970s in the usual double-blind study approach (Higby et al. 1974). Platelets could be collected by plateletpheresis in 1968 (Tullis et

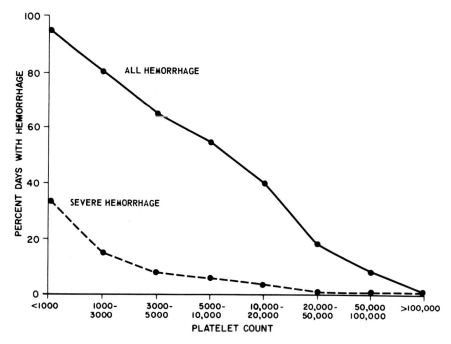

Figure 1. Relation between platelet count and hemorrhage. The incidence of hemorrhage correlates inversely with the level of circulating platelets. The lower the platelet count, the more likely it is that hemorrhage, when it occurs, will be severe. (Reproduced with permission from Gaydos, L. A., et al.: N. Engl. J. Med. 200:905–909, 1962.)

al. 1968), avoiding reliance on multiple donors for treating one patient. These methods have been continually refined. Selection of platelet donors became more sophisticated in the late 1960s with the introduction of HLA typing to match donor and recipient compatibility (Yankee et al. 1969). Nevertheless, platelet resistance remains a problem. Even platelets from HLA-identical siblings can generate resistance (Wieckowicz 1976). Increasing numbers of transfusions result in decreasing effectiveness (Table 2) (Howard and Perkins 1978, van Eys et al. 1978). Viewing this obstacle as a problem of incompatibility between donor and recipient has led to the evaluation of cross-matching techniques, such as mixed lymphocyte cultures, to supplement HLA typing. However, all such attempts have been futile to date (Wu et al. 1977, Herzig et al. 1977).

Long-term storage of platelets remains a problem. Function and physical survival to not always coincide (Kattlove 1979). We now are beginning to use frozen platelets and early success is suggested (Valeri 1979), although the results are still unsatisfactory compared to those with fresh platelets (Schiffer et al. 1976). Thus, problems remain, although the basic technology was solved long before leukemia therapy became curative. Early prophylactic platelet infusions for thrombocytopenic bleeding are effective, but infusions are not usually needed

Table 1. *Developments in Platelet Support and Leukemia Therapy*

Year	Platelet Support Technology	Leukemia Therapy
1910	Whole fresh blood found to stem hemorrhage	
1948		Amethopterin introduced
1950		Adrenal corticosteroids introduced
1953		6-Mercaptopurine introduced
1957	Platelet-rich plasma developed	
1964	Relationship between platelet count and hemorrhage established	
1965	Platelets used therapeutically	Vincristine introduced
1966		Use of vincristine plus prednisone reported
1968	Plateletpheresis introduced	Cytosine arabinoside introduced
1969	HLA matching of donor and recipient introduced	Multidrug maintenance therapy developed
1970	Platelet prophylaxis proven	
1971		L-Asparaginase introduced. Continuous complete remission demonstrated as attainable goal
1972		CNS prophylaxis demonstrated effective
1974	Frozen platelets claimed effective	Possibility of cessation of therapy recognized
1976		Prognostic factors clinically applied
1978		Objectively identified leukemia types clinically applied. Acute lymphocytic, null cell, childhood type; common ALL; pure childhood ALL recognized as curable

early in the course of leukemia therapy (Simone 1971). Only when patients deteriorate and begin the palliative-investigative downward spiral are platelet transfusions needed, so platelet therapy is still linked in pediatric oncology to therapy that holds no great expectation for cure and, thus, to therapy with a small therapeutic margin and high risk. Although it need not be, platelet therapy

Table 2. *Relationship Between Number of Prior Platelet Transfusions and Response*

Number of Prior Platelet Transfusions	Adequate Platelet Increment		Total
	No	Yes	
<3	37 (43%)	49 (57%)	86
3–9	60 (56%)	47 (44%)	107
10–19	67 (79%)	18 (21%)	85
20–29	40 (82%)	9 (18%)	49
>30	53 (91%)	5 (9%)	58
Total	257 (67%)	128 (33%)	385

From van Eys et al. (1978).

is conceptually placed with chemotherapy and radiotherapy protocols. It supports the doctor rather than the patient, in a fundamental sense. Platelet therapy did make early research in pediatric leukemia possible. In the sense that curative chemotherapy would not have developed without platelet transfusion technology, that technology ranks very high among the signal accomplishments of oncology research, but now that curative regimens are developing, the need may fade, to disappear when cancer prevention has been perfected.

SUPPORTIVE CARE AS A BASIS FOR MORE INTENSIVE THERAPY

As the technology of supportive therapy improved, the applications of such techniques became bolder. In those areas in which conventional chemotherapy still failed to control disease, predictable iatrogenesis became accepted as an inevitable consequence of therapy. Supportive therapy was relied upon as a way of widening the therapeutic margin. The term "rescue therapy" began to be used after the results with chemotherapy leveled off.

The most clear-cut example of rescue therapy is autologous marrow transplantation in solid tumors. Especially in adult cancer, but to some degree also in pediatric oncology, there are tumors that will only demonstrate prolonged but not improved survival on current chemotherapy regimens at doses tolerable to the bone marrow. Autologous marrow transplantation is becoming technically feasible, and is compatible with patient survival. It has been applied to both leukemia and solid tumor patients. Table 3 summarizes results from our institution, mostly in adults with leukemia (Dicke et al. 1979). It is more difficult to prove a marrow take in solid tumor patients because regeneration of residual marrow cannot be distinguished. Marrow regeneration can be supported after near-ablative therapy in such patients, but the resulting morbidity is very serious. As a similar example, protected environments are advocated for patients on severe marrow-suppressive regimens to avoid environmentally contracted noso-

Table 3. *Influence of Diagnosis and Pretreatment on Outcome of Bone Marrow Transplantation*

Pretreatment and Diagnosis (No. Pts.)	Complete Remissions	Remission Durations (mos.)
Bone marrow stored in first remission		
AML (11)	7	2, 3, 4, 5+, 7, 8+
ALL/AUL (5)	4	2, 2, 2, 14
Bone marrow stored in second remission		
AML (1)	0	
ALL/AUL (4)	0	
Transplantation as first treatment after relapse		
AML (9)	6	2, 4, 5+, 5+, 7, 8+
Transplantation as second treatment after relapse		
AML (3)	1	3
ALL/AUL (9)	4	2, 2, 2, 14

Adapted from Dicke et al. (1979).

comial infections. Granulocyte transfusions are on occasion being used prophy-lactically and, through antibiotics, bacteriological sterilization is being attempted.

The basic premise that more chemotherapy is necessarily better is not always valid. But quite apart from that issue, supportive therapy of the type discussed here is treatment directed and not curative in itself. The target is the protocol, not the patient's disease. This mode of supportive therapy makes clinical research into intensive regimens possible and will thus remain a vital part of our acquisition of therapeutic knowledge, but the protocols that are supported are highly experimental and therefore cannot be construed as curative. Truly effective regimens need only psychosocial support therapy. Group I Wilms' tumor patients rarely need support modalities beyond those required for any surgery in any child, while Stage IV neuroblastoma is a major consumer of supportive therapy because our results are not significantly improving. The argument for treatment-directed supportive therapy is the same as is embodied in the claim for the importance of platelet transfusion technology. They make the current therapeutic approaches possible. It is hoped that chemotherapy protocols will mature into more generally applicable regimens so that there will be less need for such drastic support. Such developments have already taken place in leukemia and Wilms' tumor therapy.

SUPPORTIVE THERAPY WITH CURATIVE INTENT

The intent of a mode of supportive therapy is not inherent in the mode of care. The total set of care for a child with cancer may span years. Within that set a complication or intercurrent illness cannot be dealt with without supportive care. For example, the use of platelets and other blood components in a patient who has tumor-induced coagulopathy is curative in intent and, in fact, life saving. A specific case will illustrate this point. Figure 2 shows the early clinical course of a child with neuroblastoma with liver destruction who had the consumptive coagulopathy associated with extensive cellular damage in liver disease. In this patient, vigorous replacement therapy turned the tide. Survival would not have been possible without this support. Autologous marrow transplantation performed by infusing stem cells, collected while in remission, into a leukemic child who is in relapse is a mode of therapy that is more curative in intent *per se* than solid tumor therapy along the same principle. The distinction between supportive care with curative intent and supportive care to allow tumor therapy is conceptual. One either concentrates his efforts on the patient himself or directs all his attention to the disease. The best pediatric oncologists ought to be pediatricians first and oncologists second.

The newest modality of supportive care in oncology is nutritional support. Pediatrics grew out of nutrition because internists did not know how to feed babies. Nutritional support is an ideal paradigm of supportive care with curative intent as long as pediatric oncologists use it as pediatricians, not just as oncologists. The optimization of care is the goal of supportive therapy, not simply

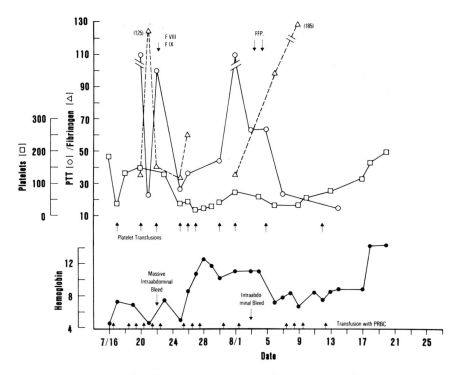

Figure 2. Clinical course of a child with neuroblastoma in liver and severe disseminated coagulopathy.

the combating of iatrogenic disease. Optimization of care implies that all the problems of the child remain the concern of the pediatrician. To use the example of thrombocytopenia again, one should react to the observation of thrombocytopenia first by evaluating the immediate need for intervention, platelet therapy, as a treatment for the symptoms. Then the etiology should be ascertained— marrow depression, myelophthisis, or consumption. The treatment should be removal of the cause. Most thrombocytopenia from marrow depression is better managed by reducing chemotherapy than by persisting in maintaining the drug dosages and instituting marrow support. Thrombocytopenia is a problem in its own right and should be so managed. If the patient is managed in a problem-oriented approach, this means it would warrant a separate problem, not a complication of the disease.

The challenge to the future is not to make nutritional care subordinate to chemotherapy, but to make it a basic mode of approach to any child. Much research needs to be done in the setting of the child with cancer to optimize the application of this modality to pediatric oncology. Therefore, this conceptual view of nutritional care in no way diminishes the clinical research challenge.

NUTRITIONAL THERAPY AS A PARADIGM FOR
OPTIMIZATION OF CARE

The diagnosis of malnutrition is based on objective data. Overt protein-calorie malnutrition is expressed in a weight/height ratio below 80% of the 50th percentile. In adults as well as children, a loss of greater than 10% body weight is prima facie evidence of overt malnutrition. The use of the weight/height ratio as a measure is necessary because children may become malnourished before actual weight loss occurs. A second criterion of malnutrition is a serum albumin value below 3.0 gm/100 ml. In pediatric cancer patients the serum albumin level is not often depressed initially because the onset of malnutrition is relatively sudden (Cohen-Teitell et al. 1979a). However, when the serum albumin level is low, the weight/height ratio may be spuriously elevated because of edema. Other criteria for diagnosis of overt malnutrition, such as tricep skinfold, skinfold thickness, midarm circumference, and creatine height index, are not well defined in children because standards are vague.

Overt malnutrition is a serious disease. Even apart from cancer, there is a high mortality. The consequences are severe: the child is listless, does not tolerate therapy well, and is susceptible to infection. Hughes et al. (1974) have pointed out that *Pneumocystis carinii* infection is closely associated with malnutrition, even in chemotherapy-suppressed patients, as can readily be demonstrated in an animal model (Figure 3). The same relationship to the nutritional state rather than the therapy is true for positive delayed hypersensitivity skin test reactivity to recall antigens in pediatric patients (Cohen-Teitell et al. 1979b).

The incidence of malnutrition ranges up to 8% in newly diagnosed cancer patients, and exceeds 35% in patients with metastatic disease. Malnutrition is not uniformly distributed among all malignant diseases. Ewing's sarcoma and metastatic neuroblastoma, in particular, predispose patients to malnutrition (van Eys 1979b).

Malnutrition is caused by inadequate intake for the caloric demands. The treatment involves providing enough calories to meet normal need, plus those calories that are required for rehabilitation. The causes of the inadequate intake must be diagnosed and treated as well. It is true that in the setting of cancer the ultimate proximal cause is the malignant disease and its treatment. However, once malnutrition is overt, it is not reasonable to allow such malnutrition to continue, because sooner or later the patient might feel better and begin eating. That may be too late for effective management of the disease malnutrition.

TREATMENT AND PREVENTION OF MALNUTRITION

The modalities of intervention available for overt, marginal, or potential malnutrition have been presented previously (van Eys 1979c). Table 4 summarizes those interventions and their indications. The more invasive interventions, continuous nasogastric infusion of elemental diets and intravenous hyperalimenta-

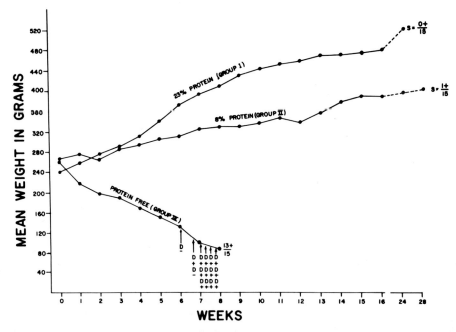

Figure 3. Mean weights of rats fed 23% protein, 8% protein, and protein-free diets. Note effects of diets on weight and incidence of *P. carinii* infection. D = spontaneous death; S = sacrificed (killed); + = *P. carinii* in lungs; − = no *P. carinii* in lungs. (Reproduced with permission from Hughes, W. T., et al.: Am. J. Dis. Child. 128:44–52, 1974. Copyright © 1974, American Medical Association.)

Table 4. *Forms of and Indications for Nutritional Support*

I. *Dietary advice and nutritional monitoring*
   All patients
II. *Supplemental diet formulas*
   1. Patients who require decreased bulk to meet caloric demand
   2. Patients who require liquid formulations for mechanical reasons
   3. Patients who require alternate formula for tube or gastrostomy feeding
III. *Elemental or other adjusted diets*
   1. Patients who have specific malabsorption problems
   2. Patients who need a transition between parenteral and oral feeding after prolonged bowel rest or recent bowel insult
   3. Patients who need specific dietary manipulation for genetic diseases or research applications
IV. *Parenteral alimentation*
   1. Patients for whom oral or enteral feeding is not possible
   2. Patients who need bowel rest
   3. Patients whose oral intake or intestinal absorption requires supplementation to meet caloric demand

Adapted from van Eys (1979c).

Table 5. *Indications for Hyperalimentation*

Circumstance	Indication
Overt malnutrition in face of inadequate intake or malabsorption	Absolute
Overt malnutrition even when intake appears adequate, but chemotherapy, radiation therapy, or surgery is planned	Absolute
Marginal malnutrition in patients who were overtly malnourished recently and who could be expected to have inadequate intake or malabsorption in the current disease episode	Relative
Objectively diagnosed, marginal malnutrition	Elective

Adapted from van Eys (1979c).

tion, are sufficiently extreme that their justification must be examined. Indications can be set for hyperalimentation (Table 5), but for hyperalimentation to be warranted, it must be shown to be safe, effective, and not counterproductive. There is no need to prove that patients on hyperalimentation have higher remission rates, live longer, or can receive more therapy. One need only prove that life is not shortened, that cancer-directed care is not impeded, and that tumor growth is not significantly and uncontrollably stimulated. Hyperalimentation treats or prevents malnutrition; it does not treat cancer or prevent its spread.

Hyperalimentation is safe in experienced hands. Those complications that occur are functions of the skill of the surgeon who places the line, the nurse who changes the dressing, and the pharmacy that prepares the fluids. Malnourished cancer patients are often desperately ill, and iatrogenic disease can be extreme in the child subjected to multiple therapies. Therefore, the incidence of complications is high concomitant with hyperalimentation. But *post hoc, ergo propter hoc* reasoning is as misleading here as it is in attributing healing powers to uncritically introduced therapeutics. M. D. Anderson Hospital is one of four institutions that executed a randomized clinical trial of hyperalimentation in pediatric patients. Complications were seen in control patients that would have been attributed to hyperalimentation in an uncontrolled trial (van Eys 1977b) (Table 6).

Sepsis need not be a problem. Our experience with catheter-related sepsis has been reported elsewhere (van Eys 1979b) (Table 7). In the controlled trial mentioned above, we found no catheter-caused sepsis. Clearly, intravenous hyperalimentation is safe in skilled hands.

Table 6. *Complications During Hyperalimentation Study*

Complication	Control Patients Randomized	Patients Receiving Hyperalimentation	
		Randomized	Nonrandomized
Congestive heart failure	2/20	0/21	3/17
Ascites	0/20	1/20	1/17

Table 7. *Intravenous Hyperalimentation at M. D. Anderson Hospital*

	1976–1977	1977–1978	Total
Number of patients	20	35	55
Number of catheter insertions	37	90	127
Catheter-related sepsis*	3%	3%	
Other sepsis†	10%	10%	

Adapted from van Eys (1979b).
* Demonstrated infected catheter (sepsis rate calculated per insertion).
† Positive blood culture, during intravenous hyperalimentation, of known etiology, and proven lack of catheter vegetations.

Table 8. *Final Outcome per Chemotherapy Episode*

Initial Status	Final Status					
	Control			IVH		
	WN	MN	Total	WN	MN	Total
WN	20	3	23	15	3	18
MN	—	2	2	12	9	21
Total	20	5	25	27	12	39

WN, well-nourished; MN, malnourished.

Furthermore, hyperalimentation is effective. In our prospective study, patients with disease metastatic to and from bone were enrolled. Even in malnourished patients who were undergoing intensive chemotherapy for metastatic disease, weight gain was usually observed. In patients not initially malnourished, hyperalimentation usually seemed to protect against weight loss (Table 8).

In our randomized trial, hyperalimentation did not impede therapy or worsen the outcome. There were no more deaths from progressive tumor growth in hyperalimentation patients than in controls. It is impossible to generate ideal data. By definition, hyperalimentation is used in sicker patients. The high infection rate is often quoted as a drawback of hyperalimentation, but when the incidences of all types of infections in patients with tumor metastatic to or from bone were compared, they were found to be associated with the patients' state of nutrition (Table 9), not with the hyperalimentation.

If one expects nutritional support to treat the tumor, one will be disappointed. Viewed as a treatment of the host, nutritional support is effective, safe, and not counterproductive. The patient will feel immeasurably better for it.

NUTRITION AS A CONCEPT OF TOTAL THERAPY

To feed a child is basic. Much of parental nurture is centered around feeding. In fact, nurture and nutriture have the same root. Unfortunately, feeding a

Table 9. *Incidence of Infection During Nutritional Support*

Patients' Treatment and Status	Infection		
	Yes	No	Total
Hyperalimentation			
Well-nourished	5	11	16
Malnourished	19	3	22
Control			
Well-nourished	7	12	19
Malnourished	1	1	2
All			
Well-nourished	13	23	36
Malnourished	20	4	24

child is so basic that few physicians are knowledgeable about nutritional management. A hospital implies shelter and food, since these very primitive physical needs of the child must be met. Therefore, most orders by physicians in the area of nutrition are negative—nothing by mouth, restricted diet—because the basic need for food is perceived as interfering with care. Positive orders, such as dietary supplementation or intravenous hyperalimentation, are much rarer and are often made only after pressure from dieticians. If nutrition is indeed basic, physicians should encourage parents and patients in a positive way. In our ward, a kitchen for parents has been installed in which the children's favorite foods can be prepared and meals can be rewarmed when hospital schedules interfere with mealtime. The kitchen is intensively used (van Eys 1977b, 1978). It is also used for dietary instruction under the supervision of our dietitian. We will have a communal dining room on the ward after our current remodeling to further integrate eating into normal care.

Nutrition is essential for survival. Therefore, any necessary nutritional intervention is part of making it possible for the child to survive. To view it any other way generates absurdities. Nutrition is supportive therapy with curative intent. It addresses the whole child, not the tumor or the side effects of therapy. When all supportive care is so viewed, we will be one step closer to curing childhood cancer.

ACKNOWLEDGMENTS

The inclusion of a large number of names on a review article requires an explanation by the senior author. Dr. Copeland was the primary mover in the introduction of parenteral nutrition for cancer patients; Dr. Taylor introduced platelet transfusions for children at M. D. Anderson Hospital and has been a major help in keeping the reports flowing in our nutrition work. Dr. Cangir has been the primary attending physician for most of the patients on our parenteral nutrition study and a strong supporter of the program. Ms. Carter supervises dietary research and was one of the dieticians supervising the kitchen on our ward. Ms. Teitell and Ms. Ortiz were the hyperalimentation nurses, without whom our results would have been much poorer.

This investigation was supported in part by contract NO1–CP–65794 from the Diet Nutrition and Cancer Program of the National Cancer Institute.

REFERENCES

Alvarado, J., I. Djerassi, and S. Farber. 1965. Transfusion of fresh concentrated platelets to children with acute leukemia. J. Pediatr. 67:13–22.

Cohen-Teitell, B., J. van Eys, and J. Herson. 1979a. Comparison of techniques of assessing malnutrition in children with cancer (Abstract). J. Parent. Ent. Nutr. 4:514.

Cohen-Teitell, B., J. Herson, and J. van Eys. 1979b. Recall antigen response in pediatric cancer patients receiving hyperalimentation. J. Parent. Ent. Nutr. 4:9–11.

Copeland, E. M., B. V. McFadyen, V. T. Lanzotti, and S. J. Dudrick. 1976. Nutritional care of the cancer patient, *in* Cancer Patient Care at M. D. Anderson Hospital and Tumor Institute, R. L. Clark and C. D. Howe, eds. Year Book Medical Publishers, Chicago, pp. 607–628.

Dicke, K. A., A. Zander, G. Spitzer, D. S. Verma, I. Peters, L. Vellekoop, K. B. McCredie, and J. P. Hester. 1979. Autologous bone marrow transplantation in relapsed adult acute leukemia. Lancet 1:514.

Freireich, E. J, 1966. Effectiveness of platelet transfusion in leukemia and aplastic anemia. Transfusion 6:50–54.

Freireich, E. J, A. Kilman, L. Gaydos, N. Mantel, and E. Frei. 1963. Response to repeated platelet transfusions for the same donor. Ann. Intern. Med. 59:277–287.

Gaydos, L. A., E. J Freireich, and N. Mantel. 1962. The quantitative relation between platelet count and hemorrhage in patients with acute leukemia. N. Engl. J. Med. 200:905–909.

Herzig, R. M., P. I. Terasaki, R. J. Trapani, G. P. Herzig, and R. G. Graw, Jr. 1977. The relationship between donor-recipient lymphotoxicity and the transfusion response using HLA-matched platelet concentrates. Transfusion 17:657–661.

Higby, D. J., E. Cohen, J. F. Holland, and L. Sinks. 1974. The prophylactic treatment of thrombocytopenic leukemia patients with platelets: A double blind study. Transfusion 14:440–446.

Howard, J. E., and H. A. Perkins. 1978. The natural history of alloimmunization to platelets. Transfusion 10:496–505.

Hughes, W. T., R. A. Price, F. Sisko, W. S. Havron, A. G. Kafalos, M. Schonland, and P. M. Smythe. 1974. Protein calorie malnutrition—A host determinant for *Pneumocystis carinii* infection. Am. J. Dis. Child. 128:44–52.

Kattlove, H. E. 1979. Platelet preservation—What temperature? A rationale for strategy. Transfusion 19:328–330.

Schiffer, C. A., D. H. Buchholz, J. Aisner, J. H. Wolff, and D. M. Wiernik. 1976. Frozen autologous platelets in the supportive care of patients with leukemia. Transfusion 16:321–329.

Simone, J. V. 1971. Use of fresh blood components during intensive combination therapy of childhood leukemia. Cancer 28:562–565.

Tullis, J. L., W. G. Eberle II, P. Baudanza, and R. Finch. 1968. Plateletpheresis: Description of a new technique. Transfusion 8:156–164.

Valeri, C. M. 1979. Hemostatic effectiveness of liquid preserved and previously frozen platelets. N. Engl. J. Med. 290:353–358.

van Eys, J., ed. 1977a. The Truly Cured Child: The New Challenge in Pediatric Cancer Care. University Park Press, Baltimore, 177 pp.

van Eys, J. 1977b. Nutritional therapy in children with cancer. Cancer Res. 37:2457–2461.

van Eys, J. 1978. Nutrition and cancer in children. Cancer Bull. 30:93–97.

van Eys, J., ed. 1979a. The Normally Sick Child. University Park Press, Baltimore, 188 pp.

van Eys, J. 1979b. Malnutrition in children with cancer: Incidence and consequence. Cancer 43:2030–2034.

van Eys, J. 1979c. Nutritional management as adjuvant in pediatric cancer therapy, *in* Care of the Child with Cancer. American Cancer Society, New York, pp. 86–92.

van Eys, J., D. Thomas, and B. Olivos. 1978. Platelet use in pediatric oncology: A review of 393 transfusions. Transfusion 18:169–173.

Wieckowicz, M. 1976. Single donor platelet transfusions: Scientific, legal and ethical considerations. Transfusion 16:193–199.

Wu, K. K., J. C. Hoak, J. A. Koepke, and J. S. Thompson. 1977. Selection of compatible platelet donors: A prospective evaluation of three cross-matching techniques. Transfusion 17:638–643.

Yankee, R. A., F. C. Grumet, and G. N. Rogentine. 1969. Platelet transfusion therapy: The selection of compatible platelet donors for refractory patients by lymphocyte HL-A typing. N. Engl. J. Med. 28:1208–1212.

Status of the Curability of Childhood Cancers,
edited by J. van Eys and M. P. Sullivan.
Raven Press, New York © 1980.

Statistical Design for Pediatrics: Past, Present, and Future

Stephen L. George, Ph.D.

Biostatistics Section, St. Jude Children's Research Hospital, Memphis, Tennessee

The impressive success in treating malignant diseases of childhood since the Second World War has been achieved through the development of new drugs and a coordinated, multimodal approach involving surgery, radiotherapy, combination chemotherapy, and supportive care, and the application of statistical experimental design concepts in controlled clinical trials of the new therapies. A history of these advances in cancer treatment would, in fact, be impossible to describe without mentioning the impact of controlled clinical trials.

The first controlled clinical trial in cancer, conducted by Frei and co-workers in the 1950s, was a randomized comparison of "continuous" and "intermittent" methotrexate in combination with 6-mercaptopurine in the treatment of acute leukemia, primarily in children (Frei et al. 1958). The trial, a cooperative study by four medical services, included general design characteristics that are still valid for trials planned today: a written protocol, stratified randomization of patients to treatment groups, and precise definitions of diagnosis, eligibility, response, toxicity, and end points.

During the past 25 years, the number and size of clinical trials of cancer treatment have grown dramatically. The National Institutes of Health (NIH) Inventory of Clinical Trials (1976) lists 459 clinical trials in cancer sponsored by the National Cancer Institute that were active in 1976. The European Organization for Research on the Treatment of Cancer (EORTC), on a smaller scale, is carrying out cooperative studies in Europe. The International Cancer Research Data Bank Program (ICRDBP) publishes summaries of treatment protocols and the Union Internationale Contre le Cancer (UICC) maintains lists of active clinical trials in cancer conducted throughout the world (ICRDBP 1976, UICC 1974).

The development and application of clinical trials in cancer in general and pediatric cancer in particular have been closely intertwined with the development of effective cancer chemotherapy over the past 30 years. The first effective anticancer drug, the antimetabolite aminopterin, was introduced by Farber and co-workers in 1947, less than 10 years before the start of Frei and co-workers' initial trial. The first clinical trials were primarily and appropriately drug evaluation trials with relatively simple designs and little consideration of other modalities. Today's trials, in contrast, are complicated, multimodal investigations involving many specialties and institutions. Pediatric studies have been particularly important since the introduction of the clinical trial into clinical research. Currently there are national study groups for Wilms' tumor, rhabdomyosarcoma, Ewing's sarcoma, and Hodgkin's disease. Clinical trials are being carried out on almost all major pediatric neoplasms in clinical cooperative groups such as the Southwest Oncology Group and Children's Cancer Study Group and at single institutions that treat large numbers of patients.

The need to consider pediatric neoplasms separately from adult neoplasms stems from the obvious fact that the types and sites of cancers seen in children, their natural history, etiology, and prognosis differ substantially from those of cancers seen in adults. Cancers in childhood are predominately leukemias, embryonal tumors, and sarcomas. Some are associated with certain congenital anomalies and defects, with the obvious implication that genetic and early developmental disorders are involved in the etiology of the disease. Adult cancers, in contrast, are primarily adenocarcinomas or carcinomas with an etiology more closely associated with environmental and social factors (e.g., dietary and smoking habits) and perhaps the aging process itself.

In recent years, with increasing therapeutic success in children with cancer, including a substantial proportion of apparent cures, an even stronger reason for considering pediatric cancer apart from adult cancer has arisen. This reason is that children, because they are biologically, psychologically, and socially immature, are at a much greater risk of long-term effects of the disease and its treatment than are adults. Adding to this risk is the fact that, if cure is achieved, more years of life are generally salvaged than is the case with adults.

In this paper I will attempt to address the impact of the improved prognosis and increased knowledge of disease behavior, especially with respect to prognostic factors, on the design, execution, and analysis of clinical trials. Examples will be given for two prototypical diseases, Wilms' tumor (WT) and acute lymphocytic leukemia (ALL). Attention will not be focused on general statistical design concepts appropriate for clinical trials since these have been discussed at length elsewhere (Hill 1971, Schwartz et al. 1970, Burdette and Gehan 1970, Armitage 1975, George 1976, 1978).

SOME BASIC STATISTICAL CONCEPTS

In the earliest trials of therapy for childhood cancer, the major end point (i.e., the variable of primary interest used to evaluate or compare therapies) was the initial proportion of short-term responses to the therapy. This was appropriate because of the relative simplicity of the treatment design and the lack of effective long-range control of the disease. Except for phase II drug studies, current trials with initial response to therapy as the major end point are rare. Even in late-stage disease, such as recurrent ALL, the response rate with multidrug chemotherapy is quite high, even though the response is usually brief. Also, the increasing proportion of patients with long disease-free intervals, or remissions, has led necessarily to more complicated treatment designs and to more long-range end points, such as lengths of remission and survival.

This shift in emphasis from response rate to measures of time (e.g., remission and survival times) has contributed to a remarkable growth during the past 15 years in research on statistical methodology appropriate for such studies, and illustrates the "spin-off" benefits of clinical trials beyond the obvious benefit of increased knowledge of specific therapeutic approaches. The topics addressed in this research have ranged from relatively simple investigations of the necessary length and size of proposed trials (George and Desu 1974) to highly theoretical investigations of the role of certain statistical models in the analysis of the types of data commonly arising in clinical trials (Cox 1972) and philosophical discussions touching on the foundations of statistical and scientific inference (Anscombe 1963). Although some of this work would likely have developed anyway, it was the widespread application of clinical trials in cancer and other diseases that provided the strongest motivation.

To simplify the remainder of the paper, it is necessary to define some elementary statistical concepts and notations. The basic statistical concept is that of a "probability distribution" of responses. In terms of lengths of remission (or any other measure of time), the survivorship function, $S(t)$, summarizes this notation:

$$S(t) = P(T > t), t \geqq 0,$$

where $S(t)$ is the probability of a length of remission longer than time t. In standard statistical theory, $S(0) = 1$ and $S(\infty) = 0$, but as will be discussed later, the latter requirement will have to be dropped if we want to incorporate cures in the model.

A more fundamental concept is that of the hazard function (or instantaneous failure rate), $\lambda(t)$ where $\lambda(t)\Delta t$ gives the approximate probability of relapse in the time interval $[t, t + \Delta t]$ conditional on the patient's remaining disease free up to time t. The survivorship function can be derived from the hazard function, and vice versa, from the relationship

$$S(t) = \exp [-\int_o^t \lambda(u)du].$$

Hypothetical examples of hazard functions are given in Figure 1. Note that the hazard function may increase, decrease, or remain constant over time. Since the hazard function represents an instantaneous failure rate, a general idea of the shape of this function may be obtained by plotting the conditional probability of relapse for specified time periods (e.g., yearly or monthly). This is illustrated in Figure 2, which gives the conditional yearly probability of death for the U.S. population for each year of life from birth through age 70. This figure shows that mortality is quite high in infants, decreases steadily through age 10 or 11, increases again up to age 20, remains relatively constant in the 20s, then begins its inexorable increase through the later years of life. From age

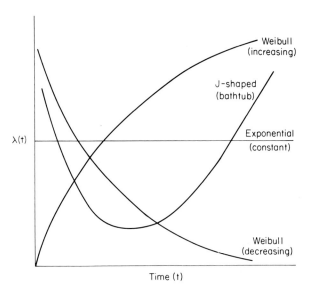

Figure 1. Typical hazard functions.

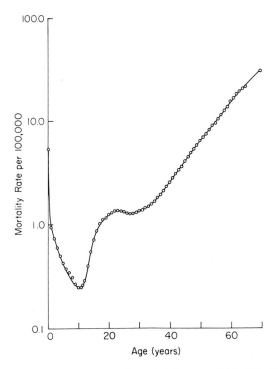

Figure 2. Mortality rate by age, U.S. population, 1976 (source: Table 100, Statistical Abstract of the U.S., 1978).

30 on the increase is very nearly exponential (linear on a log scale), with a doubling of the death rate approximately every 7 years.

DEFINITIONS OF PERIOD OF RISK AND CURE

One of the most troubling aspects of the current status of the treatment of childhood cancer is the impossibility of determining definitively that a patient has been cured. The key element in the definition of cure, the complete eradication of disease, is the primary difficulty. In some patients, despite an apparent disappearance of disease and return to health, undetectable disease remains. This lack of ability to detect occult disease has led us away from an unequivocal definition of cure to an operational definition involving a hypothetical period of risk, during which the patient is at risk of relapse but beyond which the risk is negligible. In this context, the patient may be considered cured if he or she remains disease free beyond the period of risk.

An interesting early attempt to define a period of risk was made by Collins (1958), who reasoned that, at diagnosis, a tumor could not have been growing for longer than the patient's age plus the 9-month gestation period. Thus, if the tumor is removed with no evidence of residual disease, the length of the period of risk, assuming the same growth rate as before, could be considered equal to the patient's age plus 9 months. (For example, a child diagnosed on his 3rd birthday would be at risk 3 years 9 months, or until the age of 6 years 9 months.) It now seems clear that such a concept of period of risk is not very useful in practice. In Wilms' tumor, for example, the evidence strongly indicates that, regardless of the patient's age, the period of risk is around 2 years. Nevertheless, this definition makes the important point that the period of risk varies from patient to patient, so some statistical approach is needed for the proper analysis of competing treatments.

From a statistical viewpoint, it is not necessary to identify a time beyond which the probability of relapse is zero since this may never occur. It is important, however, to identify a time beyond which the probability of relapse is so small that relapses will be extremely rare. The definition of "rare" is necessarily subjective, and will vary by disease and even, perhaps, by treatment. Also, although it seems reasonable to assume that a time exists beyond which the risk of relapse is negligible, there are no logical, statistical, or biological reasons for believing this is true for all types of cancer. It is theoretically possible that the hazard may initially decrease with time but eventually increase, although this does not seem to fit the facts now known.

For our purposes, a disease will be considered curable if the probability of disease-free survival, $S(t)$, does not approach zero for large t. That is, there is some nonzero probability that a patient will remain disease free indefinitely. It is important to note that this statistical definition of cure does not imply that the risk of relapse is zero beyond some time. For example, in the so-called Gompertz failure model, the hazard function is

$$\lambda(t) = \exp{(\lambda + \alpha t)}$$

where, if $\alpha < 0$, the function is decreasing and approaching zero, but for any finite t is always greater than zero. The survivorship function in this case approaches the limit

$$\exp\left\{\frac{\exp{\lambda}}{\alpha}\right\},$$

which is not zero. These concepts of a decreasing (but never zero) hazard function and a positive probability of cure correspond well with recent experience in many diseases. The concepts also reflect our current uncertainty over when, if ever, an individual patient may be considered cured. Actual data from clinical trials can be used to estimate $\lambda(t)$ and $S(t)$, and these, in turn, can be used in the design of new trials.

MODEL DISEASES: WILMS' TUMOR AND ACUTE LYMPHOCYTIC LEUKEMIA

The two diseases I shall use to illustrate these points are Wilms' tumor (WT), or nephroblastoma, and acute lymphocytic leukemia (ALL). They were chosen because they demonstrate the success of past clinical studies and the problems this success poses for similar studies in the future. However, they are not representative of all childhood cancers. Despite the hope raised by the treatment of these two cancers, similar diseases, such as metastatic neuroblastoma and acute nonlymphocytic leukemia, have proved much more resistant to similar therapeutic approaches.

These two diseases, the first a malignant renal tumor and the other the most common hematopoietic neoplasm in children, seem to share little in terms of etiology, natural history, and responsiveness to various therapeutic approaches. However, they are similar in that both are diagnosed predominantly in preschool children and both have been transformed in the last 25 years from incurable, inevitably fatal diseases to diseases with a relatively high probability of cure. Such progress has not been without cost. The therapies used are highly toxic, aggressive combinations of surgery (for Wilms' tumor), radiation therapy, and chemotherapy, with resultant short-range toxicity and possible long-range induction of developmental defects or even second cancers.

Because of its documented stable incidence with respect to geography, climate, environment, race, and sex, Wilms' tumor has become a benchmark disease for evaluating incidence data in different regions of the world, to the point that underreporting of cancer may be suspected if the reported incidence of WT seems too low in a specific area. Wilms' tumor is the second most common malignant solid tumor in children, with an incidence of approximately 0.75 per 100,000 per year for children under 15 years of age (Cutler and Young 1975). Approximately 380 children with new cases of Wilms' tumor are expected per year in the U.S., based on current population estimates (Statistical Abstract 1978). The disease is found predominantly (75%) in children under 5 years of age, though rarely at birth, and cases are about equally distributed between boys and girls (Rubin 1978). Prognostic factors found to be important in Wilms' tumor include histology, patient's age at diagnosis, and extent of disease, or stage. Patient's sex and race appear to be of no prognostic significance (Breslow et al. 1978).

The increased survival in patients with localized Wilms' tumor achieved with adjuvant chemotherapy provided the first solid evidence of the ability of chemotherapy to control both overt and occult metastases. The history of therapeutic advances in the treatment of Wilms' tumor, an incurable disease in the 1950s, has served as a model for treating other pediatric and adult tumors by surgery, radiotherapy, single-drug chemotherapy (actinomycin D and vincristine), scheduling and combinations of drugs, refinement of therapy, formation of a national study group to study specific therapeutic approaches on a broad scale, and careful attention to follow-up for late sequelae and complications.

Recent publications from the National Wilms' Tumor Study Group indicate that about 75% of patients without metastases at diagnosis will remain disease free at least 2 years after diagnosis (Breslow et al. 1978). Since relapses after 2 years are extremely rare, it appears that approximately three fourths of all patients with nonmetastatic Wilms' tumor can be cured of their disease. Early results from later studies are even more encouraging. The results vary by histology and patient's age, as indicated in Table 1.

Disease control is still a significant problem in patients with an unfavorable histology (10% of all patients), but current therapy appears adequate (relapse rate of less than 10%) for infants with a favorable histology. Older children have an intermediate prognosis (approximately 25% relapse).

Acute lymphocytic leukemia in childhood is an obvious choice for a model of disseminated cancer (Simone 1979), due to the impressive improvement in therapeutic results in the postwar years, the successful application of theories and discoveries from the basic sciences and animal studies to treatment regimens (especially theories on the development of drug resistance and cell kinetics), the identification of subpopulations of patients based initially on general patient characteristics and more recently on specific cell characteristics, and findings of potential importance in both biology and medicine (such as the concept of pharmacologic sanctuaries).

Table 1. *Two-Year Relapse Rate in Nonmetastatic Wilms' Tumor*

Histology	Age (Years)	Relapse Rate
Favorable	<2	9% (9/97)
Favorable	≧2	26% (44/171)
Unfavorable	All ages	71% (24/34)

From Breslow et al. (1978).

Table 2. *Relapse Rates in 6-Month Intervals from Attainment of Complete Remission, ALL*

Time Period (Months)	Standard-Risk Patients	High-Risk Patients
0–6	6% (572)*	43% (151)
6–12	14% (507)	40% (81)
12–18	12% (396)	21% (45)
18–24	10% (312)	13% (31)
24–30	7% (258)	8% (26)
30–36	8% (219)	5% (22)

From George et al. (1979).
* Effective numbers of patients at risk during the time interval.

Acute lymphocytic leukemia is the most common cancer seen in children, with an annual incidence of approximately 2.3 per 100,000 per year for children under 15 years of age (Cutler and Young 1975). The incidence of all types of leukemia is nearly 4.0 per 100,000 per year in children. Approximately 1,200 new ALL cases per year are expected in the U.S., more than three times the expected number of Wilms' tumor cases. About half of the children are under

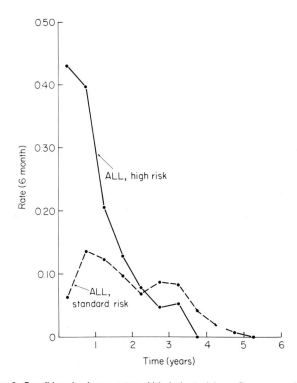

Figure 3. Conditional relapse rates, ALL (adapted from George et al. 1979).

5 years of age and approximately 60% are boys. Prognostic factors known to be of importance are initial leukocyte count, presence or absence of a mediastinal mass, CNS disease, or E-rosette formation, and the patient's age, race, and occasionally sex (George et al. 1973). It is now customary to separate patients into risk groups on the basis of these factors.

The therapeutic advances against ALL have paralleled those against Wilms' tumor (Mauer 1978). When aminopterin was introduced 30 years ago (Farber 1948), the median survival for newly diagnosed children with ALL was approximately 3 months. Today, through the effective use of prophylactic CNS therapy and combination chemotherapy given over 2½ years, the cure rate is about 50% for the standard-risk patient (i.e., WBC less than 100,000, no mediastinal mass, CNS disease, or E-rosette formation). For high-risk patients (those with one or more of the above features) the cure rate is approximately 20%. In the latter cases a cure is defined as disease-free survival at least 4 years beyond cessation of therapy (George et al. 1979).

One interesting finding is that the standard- and high-risk patients differ markedly with respect to relapse in the first 2 years of remission but not thereafter, as indicated in Table 2 and Figure 3. Another interesting finding is that the Gompertz failure model appears to fit the observed failure rates quite well through the first 2 to 3 years for both Wilms' tumor and high-risk ALL, but does not appear to describe the standard-risk ALL pattern. This is illustrated graphically in Figure 4, in which the logarithm of the relapse rate is plotted against time. Also, the relapse rates for Wilms' tumor and ALL, high-risk, appear to follow a "proportional hazards" model in that the rate of risk of relapse from one group to another is approximately constant (independent of time). Patients with ALL, high-risk, are approximately three to four times as likely to relapse as Wilms' tumor patients, regardless of time from diagnosis.

The fitted models reveal that the estimated relapse rate at 24 months is approximately .02 for Wilms' tumor patients, while for ALL patients the time at which the estimated rate reaches .02 is approximately 5 years. Thus, if one is willing to accept the same criterion of cure for both diseases, one could declare a cure for any patient who remained free from Wilms' tumor for 2 years or from ALL for 5 years.

PROBLEMS FOR FUTURE CLINICAL TRIALS

One neglected aspect of the success in treating childhood malignant diseases is the effect of this success on the design of future studies. The nonzero probability of a cure has had a profound impact on the types of studies, the outcome variables studied, and the length and size of the studies. The objective in many diseases, such as Wilms' tumor and acute lymphocytic leukemia, is no longer simply prolongation of remission or survival, but eradication of disease with minimal long-term effects.

The key features of the treatment of childhood cancers that will (or should)

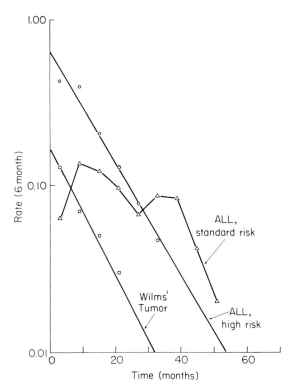

Figure 4. Fitted hazard models, WT and ALL (adapted from Breslow et al. 1978 and George et al. 1979).

have an important impact on clinical trials in the future are the increasing cure rate and its two concomitants, the possibility of late effects and the increasing knowledge of prognostic factors. These three features directly affect the feasibility of conducting any trial in some diseases, since their net effect is to require more patients, longer trials, longer and more systematic follow-up, and, of course, higher costs. I will discuss each of these features in turn.

In any disease in which there is already a substantial proportion of cures by current conventional therapy, some conservatism in altering therapy is required. If the cure rate is particularly high, as in infants with nonmetastatic Wilms' tumor, the objective of the trials should be decreasing late effects, rather than increasing the cure rate. In any case, the final results of treatment for a group of patients who are diagnosed this year will not be known until these patients have been followed beyond their period of risk, as defined previously. This period will vary by disease type and may considerably delay the final results.

The problem of late effects of the disease and its therapy arises only when that therapy becomes successful. Late effects of therapy of a disease with no long-term survivors are not important. Since success has been obtained with aggressive, multimodal therapy using radiation and combinations of drugs, it was correctly anticipated that long-term survivors would have some developmental difficulties. Since radiation and some of the drugs are themselves carcinogenic, late effects may include second neoplasms. As more children are cured of their initial disease, these problems loom as significant threats to their long-term survival. Obvious implications for future studies are that the objectives must now explicitly include the minimization of late effects and that methods for evaluating the late effects of competing therapies must be planned in the design of the trial. It is especially important that any study in which the standard therapy is reduced be designed so that the relative contribution of each therapy to disease control and to late effects can be assessed. If the numbers of patients admitted to such a study are insufficient, one runs the very real risk of falsely concluding that the reduced therapy is as good as the standard therapy in preventing relapses. The last and perhaps most important point to consider in the design of a study in which late effects may be present is that one must be prepared to follow all patients for the remainder of their lives. This follow-up must include carefully planned examinations, such as neuropsychological and endocrine function tests, possibly at yearly intervals. It cannot mean simply "keeping in touch," although even that in itself can be expensive. This simple point, taken in conjunction with the improving cure rates and the increasing numbers of patients required for a proper analysis, may dissuade some researchers from attempting to conduct trials.

One side benefit of previous clinical trials in pediatric cancer has been the increased knowledge and appreciation of factors that influence the clinical course of disease. Many diseases that were previously thought to be homogeneous entities have been shown to be very diverse. A prime example is acute lymphocytic leukemia, for which most of the numerous prognostic factors mentioned earlier have been known for some time. It has become evident in recent years that acute lymphocytic leukemia actually consists of at least two or three distinct diseases, depending on the origin of the stem cells. A tremendous amount of research is currently being invested in refining our definitions of these diseases.

All this increased knowledge is a mixed blessing for future studies. One effect of defining and redefining prognostic groupings is the fragmentation of the patient population into various subgroups. Because of the differing prognoses, different therapies are often proposed for these subgroups, creating the need for separate clinical trials for each subgroup. This practice requires more patients and creates difficulties in comparing one trial to another, since definitions may vary from trial to trial. A similar situation exists when staging definitions change from trial to trial. The original aim of clinical trials was to treat enough patients in the same way so that solid inferences concerning the effects of therapy on a large class of patients could be drawn. Today it is sometimes said that the ultimate goal of the study of prognostic factors is to enable each patient to have an individualized treatment regimen based on these factors. Although this goal is appealing, its premature application might preclude the conducting of additional, sorely needed, clinical trials.

SUMMARY

In summary, clinical trials have played a key role in the development of effective therapeutic approaches in pediatric oncology. These trials have complemented findings in the basic sciences and facilitated the practical therapeutic application of those findings in a logical and scientifically valid manner. Unfortunately, successful clinical trials of therapy for cancer in children will clearly be more difficult, time consuming, and costly in the future than those conducted in the past. Investigators undertaking trials must carefully consider the implications of curative therapy and be prepared for the arduous follow-up required. Despite these difficulties, additional clinical trials are sorely needed. Some children still die of their disease and many who survive suffer long-term disabilities. Until a method of disease prevention is available, the best hope for continued progress in disease control lies in carefully planned and executed clinical trials.

ACKNOWLEDGMENTS

This investigation was supported by grant CA21765, awarded by the National Cancer Institute, Department of Health, Education and Welfare. Ms. Jane Seifert assisted in the scientific editing.

REFERENCES

Anscombe, F. J. 1963. Sequential medial trials. J. Am. Stat. Assoc. 58:365–383.

Armitage, P. 1975. Sequential Medial Trials. 2nd ed. John Wiley & Sons, New York, 194 pp.

Breslow, N., N. Palmer, L. Hill, J. Burins, and G. J. D'Angio. 1978. Wilms' tumor: Prognostic factors for patients without metastases at diagnosis. Cancer 41:1577–1589.

Burdette, W. J., and E. A. Gehan. 1970. The Planning and Analysis of Clinical Studies. Charles C Thomas and Sons, Springfield, Ill., 104 pp.

Collins, V. P. 1958. The treatment of Wilms' tumor. Cancer 11:89–94.

Cox, D. R. 1972. Regression models and life tables. J. R. Stat. Soc. 34:187–202.

Cutler, S. J., and J. L. Young, eds. 1975. Third National Cancer Survey: Incidence Data. U.S. Government Printing Office, Washington, D.C., 454 pp.

Farber, S., L. K. Diamond, R. D. Mercer, R. F. Sylvester, and J. A. Wolff. 1948. Temporary remissions in acute leukemia in children produced by folic acid antagonist 4-aminopteroyl-glutamic acid, aminopterin. N. Engl. J. Med. 238:787–793.

Frei, E., J. F. Holland, M. A. Schneiderman, D. Pinkel, G. Selkirk, E. J Freireich, R. T. Silver, G. L. Gold, and W. Regelson. 1958. A comparative study of two regimens of combination chemotherapy in acute leukemia. Blood 12:1126–1148.

George, S. L. 1976. Practical problems in the design, conduct and analysis of cooperative clinical trials, *in* Proceedings of the IXth International Biometric Conference. Vol. 1. Biometric Society, Raleigh, N.C., pp. 227–244.

George, S. L. 1978. Design and evaluation of leukemia trials. Clin. Haematol. 7:227–243.

George, S. L., R. J. A. Aur, A. Mauer, and J. Simone. 1979. A reappraisal of the results of stopping therapy in children with acute lymphoblastic leukemia. N. Engl. J. Med. 300:269–273.

George, S. L., and M. M. Desu. 1974. Planning the size and duration of a clinical trial designed to study the time to some critical event. J. Chronic Dis. 27:15–24.

George, S. L., D. J. Fernbach, T. J. Vietti, M. P. Sullivan, D. M. Lane, M. E. Haggard, D. H. Berry, D. Lonsdale, and D. Komp. 1973. Factors influencing survival in pediatric acute leukemia: The SWCCSG experience. Cancer 32:287–298.

Hill, A. B. 1971. Principles of Medical Statistics. 9th ed. Lancet, London, 381 pp.

International Cancer Research Data Bank Program. 1976. Compilation of Clinical Protocol Summaries. U.S. Government Printing Office, Washington, D.C., 449 pp.

Mauer, A. M. 1978. Treatment of acute leukemia in children. Clin. Haematol. 7:245–258.

National Institutes of Health. 1976. Inventory of Clinical Trials. U.S. Government Printing Office, Washington, D.C.

Rubin, P., ed. 1978. Clinical Oncology for Medical Students and Physicians. 5th ed. University of Rochester, Rochester, N.Y., 327 pp.

Schwartz, D., R. Flamant, and J. Lellouch. 1970. L'Essai Therapeutique Chez l'Homme. Editions Medicales, Flammarion, Paris, 297 pp.

Simone, J. V. 1979. Childhood leukemia as a cancer research model. Cancer Res. 39:4301–4307.

Statistical Abstract of the U.S. 1978. 99th ed. U.S. Bureau of the Census, Washington, D.C., 1,057 pp.

Union Internationale Contre le Cancer. 1974. Controlled Therapeutic Trials in Cancer. UICC, Geneva, 220 pp.

STATUS OF THE CURABILITY OF SOLID TUMORS

Status of the Curability of Childhood Cancers,
edited by J. van Eys and M. P. Sullivan.
Raven Press, New York © 1980.

Status of the Curability
of Solid Tumors

Marvin M. Romsdahl, M.D., Ph.D.

*Department of Surgery, The University of Texas System Cancer Center M. D. Anderson
Hospital and Tumor Institute, Houston, Texas*

Until 20 years ago, lay persons and physicians were inclined to regard cancer as a disease afflicting adults, primarily older individuals. Adult cancer is more common than childhood neoplasia, as reflected in recent statistics indicating that only 6,000 cases of childhood cancer will be diagnosed in 1979, out of a total of 765,000 cases for all age groups (excluding nonmelanomatous skin cancer and carcinoma in situ). However, two factors have served to focus attention on cancer in children. First, progress in the management of childhood cancer is distinctly evident and, second, cancer is the leading cause of death from disease among children 3 to 14 years of age (American Cancer Society 1979).

Since favorable responses to treatment have been achieved, it seems appropriate to examine in greater depth the status of the curability of childhood cancers. As recently as 20 years ago, surgery was the only practical means of curing solid tumors in children or adults. Chemotherapy was a recent innovation, demonstrating value primarily in the management of leukemia and lymphoma. The sixties were, in retrospect, a transition period characterized by intensive investigations into the role of chemotherapy for solid tumors. During this same period, substantial technical developments permitted greater clinical application of radiotherapy. Despite remarkable efforts, by 1969 the only major change in survival rates of children with solid tumors was in Wilms' tumor (Myers et al. 1975) (Table 1). This finding, nevertheless, demonstrated the importance of treating cancers prior to their spread to other parts of the body (Farber 1969).

The seventies have been characterized by attempts to employ and expand, in different combinations and to different degrees, surgery, radiotherapy, and chemotherapy. Some hoped that immunotherapy would further increase the curability of cancers; however, it appears that a better understanding of immunology as a factor in host resistance to cancer will be necessary before this discipline can be effectively used in clinical practice.

Today, appropriate questions are, What is the status of the curability of childhood cancers? and, What progress has been made since our previous clinical conference on this subject 12 years ago? We know that approximately 6,000

Table 1. *Five-Year Survival Rates in Childhood Cancers*

Tumor Type	Rate (%)		
	1955–59	1960–64	1965–69
Brain and nervous system*	34	38	45
Neuroblastoma	27	23	22
Retinoblastoma	83	93	91
Wilms' tumor	41	42	60
Bone sarcoma	(25)†	23	22
Soft tissue sarcoma	57	(42)	36
Leukemia	1	4	5
Hodgkin's disease	(42)	(59)	66
Non-Hodgkin's lymphoma	16	17	20
All childhood cancers	29	31	34

* Excluding neuroblastoma.
† Rates in parentheses have 5–10% standard error.
From Myers et al. (1975).

new patients are now diagnosed annually with cancer, while 2,500 deaths occur annually from all types of childhood cancer, producing an overall cure rate of 39% (American Cancer Society 1979). Approximately half of these deaths are due to leukemia; the remainder are related to a broad spectrum of solid tumor types affecting areas such as the brain and nervous system, bone, kidney, and connective tissue. Five years ago Myers et al. (1975) reported a 5-year survival rate of 34% for childhood cancer in whites for 1965–69.

In the seventies, clinical characteristics of newly diagnosed cancers have been better described. Results usually are reported for defined stages or groups at initial presentation. While results based on these factors, which usually represent extent of disease, are more meaningful, they often cannot be compared with results from reports in which such staging was not done. In assessing favorable treatment results in patients with Wilms' tumor, rhabdomyosarcoma, osteosarcoma, and Ewing's sarcoma, it is important to verify that patients now being treated are indeed clinically similar to previously treated children. According to the latest figures (American Cancer Society 1979), long-term survival rates appear to be increasing. Improvements in curability are predominantly seen in the diseases listed in Table 2. Improvements in the leukemia and lymphoma groups have been primarily due to improved survival rates in patients with acute lymphoblastic leukemia and Hodgkin's disease. The 5-year survival rate (age-adjusted for normal life expectancy) for all cancers is 39% today.

It is clear that the management of solid tumors in children is more successful overall than that of solid tumors in adults. These better results among children have led to speculation about the basic nature of these tumors and the reasons they respond more to agents that are not effective against tumors in adults. In comparing the relative incidences of histologic tumor categories in children and adults, several authors (Breslow and McCann 1971, Sutow et al. 1977, Dorn and Cutler 1959, Griswold et al. 1955) have agreed that carcinomas and

Table 2. *Two- to Five-Year Survival Rates in Selected Childhood Cancers*

Tumor Type	Rate (%)
Wilms' tumor	76–92*
Osteosarcoma	55
Ewing's sarcoma	50
Rhabdomyosarcoma	68
Leukemia	3–50†
Hodgkin's disease	79–90‡
Non-Hodgkin's lymphoma	32
All cancers	39§

* Groups I–III. From Sutow (1979).
† Primarily acute lymphoblastic leukemia. From Simone (1979).
‡ Stages I–IV. From Sutow et al. (1977).
§ From American Cancer Society (1979).

adenocarcinomas account for approximately 85% of all cancers (Table 3). This is in sharp contrast to an incidence of 5% for such tumors in children under 14 years of age. The highest incidence in children are in the leukemia and lymphoma groups, sarcomas, and embryonal tumors, in that order (Sutow 1970). While this marked difference by histologic type may well be an important factor in the more favorable response to chemotherapy of childhood tumors, other undefined variables associated with younger age may also be important. For example, neuroblastoma is substantially more curable when the disease is diagnosed soon after birth, rather than later (Breslow and McCann 1971), a situation deserving of further scientific and clinical investigation.

Improvements in curability have not been seen for all types of childhood cancer. While substantial improvements in survival have been achieved for patients with Wilms' tumor, osteosarcoma, Ewing's sarcoma, and rhabdomysarcoma (Table 2), the same have not been shown for soft tissue sarcomas (other than rhabdomyosarcoma). Management of Ewing's sarcoma appears promising;

Table 3. *Distribution of Childhood and Adult Cancers*

Tumor Type	Children* (0–14 Years)	All Ages†
Leukemias/lymphomas	41	6
Sarcomas	27	3
Embryonal tumors	16	1
Neural tumors	6	2
Carcinomas and adenocarcinomas	5	85
All others	5	3

* From Sutow (1970).
† From Dorn and Cutler (1959); includes 594 children.

however, further follow-up and confirmation of preliminary results will be needed to evaluate the curability of this neoplasm (Tefft et al. 1977).

These comments should not be interpreted as expressing low expectations for cure of childhood solid tumors. The results attained are indeed substantial compared with those reported at our clinical conference 12 years ago. However, further research is still needed, especially in certain tumor types, to achieve our ultimate goal of curing children with solid tumors.

As we continue to improve the curability of childhood solid tumors, we will have to cope with the problems that confront long-term survivors. The intensity of therapy, the long lifespans of successfully treated individuals, and the use of a combined modality approach all contribute to those problems. Ultimately, it will be highly desirable to ascertain the minimal therapy required to achieve long-term survival.

Physical deformity is a predictable outcome of surgery, particularly radical surgery, while radiotherapy can be expected to affect later development, fertility, and certain organ functions. Surgery combined with radiotherapy may not profoundly reduce anticipated complications, and the addition of chemotherapy to radiotherapy may well lead to unpredictable long-term sequelae. Currently chemotherapy, usually in some combination, has improved survival rates for childhood cancer (Sutow et al. 1977). Truly, much must be learned to optimize the use of chemotherapy and radiotherapy, either simultaneously or sequentially, so as to maximize their antitumor effect while reducing potential undesirable side effects. We know that Adriamycin is associated with cardiac toxicity, cyclophosphamide with bladder injury, methotrexate with hepatic and renal toxicity, and bleomycin with pulmonary fibrosis. Reproductive performance and function are affected by radiotherapy and chemotherapy, the latter most likely with alkylating drugs. The carcinogenic potential of current treatment modalities is great and requires further study (Meadows et al. 1975, Jaffe 1976). It is of paramount importance that long-term follow-up studies include data on all potential sequelae to correctly ascertain factors that may dictate modifying our management programs.

Although environmental factors have been correctly implicated in certain adult solid tumors, and are presumed to be important in others, environmental carcinogens cannot be implicated in most childhood cancers because of children's limited exposure. The early peak ages of occurrence of certain tumors, especially neuroblastoma, Wilms' tumor, hepatoblastoma, retinoblastoma, and rhabdomyosarcoma, suggest that exposures to carcinogens were brief, or that the mutagenic event occurred during fetal development. These considerations remind us that reductions in mortality from neoplasms in this age group are not likely to be achieved by programs in prevention (Holmes and Holmes 1975). Our greatest hope appears to be to maximize efforts to gain biological information as a basis for implementing rational therapy regimens.

Developments in the management of solid tumors have been significant. Progress, as measured by increased curability, is the standard most visible to the public and has been truly impressive for several tumor types. The impact of these favorable results has led to measurable increases in survival. It is more difficult to ascertain quantitatively our progress toward lessening the adverse impact of childhood cancer on our communities. Data now available strongly suggest that long-term survivors of childhood cancer adjust well to employment and school, as well as to marriage (Maurer et al. 1977). This strengthens our commitment to further increasing the curability of childhood cancer.

It is not possible in this session to address all or even most of the special problems associated with solid tumors in children. Presentations will be made on the three major treatment modalities, chemotherapy, surgery, and radiotherapy, and their roles in the management of childhood solid tumors. Presentations on the management of bone cancer, neuroblastomas, and brain tumors will follow. One speaker will discuss the role of pathology in the management of bone cancer. It is refreshing to witness the recognition by medical oncologists of the important contributions of this specialty and its integration into the practical aspects of patient management. It is hoped that these presentations, combined with those by other participants at this clinical conference, will direct us toward even more effective means of curing childhood cancers.

REFERENCES

American Cancer Society. 1979. Cancer Facts and Figures. American Cancer Society, New York, 20 pp.

Breslow, N., and B. McCann. 1971. Statistical estimation of prognosis for children with neuroblastoma. Cancer Res. 31:2098–2103.

Dorn, H. F., and S. J. Cutler. 1959. Morbidity from Cancer in the United States. Public Health Monogr. No. 56, Public Health Service Pub. No. 590. U.S. Government Printing Office, Washington, D.C., 207 pp.

Farber, S. 1969. The control of cancer in children, *in* Neoplasia in Childhood (The University of Texas System Cancer Center Twelfth Annual Clinical Conference on Cancer 1967). Year Book Medical Publishers, Inc., Chicago, pp. 321–327.

Griswold, M. H., C. S. Wilder, S. J. Cutler, and E. S. Pollack. 1955. Cancer in Connecticut, 1935–1951. Connecticut State Department of Health, Hartford, Conn.

Holmes, H. A., and F. F. Holmes. 1975. After ten years, what are the handicaps and life styles of children treated for cancer? An examination of the present status of 124 such survivors. Clin. Pediatr. 14:819–823.

Jaffe, N. 1976. Late side effects of treatment: Skeletal, genetic, central nervous system and oncogenic. Pediatr. Clin. North Am. 23:233–244.

Maurer, A. M., J. V. Simone, and C. B. Pratt. 1977. Current progress in the treatment of the child with cancer. J. Pediatr. 91:523–539.

Meadows, A. T., G. J. D'Angio, A. E. Evans, C. C. Harris, R. W. Miller, and V. Miké. 1975. Oncogenesis and other later effects of cancer treatment in children. Radiology 114:175–180.

Myers, M. H., H. W. Heise, F. P. Li, and R. W. Miller. 1975. Trends in cancer survival among U.S. white children, 1955–1971. J. Pediatr. 87:815–818.

Simone, J. V. 1979. Leukemia, *in* Care of the Child with Cancer. American Cancer Society, New York, pp. 50–55.

Sutow, W. W. 1970. Drug therapy and curability of childhood cancer. Postgrad. Med. 48:173–177.

Sutow, W. W. 1979. Wilms' tumor—Retrospect and prospect, *in* Care of the Child with Cancer. American Cancer Society, New York, pp. 62–70.

Sutow, W. W., T. J. Vietti, and D. J. Fernbach, eds. 1977. Clinical Pediatric Oncology. 2nd ed. C. V. Mosby Co., St. Louis, 751 pp.

Tefft, M., B. M. Chabora, and G. Rosen. 1977. Radiation in bone sarcomas. Cancer 39:806–816.

Status of the Curability of Childhood Cancers,
edited by J. van Eys and M. P. Sullivan.
Raven Press, New York © 1980.

Chemotherapy as a Curative Intervention in Malignant Solid Tumors in Children

W. W. Sutow, M.D.

Department of Pediatrics, The University of Texas System Cancer Center M. D. Anderson Hospital and Tumor Institute, Houston, Texas

Chemotherapy constitutes an important and significantly effective arm of multimodal intervention in the management of childhood cancer today. This review will attempt to present a perspective of the current status of chemotherapy, to provide a brief historical survey of the development of some key concepts in chemotherapy, and to examine a few projections that seem justified. Accordingly, the discussion will be general, emphasizing the philosophy of cancer treatment more than the tactics, the principles more than the actual schemas. The precise statistics and the intricate details of management will be presented in subsequent chapters dealing with specific tumors.

Mortality tables continue to demonstrate the medical significance of cancer in children. Table 1 lists Public Health Service data for 1973 showing the causes of death in children 1 through 14 years of age. Almost half of the deaths were due to accidents, homicides, and suicides. The second leading cause of death overall and the leading medical cause of death was cancer. Eleven percent of children who died died of cancer.

The same mortality data can be rearranged to indicate the relative frequency of cancer deaths in various age groups (Table 2). In children under 5 years of age, 1.5% of all deaths were due to cancer. In the age groups 5 through 9 years and 10 through 14 years, 14.5% and 11.8%, respectively, of the deaths

Table 1. *Causes of Death in Children 1–14 Years Old*

Rank Order	Cause	% of All Deaths	Death Rate per 100,000
1	Accident	46.4	23.7
2	Cancer	11.0	5.6
3	Congenital malformation	8.0	4.1
5	Homicide	2.9	1.5
11	Benign neoplasm	0.8	0.4
15	Suicide	0.6	0.3

From U.S. Vital Statistics, 1973 (1975).

69

Table 2. *Cancer Deaths in Children by Age*

Age (Years)	Cancer Deaths as % of Total
Under 1	0.2
1 to 4	8.0
5 to 9	14.5
10 to 14	11.8
15 to 19	6.0

From U.S. Vital Statistics, 1973 (1975).

Table 3. *Relative Frequency of Solid Tumors (Seer Program, 1973–76)*

Tumor Type	% of All Tumors	Frequency Relative to Wilms' Tumor
Central nervous system	33.1	3.22
Neuroblastoma	14.1	1.37
Wilms' tumor	10.3	1.00
Other soft tissue sarcoma	5.7	0.55
Rhabdomyosarcoma	5.5	0.54
Osteosarcoma	4.6	0.45
Retinoblastoma	4.5	0.43
Gonadal/germ cell	3.7	0.36
Ewing's sarcoma	3.2	0.31
Liver	2.4	0.23
Miscellaneous	13.1	1.28

From Young et al. (1978).

were due to cancer. In mid- and late adolescence, 15 through 19 years, the fraction of cancer deaths dropped to 6%.

What are the malignant solid tumors of childhood? The relative frequencies of childhood solid tumor types are shown in Table 3. Since Wilms' tumor appears to occur at a constant frequency throughout the world, a number of investigators have suggested using it as the index tumor in showing the relative frequencies of other tumors (Innis 1973, Editorial 1973). In the United States, for each case of Wilms' tumor there were 3.2 cases of brain tumors, 1.4 cases of neuroblastomas, and about 0.5 cases each of rhabdomyosarcomas and osteosarcomas in the period covered by the table (Young et al. 1978).

HISTORY OF CHEMOTHERAPY

The chronological sequence of steps in the development of curative chemotherapy was summarized recently by Zubrod (1978) in an address to the American Association for Cancer Research. The age of modern cancer chemotherapy probably began with the wartime studies of nitrogen mustards in the 1940s.

By the late 1950s clinical cancer chemotherapy was usually concerned with the management of metastatic cancer. In the early 1960s combination drug programs were developed. By the end of the 1960s adjuvant chemotherapy regimens for nonmetastatic cases were being used widely, particularly for such pediatric cancers as Wilms' tumor, rhabdomyosarcoma, and osteosarcoma. In the 1970s the investigative clinical activities appeared to emphasize selective toxicity, a phrase borrowed from terminology for chemotherapy of infectious diseases.

The introduction of key drugs into clinical oncology began in the early 1940s, when the nitrogen mustards were developed. By 1955 the use of actinomycin D (AMD) was increasing. From 1957 to 1962 the clinical capabilities of another alkylating agent, cyclophosphamide (CYT), were explored and established. From about 1962 to 1965 the vinca alkaloids, particularly vincristine (VCR), were investigated. Adriamycin (ADR), a relatively recent antibiotic, became an important component of chemotherapy around 1969. The use of methotrexate to treat leukemia began more than 30 years ago, about 1948. Interest in the drug underwent a resurgence with the application of high-dose regimens (HD-MTX) in the treatment of osteosarcoma beginning about 1972. Djerassi and his colleagues (with investigations going back at least to 1968) deserve much of the credit for this new look at an old drug (Djerassi 1975).

Table 4 shows the relationship between a spectrum of tumors and a spectrum of drugs. The table permits a quick reading of the drugs considered to have activity against specific tumors. For example, for Wilms' tumor both AMD and VCR are used in primary regimens, and CYT and ADR are noted to have definite clinical effect. For rhabdomyosarcoma four drugs, AMD, CYT, ADR, and VCR, are used in primary regimens. In osteosarcoma the key drugs in adjuvant chemotherapy are CYT, ADR, and HD-MTX.

Reading across the table reveals the overall usefulness of each drug against various tumors. For example, AMD is included in the primary regimens for Wilms' tumor, rhabdomyosarcoma, and Ewing's sarcoma, while CYT has been

Table 4. *Chemotherapy Profile of Various Drugs*

Drug	Tumor					
	WT	RHBD	OST	ES	CNS	NB
AMD	*	*	—	*	—	±
CYT	+	*	*	*	—	*
ADR	+	*	*	*	—	*
HD-MTX	—	—	*	—	+	—
VCR	*	*	±	*	+	*
DTIC	—	—	—	+	—	*

WT, Wilms' tumor; RHBD, rhabdomyosarcoma; OST, osteosarcoma; ES, Ewing's sarcoma; CNS, brain tumor; NB, neuroblastoma; *, in primary regimen; +, clinically effective; ±, possibly effective; —, not effective or unknown.

incorporated in chemotherapy regimens for rhabdomyosarcoma, osteosarcoma, Ewing's sarcoma, and neuroblastoma. The two other drugs used widely in pediatric oncology are ADR and VCR.

STRATEGY OF THERAPY

The evolution of a strategy for chemotherapy in pediatric oncology can be discussed under several well-established headings. The transition from use of single agents to multiple-agent therapy to multidisciplinary regimens, in retrospect, was logical. It was based on progressively improving results.

Similarly, the shift in emphasis from palliative treatment of metastatic disease to more intensive approaches with curative intent to adjuvant chemotherapy in presumably nonmetastatic cases again resulted from increasingly effective chemotherapeutic programs. Dose and schedule changes have yielded exciting breakthroughs, exemplified by pulse-VAC regimens in rhabdomyosarcoma and HD-MTX administration in osteosarcoma. One of the most significant developments in chemotherapy has been the ability to channel efforts away from concentration on increasing the effectiveness of therapy toward the refinement of therapy without sacrifice of treatment results.

Another area of clinical investigation that has become better delineated has been the identification of factors that can predict the probable outcome of therapy and the behavior of the disease. As a result, therapeutic decisions are being based on consideration of these factors. Already established for a number of solid tumors are such probable determinants of outcome as the age of the patient, site of the primary lesion, histopathology of the tumor, extent of the disease, and the pattern of metastases. With the development of effective chemotherapy, the clinical investigator is now armed with weapons of sufficient firepower to warrant testing conceptual innovations.

Childhood Rhabdomyosarcoma

The chemotherapeutic interventions in childhood rhabdomyosarcoma illustrate the ways in which chemotherapy has been integrated into treatment programs for childhood solid tumors.

Current survival rates in childhood rhabdomyosarcoma are indicated by the results of the First Intergroup Rhabdomyosarcoma Study (IRS-I). Both the 'disease-free and overall survival rates are shown for clinical groups I, II, III, and IV in Table 5. Today the 2-year disease-free survival rate is 80% in group I rhabdomyosarcoma patients and 75% in group II patients. Similarly, the 2-year overall survival rate can be as high as 80% in group III patients.

Two major changes in the philosophy of therapy for rhabdomyosarcoma have involved rhabdomyosarcomas arising in genitourinary sites and rhabdomyosarcomas arising in certain parameningeal sites.

The results of IRS-I demonstrated that children with genitourinary rhabdo-

Table 5. *Rhabdomyosarcoma Patient Survival in IRS-I*

Clinical Group	No. of Patients	No. Surviving	2-Year Survival Rate (%)
Disease-free survival			
I	72	62	86
II	128	96	75
III	142	06	67
IV	51	17	33
Overall survival			
I	73	68	93
II	130	101	78
III	238	155	65
IV	113	45	40

From Maurer et al. (1980).

myosarcoma primaries had consistently better survival rates than children with rhabdomyosarcomas of other sites (Gehan et al. 1980). This seemed to hold true regardless of the stage or extent of disease (Table 6).

Although the results were excellent in children with genitourinary rhabdomyosarcoma, the high survival rate was attained in many patients at the cost of radical exenterative surgery and subsequent loss of bladder and rectal functions. More recently, with the availability of consistently effective chemotherapy, a change in therapeutic attitude has been fostered in a number of institutions (Rivard et al. 1975, Kumar et al. 1976, Hays and Ortega 1977, Flamant et al. 1979, Ortega 1979). This change has involved the use of preoperative chemotherapy and conservative surgery. Resection of tumor, rather than exenteration, preserves bladder and bowel functions.

Table 6. *Number of Patients Surviving 2 Years by Primary Site and Group*

Primary Site	Clinical Group							
	I		II		III		IV	
	No.	(%)	No.	(%)	No.	(%)	No.	(%)
Disease-free survival								
Genitourinary	36	(92)	28	(79)	27	(54)	27	(39)
Extremities	19	(62)	30	(63)	21	(24)	27	(3)
Head and neck			29	(82)	97	(53)	21	(10)
Orbit			15	(93)	36	(68)		
Overall survival								
Genitourinary	36	(95)	28	(78)	27	(87)	27	(57)
Extremities	19	(73)	31	(75)	21	(50)	27	(25)
Head and neck			30	(88)	97	(58)	21	(48)
Orbit			15	(93)	36	(83)		

From Gehan et al. (1980).

In the Second Rhabdomyosarcoma Study (IRS Committee 1978), the efficacy of conservative surgery with chemotherapy in maintaining good disease control and survival is being investigated. The institutions participating in this study of tumors of certain pelvic sites use primary chemotherapy. Patients in groups I, II, and III with rhabdomyosarcoma of the prostate, bladder, uterus, and vagina are treated initially with multiagent vincristine, actinomycin D, and cyclophosphamide (VAC) chemotherapy. They are reevaluated at 8 weeks to determine if there has been a response or if the disease is increasing. If no regression has occurred by 8 weeks, definitive surgery is carried out at that time. If a response has occurred, chemotherapy is continued for 8 more weeks and definitive surgery is performed on week 16. It is anticipated that most patients will have enough tumor regression so that conservative surgery will suffice.

The ability of chemotherapy to produce consistent and substantial regression of tumor masses was demonstrated in IRS-I (Tefft et al. 1977, Maurer et al. 1980). In that study, patients in clinical groups III and IV (gross residual disease or metastases) received chemotherapy for 5 weeks before the administration of radiation therapy. The frequencies of response are shown in Table 7. Regimen E was a three-drug pulse-VAC regimen, and regimen F a four-drug treatment with pulse-VAC plus Adriamycin. There were responses in 80% of the patients and complete regressions in about 50%, regardless of clinical group and type of chemotherapy.

The second change in therapeutic attitude related to rhabdomyosarcomas originating in the so-called parameningeal sites, including the nasopharynx, nasal cavity, paranasal sinuses, and middle ear (Gerson et al. 1978, Tefft et al. 1978, Chan et al. 1979, Raney et al. 1980).

Between 1972 and 1976, 161 children with rhabdomyosarcoma of the head and neck were registered in IRS-I (Tefft et al. 1978). Of this number, 40% had tumors involving a parameningeal site. Of the 57 patients with parameningeal tumors at the time of the analysis, 20 (35%) developed intracranial extension, that is, meningeal spread or breakthrough. Of greatest importance was the uniformly fatal outcome in such patients.

In IRS-II (IRS Committee 1978), patients at risk of meningeal complications have been identified early. They undergo careful evaluation at the time of entry on the study. Special attention is paid to warning signs, such as tumor cells

Table 7. *Tumor Regression after Preradiotherapy Chemotherapy*

Clinical Group	Regimen	No. of Patients	Response Rate (%)	
			Complete	Partial
III	E	48	53	29
	F	47	47	34
IV	E	26	50	31
	F	30	43	40
Total		151	48	33

Table 8. *Chemotherapy Interventions for Wilms' Tumor and Osteosarcoma*

Wilms' tumor	Osteosarcoma
Adjuvant therapy	Adjuvant therapy
Refinement of therapy	Metastatic therapy
Radiotherapy	Preoperative chemotherapy
Chemotherapy	Development of limb-sparing procedures
Management of metastases	
Preoperative chomothorapy (?)	

in the cerebrospinal fluid, cranial nerve dysfunction, erosion of the base of skull, or enlargement of neural foramina.

If the evaluation is negative, no change in the therapy plan is made and the radiation treatment field is reviewed carefully. However, if the evaluation is positive, radiation therapy is administered to the craniospinal meninges and intrathecal chemotherapy is given. This chemotherapeutic approach is similar to that used for central nervous system disease in acute leukemia.

For comparison, some goals of the current approaches to Wilms' tumor and to osteosarcoma are listed in Table 8.

Treatment of Metastases

The occurrence of metastases during or after primary treatment is discouraging, but with the recent availability of effective multimodal programs, a metastatic relapse now need not presage a fatal outcome (Table 9).

Experience at M. D. Anderson Hospital (MDAH) in treating patients with metastatic rhabdomyosarcoma has not been good, with a 13% 2-year survival rate in 46 patients (Okamura et al. 1977). In IRS-I, 51 patients were in group IV (metastases at diagnosis). Their survival rate was 33% at 2 years (Maurer et al. 1980).

In the First National Wilms' Tumor Study (NWTS-I), 45% of 103 patients

Table 9. *Two-Year Survival after Development of Metastases*

Disease	No. of Patients Treated	Survival Rate (%)
Rhabdomyosarcoma		
MDAH	46	13
IRS, group IV	51	33
Wilms' tumor (NWTS)		
Metastatic cases	103	45
Group IV	84	56
Osteosarcoma		
MDAH	44	39

From Okamura et al. (1977), Maurer et al. (1980), Sutow et al. (1979), Perez et al. (1978), and Sutow et al. (1980).

who developed metastases during the study were alive 2 years later (Sutow et al. 1979). The group IV patients, who were metastatic at the time of diagnosis, had a 2-year survival rate of 56%. Forty-four osteosarcoma patients with metastases who were treated after 1970 had a 39% 2-year survival rate (Perez et al. 1978, Sutow et al. 1980).

Examination of survival patterns in metastatic disease has led to the recognition of several prognostic factors, including the interval between diagnosis and development of metastases, site of metastases, premetastatic factors, and postmetastatic therapy.

Postmetastatic survival was examined in 106 patients with osteosarcoma treated at MDAH (Sutow et al. 1980). Of 62 treated before 1970, four survived 2 years. The 44 treated after 1970 had a significantly better 2-year survival rate, 39%. (Adriamycin and HD-MTX treatments became available after 1970.)

Another factor that seems to influence postmetastatic survival is the length of time from diagnosis to development of metastases. In one study, this interval was used to divide patients into three categories. In the "early" group were those who had metastases at diagnosis, in the "mid" category those who developed metastases during the 1st year, and in the "late" category those who developed metastases after 13 months. The survival curve for those treated after 1970 who were metastastic at diagnosis was very poor, with seven of eight dying within 1 year from development of metastases. The middle group had a better survival rate, with 10 of 29 alive 2 years later. By far the best survival was recorded for the late metastasizers, six of seven of whom were surviving more than 2 years.

That the MDAH series does not represent an unique experience is indicated by data from two other institutions for patients treated after 1970. Researchers at Sidney Farber Cancer Center have reported a 2-year survival rate after metastases of 41% in 39 patients (Jaffe et al. 1976, 1977), and those at Memorial Sloan-Kettering Cancer Center a survival rate of 60% in 45 patients (Rosen et al. 1978).

The evaluation of survival after metastases in Wilms' tumor has generated even more informative data (Sutow et al. 1979). In NWTS-I, 84 patients were registered as group IV. Another 103 patients developed metastatic disease while on study. The 3-year survival rate was 58% for the group IV patients and 44% for those who were initially in groups I, II, and III. The results suggest that prior exposure to active drugs (as was the case with group I, II, and III patients, but not group IV) may be detrimental.

Significantly related to postrelapse survival in group I–III patients were histology, time to relapse, and site of metastasis. Unfavorable histology, early relapse, and metastases to sites other than the lungs were bad prognostic factors. Group I patients who relapsed had better postrelapse survival rates than relapsed group II and III patients, the difference deriving largely from the fact that metastases were limited to the lungs in most group I patients. The administration of actinomycin D, vincristine, or both during the premetastatic phase in group II and III patients did not correlate with postmetastastic survival.

CURRENT ACHIEVEMENTS OF CHEMOTHERAPY

The current achievements with chemotherapeutic intervention in malignant solid tumors of childhood can be summarized as follows:

1. *Definite improvement in cure rate with primary therapy.* For some tumors it seems reasonable to credit chemotherapy with having brought about a definite improvement in the cure rate. The tumors in which this has occurred include Wilms' tumor, rhabdomyosarcoma, and osteosarcoma.

2. *Probable or possible improvement in cure rate with primary therapy.* In another category are those tumors in which improvement in cure rate appears probable or possible. In this category available data do not permit a definitive statement. For example, in Ewing's sarcoma an improvement in cure rate is suggested, but the duration of follow-up in a tumor notorious for late relapses seems too short in most studies for definite statements of success. Neuroblastoma is an enigma. To what degree chemotherapy has changed the cure rate is difficult to establish satisfactorily. Germ cell tumors are also in this category. Because of the relatively good results being reported, these tumors seem responsive to several drug combinations. Some of the good outcome may be attributable to chemotherapy.

3. *Definite improvement in cure rate from postmetastatic therapy.* Successful postmetastatic therapy has been used in Wilms' tumor and to some degree in osteosarcoma. For most other tumors, the cure rates after metastases appear not to have been influenced as yet. It is noteworthy that postmetastatic survival in childhood rhabdomyosarcoma, a chemosensitive tumor, remains unsatisfactory.

4. *Attainment of optimum cure rate permitting refinement of therapy.* In two major tumors the chemotherapeutic regimens have become so effective that refinement of therapy has been achieved or is being investigated.

Refinement of therapy in Wilms' tumor was attained, first, by omitting postoperative irradiation of the tumor bed in stage I patients and, second, by reducing the duration of chemotherapy in stage I patients. In NWTS-III the possibility of further refinement of therapy is being investigated. The study is assessing the effectiveness of chemotherapy after reduction in duration from 15 months to 6 months to 3 months. During the conventional 15-month therapy with VCR and AMD, the patient receives 18 doses of VCR and seven of AMD. As the duration of therapy is shortened to 6 months and then 3 months, the amount of drug given is correspondingly decreased from 18 to 12 to 10 doses of VCR and from seven to four to two courses of AMD.

In rhabdomyosarcoma, therapy has been refined in three areas (Maurer et al. 1980). First, IRS-I demonstrated that postoperative irradiation can be omitted in group I patients receiving chemotherapy. Second, the study showed that adjuvant two-drug therapy with VCR and AMD was as effective as three-drug VAC therapy in group II patients. The omission of cyclophosphamide from any combination regimen is a significant advantage, as considerable toxicity and morbidity are eliminated. Third, the use of chemotherapy in rhabdomyosarcoma is permitting refinement of another modality, surgery. As described above, the capacity of preoperative therapy to produce tumor regression may permit conservative surgery in certain pelvic sites.

5. *Identification of clinical areas for further intensive therapeutic investigations.* Progress has been slow in the treatment of brain tumors and advanced stages of neuroblastoma. In most solid tumors the treatment for metastatic disease remains unsatisfactory. One recent advance in pediatric oncology has been the recognition of prognostic factors, which allow the prediction of the likelihood of a successful outcome after treatment. Specifically, the identification of prognostically unfavorable subsets of patients has indicated the clinical areas in need of intensified therapy. In Wilms' tumor, this would include patients whose tumors are of an unfavorable histologic type. In rhabdomyosarcoma, it would include patients with tumors of the extremities and parameningeal sites.

OBSTACLES TO CURE

The mere fact that survival or cure rates for most solid tumors are not completely satisfactory indicates that many obstacles to cure exist. Table 10 lists some of these obstacles, based on Zubrod's discussion (1978). Tumor heterogeneity is one obstacle. In addition to specific pathologic entities, even tumors in a given diagnostic category may vary. Within rhabdomyosarcoma, for example, there are embryonal, alveolar, botryoid, and other cell types. In Wilms' tumor, prognostically good and bad histologic characteristics have been recognized.

Cumbersome methodology and slow pace characterize clinical investigations in general. Among children, the number of patients with a given type of solid tumor is small, so accumulation of meaningful numbers of patients requires a long time. Multi-institutional collaborative studies are conceptually attractive but there are many operational snags.

Time is required to develop an acceptable protocol and to set up the mechanism to conduct the study; 2 or even 3 years are usually needed. For most pediatric solid tumors, 3 to 4 years of patient entry are required to register sufficient numbers to satisfy the statistical prerequisites. A follow-up period of 2 years or longer is necessary from the date of last patient entry. Thus, 8 or 9 years are required to design, conduct, and complete a major study, and there is a

Table 10. *Obstacles to Cure of*
Solid Tumors

1. Tumor heterogeneity
2. Cumbersome methodology
3. Slow pace of clinical studies
    a. Conduct of studies
    b. Assessment of results
4. Iatrogenic factors
    a. Communication
    b. Collaboration

danger that the question being asked may have lost its importance 8 to 9 years later because new means of therapy have been discovered.

Have improvements in the effectiveness of chemotherapeutic interventions for solid tumors plateaued? Has the available technology reached the trade-off point? That is, to gain additional benefit, will the treatment regimens need to be so complex that the difficulty of following the treatment schema and the severity of the side effects of therapy outweigh added benefits of therapy? For some tumors, such as Wilms' tumor, for which the 2-year survival rate is 90% or 95%, the risk-versus-benefit equation can be approached deliberately. But in other tumors for which we are striving to reach even a 50% or 75% cure rate, we cannot settle yet for a trade-off.

REFERENCES

Chan, R. C., W. W. Sutow, and R. D. Lindberg. 1979. Parameningeal rhabdomyosarcoma. Radiology 131:211–214.

Djerassi, I. 1975. High-dose methotrexate and citrovorum factor rescue: Background and rationale. Cancer Chemother. Rep. 6:3–6.

Editorial. 1973. Nephroblastoma: An index reference cancer. Lancet 2:651.

Flamant, F., D. Chassagne, J. M. Cosset, A. Gerbaulet, and J. Lemerle. 1979. Embryonal rhabdomyosarcoma of the vagina in children: Conservative treatment with curietherapy and chemotherapy. Eur. J. Cancer 15:527–532.

Gehan, E. A., F. N. Glover, H. M. Maurer, W. W. Sutow, D. M. Hays, W. Lawrence, Jr., W. Newton, Jr., and E. H. Soule. 1980. Prognostic factors in children with rhabdomyosarcoma, in Proceedings of Symposium on Sarcomas of Soft Tissue and Bone in Childhood. Natl. Cancer Inst. Monogr. (in press).

Gerson, J. M., N. Jaffe, M. Donaldson, and M. Tefft. 1978. Meningeal seeding from rhabdomyosarcoma of the head and neck with base of skull invasion: Recognition of the clinical evolution and suggestions for management. Med. Pediatr. Oncol. 5:137–144.

Hays, D. M., and J. Ortega. 1977. Primary chemotherapy in the management of pelvic rhabdomyosarcoma in infancy and early childhood, in Adjuvant Therapy of Cancer, S. S. Salmon and S. E. Jones, eds. North-Holland Publishing Co., Amsterdam, Oxford, New York, pp. 381–387.

Innis, M. D. 1973. Nephroblastoma: Index cancer of childhood. Med. J. Aust. 2:322–323.

Intergroup Rhabdomyosarcoma Study Committee. 1978. Protocol for Intergroup Rhabdomyosarcoma Study–II, p. 88.

Jaffe, N., E. Frei III, D. Traggis, and H. Watts. 1977. Weekly high-dose methotrexate-citrovorum factor in osteogenic sarcoma: Presurgical treatment of primary tumor and of overt pulmonary metastases. Cancer 39:45–50.

Jaffe, N., D. Traggis, J. R. Cassady, R. M. Filler, H. Watts, and E. Frei. 1976. Multidisciplinary treatment for macrometastatic osteogenic sarcoma. Br. Med. J. 2:1039–1041.

Kumar, A. P. M., E. L. Wrenn, Jr., I. D. Fleming, H. D. Hustu, and C. B. Pratt. 1976. Combined therapy to prevent complete pelvic exenteration for rhabdomyosarcoma of the vagina or uterus. Cancer 37:118–122.

Marcove, R. C., V. Miké, J. V. Hajek, A. G. Levin, and R. V. P. Hutter. 1970. Osteogenic sarcoma under the age of twenty-one: A review of one hundred and forty-five operative cases. J. Bone Joint Surg. 52A:411–423.

Maurer, H. M., M. Donaldson, E. A. Gehan, D. Hammond, D. M. Hays, W. Lawrence, Jr., R. Lindberg, W. Newton, A. Ragab, R. B. Raney, F. Ruymann, E. H. Soule, W. W. Sutow, and M. Tefft. 1980. The Intergroup Rhabdomyosarcoma Study—Update 1978, in Proceedings of Symposium on Sarcomas of Soft Tissue and Bone in Childhood. Natl. Cancer Inst. Monogr. (in press).

Okamura, J., W. W. Sutow, and T. E. Moon. 1977. Prognosis in children with metastatic rhabdomyosarcoma. Med. Pediatr. Oncol. 3:243–251.

Ortega, J. A. 1979. A therapeutic approach to childhood pelvic rhabdomyosarcoma without pelvic exenteration. J. Pediatr. 94:205–209.

Perez, C., J. Herson, J. C. Kimball, and W. W. Sutow. 1978. Prognosis after metastases in osteosarcoma. Cancer Clin. Trials 1:315–320.

Raney, R. B., Jr., H. M. Donaldson, W. W. Sutow, R. D. Lindberg, H. M. Maurer, and M. Tefft. 1980. Special considerations related to primary site in rhabdomyosarcoma: Experience of the Intergroup Rhabdomyosarcoma Study, *in* Proceedings of Symposium on Sarcomas of Soft Tissue and Bone in Childhood. Natl. Cancer Inst. Monogr. (in press).

Rivard, G., J. Ortega, R. Hittle, R. Nitschke, and M. Karon. 1975. Intensive chemotherapy as primary treatment for rhabdomyosarcoma of the pelvis. Cancer 36:1593–1597.

Rosen, G., A. G. Huvos, C. Mosende, E. J. Beattie, Jr., P. R. Exelby, B. Capparos, and R. C. Marcove. 1978. Chemotherapy and thoractomy for metastatic osteogenic sarcoma: A model for adjuvant chemotherapy and the rationale for the timing of thoracic surgery. Cancer 41:841–849.

Sutow, W. W., J. Herson, and C. Perez. 1980. Survival after metastasis in osteosarcoma, *in* Proceedings of Symposium on Sarcomas of Soft Tissue and Bone in Childhood. Natl. Cancer Inst. Monogr. (in press).

Sutow, W. W., N. Breslow, N. F. Palmer, G. J. D'Angio, and J. R. Takashima. 1979. Prognosis after relapse in children with Wilms' tumor: Results from the First National Wilms' Tumor Study (NWTS-I). Proc. Am. Assoc. Cancer Res. 20:68.

Tefft, M., C. H. Fernandez, and T. E. Moon. 1977. Rhabdomyosarcoma: Response with chemotherapy prior to radiation in patients with gross residual disease. Cancer 39:665–670.

Tefft, M., C. Fernandez, M. Donaldson, W. Newton, and T. E. Moon. 1978. Incidence of meningeal involvement by rhabdomyosarcoma of the head and neck in children: A report of the Intergroup Rhabdomyosarcoma Study (IRS). Cancer 42:253–258.

Vital Statistics of the United States, 1973, vol. 2 (Mortality), Part B. 1975. U.S. Department of Health, Education and Welfare, Public Health Service, National Center for Health Statistics, Rockville, Md., 693 pp.

Young, J. L., Jr., H. W. Heise, E. Silverberg, and M. H. Myers. 1978. Cancer Incidence, Survival and Mortality for Children under 15 Years of Age. American Cancer Society, New York, 16 pp.

Zubrod, C. G. 1978. Selective toxicity of anticancer drugs: Presidential address. Cancer Res. 38:4377–4384.

Status of the Curability of Childhood Cancers,
edited by J. van Eys and M. P. Sullivan.
Raven Press, New York © 1980.

Improved Curability and Changing Concepts in Pediatric Cancer Surgery

Philip R. Exelby, M.D.

Department of Surgery, Memorial Sloan-Kettering Cancer Center, New York, New York

The past decade has seen great advances in the management of cancer in children. The development of multidisciplinary treatment has improved survival rates and influenced the role of surgery in the primary treatment of solid tumors. In the background of multidisciplinary treatment, the position of surgery must be continually reevaluated. At the same time, the principles of good cancer surgery must be followed, and surgery integrated carefully with the other modalities of treatment. Improvements in chemotherapy and radiation therapy have made possible less radical surgery with attention to preservation of limbs and vital pelvic structures not involved with disease. Less radical surgery does not necessarily mean a less complicated procedure for the surgeon or the patient. In fact, modern cancer surgery in children has become extremely complex, and the newer procedures are often more difficult technically and require more attention to basic surgical principles and extremely detailed postoperative care and follow-up. In addition, surgery is often carried out in areas of the body that have received large doses of radiation in patients whose physiological status and healing powers have been changed by multiple-drug chemotherapy. The increased technical difficulty of the procedures carried out in a setting unfavorable for major surgery means that planning of the correct procedure and timing of the procedure have become extremely important. The present aim of surgery is to remove the tumor by a well-planned cancer operation preserving anatomical and physiological function in the child as much as possible.

PRIMARY TREATMENT

Primary surgical treatment has classically involved a radical surgical extirpation of the primary tumor and its immediate regional lymph draining area. Over the past decade it has been possible to develop limb-saving procedures for diseases such as osteogenic sarcoma and rhabdomyosarcoma of the extremities and to spare pelvic organs in children with sarcoma botryoides of the bladder, prostate, uterus, and vagina (Rosen et al. 1976, Morton et al. 1976). After the initial success of multidisciplinary treatment in some solid cancers in children, there has been a tendency toward less than adequate primary surgical treatment. There is increasing evidence that surgery must accomplish gross total removal of the tumor to achieve a cure. When gross tumor removal is achieved by surgery, it seems that microscopic residual tumor, such as tumor close to the margins of resection, can be successfully treated by irradiation and chemotherapy. This does not mean that surgery should be planned to achieve only partial resection of the tumor when total removal is possible. Inadequate surgery is still a major cause of treatment failure.

SURGERY AFTER CHEMOTHERAPY, RADIATION THERAPY, OR BOTH

A recent development in multidisciplinary management has been the timing of surgery to follow chemotherapy, radiotherapy, or both, or a "sandwiching" of surgery between the different modalities of treatment. It has long been known that radiation therapy and chemotherapy can shrink a primary tumor and make a surgical procedure easier. It was always feared, however, that leaving the primary tumor in place for several months during chemotherapy might jeopardize the life of the patient if metastatic spread took place during this interval. The work of Rosen and co-workers (1979) with osteogenic sarcoma has convinced many surgeons that a prolonged course of chemotherapy prior to ablation of the primary tumor not only facilitates a less radical procedure, but also reduces the incidence of metastatic disease and enhances survival. In addition, pretreatment with chemotherapy prior to surgical removal of the tumor enables the pathologist and oncologist to see the effect of chemotherapy on the tumor under the microscope. There is increasing evidence that tumor response to chemotherapy, estimated histologically by the pathologist, may be the most important prognostic factor in future management of the tumor. Surgery after chemotherapy, radiation therapy, or both, is becoming standard in such tumors as pelvic rhabdomyosarcoma, neuroblastoma, bilateral Wilms' tumor, and non-Hodgkin's lymphoma. Surgery after chemotherapy, radiotherapy, or both, must be very carefully planned with the chemotherapist and radiotherapist and demands experienced judgment by the surgeon in the choice of procedure and correct timing.

SECOND-LOOK PROCEDURES

There is an increasing use of second-look procedures in childhood cancer surgery. Currently these procedures are used in patients with abdominal non-Hodgkin's lymphoma, in whom resection of residual disease is often possible after massive reduction of tumor volume by chemotherapy. Second-look surgery in this disease is carried out in the middle of intensive chemotherapy with marked myelosuppression, and the timing of the surgery is critical. Second-look surgery is also carried out on patients with bilateral Wilms' tumor, in whom conservative resection of bilateral tumors can be performed after reduction of tumor volume by radiotherapy and chemotherapy. Neuroblastoma, which is nonresectable at first surgical exploration, can often be resected in a second procedure after chemotherapy, radiotherapy, or both. Second-look procedures have improved our understanding of the natural history and response to treatment of these tumors. It has become apparent, for instance, that chemotherapy alone will eradicate gross disease in many abdominal lymphomas. Neuroblastoma, when excised in a second procedure, often shows maturation into ganglioneuroblastoma and ganglioneuroma. This maturation into a more firm, nonhemorrhagic tumor, often encapsulated, means a much simpler, safer resection.

SURGERY FOR METASTATIC DISEASE

Failure of treatment in childhood solid cancers is commonly due to uncontrolled metastatic lung disease. Aggressive resection of pulmonary metastatic osteogenic sarcoma was advocated by Martini and co-workers at Memorial Hospital in 1971. At that time surgery offered the only chance of survival to this unfortunate group of patients. Multiple thoracotomies, with removal of more and more tumor nodules at each, produced a 45% 2-year survival. Over one third of the children and adolescents so treated are still alive. With the development of more successful chemotherapy protocols for osteogenic sarcoma, resection of pulmonary metastases became a standard part of management. Osteogenic sarcoma is particularly suited to pulmonary wedge resection, since tumor osteoid allows palpation of very small tumors. It appears that chemotherapy can control micrometastases, since these small resected lesions below 30 μm in diameter usually contain no tumor cells, only osteoid shell. Even though chemotherapy has a marked effect on metastatic osteogenic sarcoma in the lung, thoractomy usually demonstrates persistent tumor even when X rays and computerized transaxial tomography scans are normal. Aggressive removal of all palpable lesions at multiple thoracotomies will salvage over 40% of children with metastatic osteosarcoma in lung (Rosen et al. 1978). The multiple wedge resections are well tolerated and the quality of the patient's life can be good even after several thoracotomies. Even with modern chemotherapy, the outlook for the child with metastatic lung osteogenic sarcoma is dismal unless the lesions are removed surgically.

Experience with resection of lung metastases from other childhood cancers is limited to tumors that have failed to respond to chemotherapy and radiation therapy. Surgical removal should be attempted in cases of Wilms' tumor in the lung that have failed to respond to the best and maximum tolerable chemotherapy. Of 10 patients at Memorial Hospital in whom this was the case, five are long-term survivors, one after three thoracotomies. Rhabdomyosarcoma, Ewing's sarcoma, and metastatic germ cell tumors metastatic to the lung are more difficult to control surgically. The nodules are soft and difficult to palpate in the lung, and small tumors are easily missed by the surgeon. We have only a few survivors with these tumors and advise thoracotomy for solitary or few nodules when chemotherapy and radiation therapy have nothing more to offer.

STAGING

Surgical staging is now important in diseases, such as Hodgkin's disease, in which the primary treatment is nonsurgical (Hays et al. 1972). Over the past 10 years, most centers have carried out staging laparotomies for abdominal Hodgkin's disease, enabling radiation therapy to be delivered only to areas of disease, sparing the normal growing tissues of the child. Regional node dissections in paratesticular and pelvic rhabdomyosarcoma have made treatment planning easier by accurate staging of disease. The role of node dissection in diseases such as Wilms' tumor, rhabdomyosarcoma in the extremities, and other soft tissue sarcomas remains controversial and requires further evaluation. Staging of tumor is not accurate without careful node dissections.

SUPPORTIVE SURGERY

Surgical procedures are now used extensively to assist the radiation therapist and chemotherapist in delivering the most intensive treatment. Insertions of gastrostomy feeding tubes, central lines for total parenteral nutrition, and arteriovenous shunts for chemotherapy are examples of such procedures. We have induced pneumothorax in children who require chest wall irradiation to protect the underlying lung from the adverse effects of radiation (Exelby 1974). Transposition of ovaries out of the field of pelvic irradiation (Nahhas et al. 1971), moving of testes into the thigh during irradiation of the scrotum, and displacement of pelvic viscera by prosthetic devices are other examples of supportive surgery.

MANAGEMENT OF COMPLICATIONS

Surgeons have become increasingly involved in the management of complications of multidisciplinary treatment. Interstitial pneumonia is commonly seen in the course of treatment of leukemias and lymphomas in children. Lung biopsy by needle or open wedge is often urgently needed for correct diagnosis (Adeyemi et al. 1979). Insertion of chest tubes for release of pneumothorax caused by chemotherapy for metastatic disease in the lung, insertion of abdominal catheters for dialysis in cases of anuria in the initial phase of treatment of non-Hodgkin's lymphoma, and the surgical treatment of abdominal complications of chemotherapy have become commonplace over the past decade.

The surgeon must be part of the total management team throughout the treatment of any child with cancer. In solid tumors, the surgeon must examine the child frequently during treatment to detect recurrent disease and to monitor the effect of chemotherapy and radiotherapy on surgical scars and defects. The surgeon should be responsible for the follow-up of urinary diversion conduits, limb prostheses, and growth deformities related to previous surgical procedures, in addition to detection of early complications of treatment and possible recurrence. No longer is the surgeon responsible simply for removal of the primary tumor prior to handing the patient over to his oncologic and radiotherapeutic colleagues. The surgeon must work closely with the radiation therapist and chemotherapist during the initial evaluation, throughout the treatment, and in careful follow-up of the results of multidisciplinary treatment for many years after the disease is controlled.

WILMS' TUMOR

Advances in surgery in the 1950s gave the first indication that improvements in survival in childhood cancer were possible. New developments in anesthesia and in surgical procedures for removing Wilms' tumor prolonged survival in patients with this disease prior to the introduction of chemotherapy. In the United States, surgery is used as the primary treatment for unilateral Wilms' tumor (D'Angio et al. 1976). In Europe, a study of the use of preoperative radiotherapy and chemotherapy has shown little difference between the two modalities in terms of overall survival (Lemerle et al. 1976). There is evidence, however, that preoperative chemotherapy and radiotherapy reduce tumor rupture and spillage during surgery.

Leape et al. (1978) reviewed the surgery carried out in the First National Wilms' Tumor Study. They emphasized that gentle handling, adequate exposure, thorough exploration, and complete excision are still very important in the surgical management of Wilms' tumor. They noted that spread to lymph nodes significantly altered the prognosis in patients with Wilms' tumor. When hilar nodes were involved the survival rate dropped to 56.7%, and if periaortic nodes also contained tumor, tumor-free survival was only 33%. Further analysis of their data showed that an unfavorable histology in association with positive lymph nodes had a very marked effect on survival. They noted that tumor was present in the renal vein or vena cava in 37 of the 606 patients, but that this was not an unfavorable prognostic finding if the tumor was successfully removed. The data from the National Wilms' Tumor Study provided no evidence that lymph node resection alters the outcome in patients with Wilms' tumor. However, lymph nodes were not removed systematically in this study, and only 245 of the 606 patients had lymph node tissue available for histologic analysis. It may be that formal lymph node tissue dissection offers the only chance of cure in those patients with unfavorable histology when tumor has already infiltrated the lymph nodes.

The authors concluded that factors unfavorably affecting the outcome in Wilms' tumor patients are large tumor, lymph node involvement, capsular infiltration, and metastatic spread beyond the renal bed, such as to the liver. While preoperative rupture did not affect the overall survival, it necessitated more aggressive treatment. Operative spill during the procedure did, however, increase the incidence of abdominal recurrence. Surprisingly, features that did not affect prognosis included ligation of the renal artery and vein at the beginning of the procedure. It seemed that when ligation of the main vessels occurred just before removal of the tumor, the prognosis was the same. Invasion of the vena cava or renal vein did not appear to affect prognosis. This and other studies suggest that careful surgery should still be carried out in Wilms' tumor. The incision should be a wide transperitoneal exposure, usually a long transverse incision that allows examination of the opposite kidney. There should be a thorough exploration of the abdomen, certainly removal of any suspicious lymph nodes, and perhaps a formal lymph node dissection when an unfavorable histology is suspected. The opposite kidney should be carefully palpated for involvement. The procedure carried out should be a formal radical nephrectomy with removal of a generous length of ureter. If a formal lymph node dissection is not performed, sampling and labeling of representative lymph nodes will be of benefit in staging and future management.

Bishop and co-workers (1977) reviewed the treatment of bilateral Wilms' tumor in the National Wilms' Tumor Study. Treatment of these tumors was left largely to the various institutions, but the children received similar chemotherapy. Simultaneous bilateral Wilms' tumors were noted in 33 of the 606 children studied (5.4%). In these patients the second tumor was diagnosed at the same time as the primary tumor. In addition, disease in the opposite kidney was later detected in 20 patients (3.3%), for an overall incidence of bilateral Wilms' tumors of 8.7%. Thirty of the 33 patients with simultaneous bilateral Wilms' tumors were available for detailed study. Twenty-six of these 30 patients, or 87%, were surviving disease free more than 2 years after diagnosis. All the children had received actinomycin D and vincristine according to the National Wilms' Tumor Protocol. Some children had also received Adriamycin. All but two children who had all tumor excised received radiotherapy, 11 to both kidneys, eight to the single remaining kidney, and eight to the remaining kidney and renal fossa on the nephrectomized side. Dosage delivered was between 1,000 and 2,000 rad.

Of great interest is the wide variation in the surgery employed in these patients. Four children underwent unilateral nephrectomies on the more involved side and partial resection of the opposite kidney with complete removal of tumor at surgery. All these children survived. Fifteen children underwent unilateral nephrectomies at the time of initial surgery, one had incomplete removal of the tumor on the opposite side, and seven underwent biopsies only. All these children also survived. In the remaining seven children the opposite side was only inspected; two subsequently had all known tumor excised at second look and survived. Two of the remaining five who had no further surgery died of their disease. Eleven children had single or bilateral biopsies during the initial surgery without any attempt to remove primary tumor from either side. One of these had all tumor removed at second look and survived. Nine were left with residual tumor after second look, but only one of these died. The 11th underwent a bilateral nephrectomy and renal transplantation for persistent disease 18 months after diagnosis and subsequently died of tumor.

In this group, therefore, only seven of the 30 patients studied had all their tumor excised, four initially and three subsequently, and all survived. However, 19 of the remaining 23 patients who were known to have residual tumor after surgery survived. It seems clear that bilateral Wilms' tumors are not aggressive lesions, are usually of the favorable histologic type, and may not require complete surgical removal. Surgery for bilateral tumors should be conservative and preserve as much renal parenchyma on one or both sides as possible. The surgeon should realize that cure may be achieved without removal of any tumor or kidney tissue.

In summary, surgery remains the primary modality of treatment for Wilms' tumor. The surgery must be precise, carried out through a good exposure, and include a radical nephrectomy for unilateral disease. An opening into the tumor by wedge or needle biopsy should not be performed, but nephrectomy carried out on the basis of diagnostic inspection. Spilling of tumor in patients with an unfavorable histologic type may be a fatal surgical error. The use of lymph node dissections with nephrectomy remains controversial, and prospective trials should probably first be performed at institutions wishing to carry out this procedure. Currently the evidence suggests that formal lymph node dissections may benefit patients with tumors of unfavorable histology that have already spread to the lymph nodes. The surgical management of bilateral Wilms' tumors must still be individualized. If all gross tumor can be removed and enough normal kidney preserved, surgery still appears to offer the best chance of cure with the least amount of subsequent radiation therapy and chemotherapy. It must be remembered, however, that children with bilateral Wilms' tumors have survived with a good quality of life with no resection other than biopsy of their tumors.

In the future it may be possible to do less radical surgery and to reduce the dosage of radiation therapy and dosage and length of treatment with chemotherapy. At the present time, however, the basic principles of cancer surgery must be followed in managing this tumor. Various innovative procedures have been described in recent years to improve the resectability of Wilms' tumor, to increase the safety of removal of large tumors, and to conserve as much kidney parenchyma as possible. Harrison and co-workers (1978) have described embolization of the renal artery prior to radical nephrectomy. With this procedure, carried out immediately prior to surgery, a catheter is introduced into the renal artery and Gelfoam particles are injected to block off the renal artery and reduce vascularity. This procedure decreases the amount of blood lost during surgery and shrinks the tumor by emptying the vascular spaces, thus increasing resectability. Early cessation of blood flow through the tumor may also reduce the incidence of spillage of tumor cells into the renal vein during surgical manipulation. Bench surgery, particularly for bilateral Wilms' tumor, has been described by Anderson and Altman (1976). This procedure involves removal of the kidney from its vascular pedicle, resection of the tumor, and preservation of as much normal kidney as possible while the kidney is perfused outside the body. The kidney is then placed back into the patient as an autograft. Schullinger and co-workers (1977) have described cardiac angiography through the right heart in selected cases in which there was extensive venacaval involvement with tumor. Removal of the Wilms' tumor and its extension into the right atrium was successfully accomplished using cardiac bypass. While these innovations are important, they represent advanced techniques for use in a few special cases and are supplements to, rather than substitutes for, good cancer surgery.

EMBRYONAL RHABDOMYOSARCOMA

Embryonal rhabdomyosarcoma is the commonest soft tissue sarcoma in children and includes a very complex group of tumors in terms of surgical management because of its different sites of origin. A discussion of the surgical management of embryonal rhabdomyosarcoma must take into account its different types of biological behavior in different organs of the body. The tumor has two clinical varieties: the solid embryonal rhabdomyosarcoma seen in muscle groups on the extremities, trunk, and parts of the head and neck, and the so-called sarcoma botryoides, which are grape-like lesions that form in the hollow viscera, such as the bladder, vagina, external ear, bile ducts, and nasopharynx.

The surgeon recognizes these two forms of the tumor as differing in appearance and in requirements for complete surgical removal. The solid tumors tend to be compressed by surrounding muscle bulk, fascia, or connective tissue and, as palpated, are often confined to an area that is easily visible. A wide local excision of such a tumor in the extremity or the trunk can often be carried out with minimal sacrifice of normal tissue and with gross total removal of the tumor. The sarcoma botryoides variety, on the other hand, presents as polyps growing out under a normal mucosa, and the extent of the tumor, which may be only three or four cell layers thick, may be very difficult to determine since surrounding tissues appear normal, although infiltrated extensively by tumor. Historically the surgical treatment for sarcoma botryoides was a very radical procedure, usually involving some form of exenteration in the pelvis. On the other hand, more conservative wide resections or muscle group resections in the extremities or the trunk are well-established curative procedures. Surgery for embryonal rhabdomyosarcoma of the extremities, trunk, or chest wall now usually involves a wide local resection with a margin of normal tissue beyond the tumor.

The need for resection of regional lymph nodes in these extremity and trunk tumors is controversial. In our experience, approximately 25% of limb rhabdomyosarcomas involve regional lymph nodes at the time of diagnosis. We have favored carrying out a formal superficial groin or axillary node dissection, depending on the site of the primary tumor. In lower-extremity lesions in which there is obvious gross involvement of the superficial lymph nodes in the groin, we have also extended the dissection into a deep groin or common iliac node dissection. If carefully carried out, these procedures carry little morbidity, certainly improve the staging of the disease, and probably increase curability.

After the initial success of irradiation and chemotherapy in the management of embryonal rhabdomyosarcoma, there has been a tendency to do less than adequate surgery for these tumors in the extremities. Evidence from the Intergroup Rhabdomyosarcoma Study (Hays et al. 1977) suggests that gross total removal of tumors in the extremities and trunk offers the best chance of cure. When gross tumor is left behind in extremity lesions, the cure rate falls off dramatically. The Intergroup Rhabdomyosarcoma Study did not routinely include regional node dissections and very few of these were carried out in extremity lesions in the study. At our institution we have always performed gross total removal of rhabdomyosarcoma of the extremities, as well as regional node dissection, and we irradiate the tumor bed only when microscopic disease is left behind. With this approach and chemotherapy in all cases, the survival of patients with extremity lesions at our institution is approximately 80% at 2 years.

While amputation is rarely indicated in embryonal rhabdomyosarcoma of the extremities, it may be preferred, in selected cases, to leaving gross tumor behind after a partial resection. Certainly the surgeon should not operate on a child with rhabdomyosarcoma of the extremities with the intention of removing only part of the tumor. It is possible now, through various limb-saving techniques, to carry out radical surgical removal of tumors in the extremities and replace sacrificed tissue, such as bone, by prosthetic devices.

In head and neck rhabdomyosarcomas, the response to irradiation of the primary tumor has been good. Orbital lesions, in particular, appear to be very sensitive to irradiation and these tumors can be eradicated while preserving the eye. Surgery is used for tumors in those locations when removal can be safely accomplished without causing severe anatomic defect. Such tumors include lesions of the cheek, exophytic lesions of the neck, and small lesions of the maxilla that can be removed by a partial maxillectomy. These procedures, if carried out properly, can eradicate tumor completely, sparing the child the need for irradiation of the growing tissues of the face. Probably less than 10% of all head and neck lesions fall into this category and each case must be approached individually to determine the best primary treatment. In head and neck tumors there is a place for preoperative chemotherapy and irradiation, followed by conservative resection of the primary tumor. We have used this approach in several patients with head and neck primaries who would normally have required radical surgery or radical radiation therapy. By combining the two with careful planning and timing, it has been possible to reduce the dosage of radiation and to carry out a good surgical procedure while preserving the appearance of the child.

In chest wall rhabdomyosarcoma, it is now possible to resect several ribs in continuity with a moderate-sized chest wall lesion and replace the chest wall with various forms of prosthetic mesh. The introduction of improved prosthetic material, such as Marlex, has enabled large resections of chest wall to be carried out and stability of the chest maintained postoperatively by sewing a double layer of a prosthetic material. Excellent cosmetic and functional results are now possible after total removal of chest wall tumors. When it is possible to remove the tumor complete, the patient can be spared irradiation of the chest wall and underlying lung.

In some instances when the tumor of the chest wall is large and nonresectable, we have induced artificial pneumothorax to enable large-dose radiation therapy to be given to the chest wall while protecting the underlying lung. Introduction of a catheter and insertion of air into the pleural cavity can totally collapse the lung with very little discomfort to the child. It has been our policy to compress the lung for 5 days for the duration of radiation therapy to the chest wall and then reexpand the lung for a weekend of rest prior to repeating the procedure the following week. This procedure has been well tolerated by the children and has enabled doses of 6,000 rad to be delivered to large areas of the chest wall while protecting the lung. If carried out properly, there is no disturbance of pulmonary function after such a procedure.

A large proportion of embryonal rhabdomyosarcomas in children occur in the genitourinary tract, either the bladder, prostate, vagina, uterus, or paratesticular structures. These tumors have responded well to multidisciplinary treatment (Exelby et al. 1978), but surgical management remains controversial. Paratesticular tumors, which are seen largely in teen-age boys, are treated almost everywhere by radical orchiectomy with or without hemiscrotectomy. There has been considerable debate as to whether a retroperitoneal node dissection should be carried out in this group of tumors. It has been our policy to carry out a modified bilateral retroperitoneal node dissection as described by Whitmore (1973). Careful retroperitoneal node dissections in 36 patients treated for embryonal rhabdomyosarcoma showed retroperitoneal node involvement in 24, or 67%. As in extremity lesions, it seems that a retroperitoneal node dissection is important in arriving at a correct staging, and almost certainly contributes to improved survival in children with nodal involvement. With improved chemotherapy and irradiation, it is now possible to salvage children with large primary tumors that have already spread to retroperitoneal nodes, a hopeless situation 10 years ago. In the past 10 years, the only failures of treatment have been in three children with bulky retroperitoneal nodes that could not be completely excised surgically.

It is our feeling that a retroperitoneal node dissection is an important part of the management of paratesticular rhabdomyosarcoma. The argument against the retroperitoneal node dissection has been the impairment of sexual function caused by this procedure. However, if the procedure is carried out as described by Whitmore, there is minimal impairment of sexual function. Potency, erection, orgasm, and sexual enjoyment are possible in almost all cases. However, there has been a lack of fluid ejaculate and consequent infertility in approximately 50% of these patients.

The surgical management of pelvic rhabdomyosarcoma originating in the bladder, prostate, uterus, vagina, or pelvic wall remains much more controversial. The problem is that a curative surgical procedure often involves a radical exenterative procedure. In bladder and prostate lesions, surgical eradication usually means a radical cystectomy and prostatectomy with a urinary diversion by sigmoid or ileal conduit. These procedures, in combination with radiation therapy when there is microscopic residual disease and with chemotherapy in all cases, have produced very high cure rates in these tumors, which were previously almost untreatable. However, the defect to the child growing up without a bladder is considerable, and is compounded by severe impairment of sexual function.

It is obvious that any procedure that could preserve bladder/prostate function and still eliminate the tumor would be more desirable. At the present time it seems possible in selected cases to carry out less radical procedures. Hardy and co-workers (1978) have described a prostate tumor treated by chemotherapy and irradiation and then excised by a standard prostatectomy in which the continuity of the lower tract was preserved by bringing the urethra up to the bladder neck. This child is doing well and has good urinary function. Kumar and colleagues (1976) have performed partial cystectomies for these tumors, and this procedure may well be useful when tumors are located on the dome of the bladder or anterior wall. The problem is that most of these tumors involve the prostate and base of the bladder and their extent is very difficult to determine. When the tumor involves an extensive amount of the posterior wall and base of the bladder or the bladder neck and prostate, saving the bladder may be impossible if the tumor is to be controlled.

We recently began using surgery and brachytherapy for prostate/base of bladder lesions. We carry out an abdominal exploration in addition to cystoscopy and multiple biopsies from below. During laparotomy, a pelvic node dissection is performed bilaterally, after which the bladder, bladder neck, and prostate are isolated. If the tumor appears to be localized to the bladder neck and prostate, ^{125}I seeds are implanted. Our radiotherapy department now has extensive experience treating adult prostate cancers in this fashion, and has controlled the primary tumor and preserved bladder and sexual function. We follow these children carefully by endoscopic examinations and biopsies of the area of tumor involvement. One child treated in this fashion developed widespread distant metastases, but local control of the tumor was apparently maintained. Two other children are now being treated in this way, in one of whom a primary prostate lesion has been controlled for 15 months with no evidence of tumor. Bladder function in this boy, who originally presented with complete retention of urine, now appears excellent. He seems to have normal urinary function and his bladder capacity, after an initial diminution, has increased to normal. His prostate has decreased in mass from 200 gm to normal and repeated multiple biopsies by cystoscope have shown no tumor. In addition, sexual function in this adolescent appears to be completely satisfactory. This approach is suitable only for localized tumors in this region, and the great majority of our patients are still being treated by cystectomy and prostatectomy.

Embryonal rhabdomyosarcoma of the uterus or vagina has also been treated by pelvic exenteration. With modern treatment, we have not had to perform an exenterative procedure for rhabdomyosarcoma of the vagina or uterus in the past 6 years. It appears that these tumors in young girls are much more sensitive to irradiation and chemotherapy and that survival can be achieved with limited surgery.

NEUROBLASTOMA

Modern multidisciplinary treatment, so successful in many childhood cancers, has had little impact on the overall survival of children with neuroblastoma. However, different chemotherapy regimens with or without radiation therapy in recent years have produced encouraging initial responses. Shrinking of the primary tumor, maturation of the tumor to a more benign ganglioneuroblastoma or even ganglioneuroma, and prolongation of patient survival have been seen consistently. Some innovative changes in the surgical management of neuroblastoma have been made possible by these chemotherapy responses. Delayed primary resection and second-look operations in inoperable abdominal tumors have increased our knowledge of the behavior of neuroblastoma and its response to chemotherapy. The same can be said of the use of surgery in the delayed removal of the primary tumor in stage IV neuroblastoma. Combined thoracic and neurosurgical resection of "dumbbell" tumors of the mediastinum is a technical advance that has improved results in a few special cases.

ABDOMINAL NEUROBLASTOMA

Surgical removal of a resectable primary neuroblastoma remains the treatment of choice for all primary tumors in all age groups, tumor locations, and stages of disease. Less than 20% of children with abdominal neuroblastoma have resectable lesions when first seen. The resectable tumors are usually adrenal gland primaries, stage I or II, or the rarer tumors originating in the pelvis or organ of Zuckerkandl. In stage IV tumors, a small adrenal primary can often be easily resected. The great majority of primary neuroblastomas are large, friable, hemorrhagic, infiltrating tumors spreading around the midline structures. These tumors may originate in the upper lumbar ganglia or either adrenal gland and spread to involve the porta hepatis, aorta, vena cava, and even the pancreas and spleen. Often the site of origin of these tumors cannot be determined and the normal anatomic structures in the upper abdomen are buried in tumor. In the past, heroic resection efforts yielded occasional good results, but more often severe operative and postoperative complications and only partial removal of the tumor.

Although current chemotherapy has had little impact on survival rates, it has lengthened survival time and produced significant changes in the primary tumor. Massive, hemorrhagic, unresectable tumors can be changed into smaller encapsulated, resectable lesions by several weeks or months of chemotherapy. This response to chemotherapy has influenced several surgeons to institute delayed primary resection or second-look resection procedures (Grosfeld et al. 1978a,b).

Our present policy toward nonmetastatic abdominal neuroblastoma is to perform an early initial laparotomy. Evaluation of operability can usually be determined quickly since the tumors fall into two distinct groups: localized, unilateral lesions not infiltrating surrounding structures, and large, hemorrhagic, infiltrating lesions. The localized lesions can usually be resected without difficulty in a curative operation. No attempt is made to resect the large, infiltrating lesions, but representative biopsies are taken and the abdomen is closed. Chemotherapy is given for approximately 4 months and then a second-look procedure is carried out. The aim of the second operation is gross total removal of the tumor. If the tumor is nonresectable at second look, as much tumor is removed as possible and residual tumor marked with metal clips for subsequent radiation therapy. We have treated eight large nonresectable celiac axis tumors in this fashion. All patients had residual neuroblastoma after chemotherapy, but most had large tumor conversion to ganglioneuroblastoma and ganglioneuroma. In six children the tumor was completely resectable at the second-look procedure, and four of these children are surviving. Two had only partial resections at the second-look procedure; one died of tumor and the other, an infant, is alive more than 18 months off treatment.

In stage IV disease with abdominal primaries, the diagnosis is established, if possible, without laparotomy. Chemotherapy is then given, followed by a delayed laparotomy after 4 months, at which time resection of the primary tumor is attempted. Although there have been good responses to chemotherapy by stage IV tumors and most are resectable at delayed laparotomy, all the children thus treated ultimately died of metastatic disease.

In summary, delayed or second-look laparotomy has produced good data on tumor response to chemotherapy. Even when the clinical and radiological response to chemotherapy appears complete, a tumor can usually be found at the second-look procedure. The tumor may be largely ganglioneuroma, although viable neuroblastoma cells are usually found in the specimen. In patients with stage III tumors, resection at second-look operation has improved survival. In those with stage IV tumors, delayed resection of the primary tumor appears to have little effect on overall survival.

We have had some experience in the combined resection of mediastinal "dumbbell" tumors that cause cord compression. These tumors in children are often largely ganglioneuromas, and carry a better prognosis than abdominal neuroblastomas. However, the threat of cord compression and the small potential for metastatic spread necessitate careful two-team surgical resection. Gross removal can be accomplished in these tumors with a patient survival rate approaching 100% and avoidance of spinal radiation therapy.

SUMMARY

Modern multidisciplinary treatment has changed the prognosis for the child with cancer. The major role of surgery is still resection of the primary tumor preserving physiological function and normal appearance as much as possible. Less extensive but often more complicated procedures are now carried out on sicker children. Surgery for metastatic tumors, delayed and second-look procedures, and many supportive operations are now used to cure more children and improve the quality of their survival. The surgeon, chemotherapist, and radiation therapist must be flexible and continue to work together toward these goals. The long-term effects of chemotherapy and radiation therapy may offer threats to the quality of life as great as those posed by radical surgery. Reduction of the amount of chemotherapy and radiation therapy may be as important as less radical surgery in many patients. The surgeon dealing with childhood cancer must understand the disease and the child. The first operation performed on a child with cancer often determines the course of disease. It should not be necessarily radical or conservative—it should be the correct procedure.

REFERENCES

Adeyemi, S. D., S. H. Ein, J. S. Simpson, and P. Turner. 1979. The value of emergency open lung biopsy in infants and children. J. Pediatr. Surg. 14:426–427.

Anderson, K. D., and R. P. Altman. 1976. Selective resection of malignant tumors using bench surgical techniques. J. Pediatr. Surg. 11:881–882.

Bishop, H. C., M. Tefft, A. E. Evans, and G. J. D'Angio. 1977. Survival in bilateral Wilms' tumor—Review of 30 National Wilms' Tumor Study cases. J. Pediatr. Surg. 12:631–638.

D'Angio, G. J., A. E. Evans, N. Breslow, B. Beckwith, H. Bishop, P. Feigl, W. Goodwin, L. L. Leape, L. F. Sinks, W. Sutow, M. Tefft, and J. Wolff. 1976. The treatment of Wilms' tumor: Results of the National Wilms' Tumor Study. Cancer 38:633–646.

Exelby, P. R. 1974. Management of embryonal rhabdomyosarcoma in children. Surg. Clin. North Am. 54:849–857.

Exelby, P. R., F. Ghavimi, and B. Jereb. 1978. Genitourinary rhabdomyosarcoma in children. J. Pediatr. Surg. 13:746–752.

Grosfeld, J. L., T. V. N. Ballantine, and R. L. Baehner. 1978a. Experience with "second-look" operations in pediatric solid tumors. J. Pediatr. Surg. 13:275–280.

Grosfeld, J. L., M. Schatzlein, T. V. N. Ballantine, R. M. Weetman, and R. L. Baehner. 1978b. Metastatic neuroblastoma: Factors influencing survival. J. Pediatr. Surg. 13:59–65.

Hardy, B., D. Green, and J. Folkman. 1978. Radical prostatectomy in an 18-month-old boy (Abstract) in Proceedings of the American Pediatric Surgical Association 9th Annual Meeting, p. 75.

Harrison, M. R., A. A. de Lorimier, and W. O. Boswell. 1978. Preoperative angiographic embolization for large hemorrhagic Wilms' tumor. J. Pediatr. Surg. 13:757–758.

Hays, D. M., R. E. Hittle, H. Isaacs, Jr., and M. R. Karon. 1972. Laparotomy for the staging of Hodgkin's disease in children. J. Pediatr. Surg. 7:517–527.

Hays, D. M., W. W. Sutow, W. Lawrence, Jr., T. E. Moon, and M. Tefft. 1977. Rhabdomyosarcoma: Surgical therapy in extremity lesions in children. Orthop. Clin. North Am. 8:883–902.

Kumar, A. P. M., E. L. Wrenn, Jr., I. D. Fleming, H. O. Hustu, and C. B. Pratt. 1976. Combined therapy to prevent complete pelvic exenteration for rhabdomyosarcoma of the vagina or uterus. Cancer 37:118–122.

Leape, L. L., N. E. Breslow, and H. C. Bishop. 1978. The surgical treatment of Wilms' tumor: Results of the National Wilms' Tumor Study. Ann. Surg. 187:351–356.

Lemerle, J., P. A. Voute, M. F. Tournade, J. F. M. Delemarre, B. Jereb, L. Ahstrom, R. Flamant, and R. Gerard-Marchant. 1976. Preoperative versus postoperative radiotherapy, single versus multiple courses of actinomycin D, in the treatment of Wilms' tumor. Cancer 38:647–654.

Martini, N., A. G. Huvos, V. Miké, R. C. Marcove, and E. J. Beattie, Jr. 1971. Multiple pulmonary resections in the treatment of osteogenic sarcoma. Ann. Thorac. Surg. 12:271–280.

Morton, D. L., F. R. Eilber, C. M. Townsend, Jr., T. T. Grant, J. Mirra, and T. H. Weisenberger. 1976. Limb salvage from a multidisciplinary treatment approach for skeletal and soft tissue sarcomas of the extremity. Ann. Surg. 184:268–278.

Nahhas, W. A., L. Z. Nisce, G. J. D'Angio, and J. L. Lewish, Jr. 1971. Lateral ovarian transposition: Ovarian relocation in patients with Hodgkin's disease. Obstet. Gynecol. 38:785–788.

Rosen, G., A. G. Huvos, C. Mosende, E. J. Beattie, Jr., P. R. Exelby, B. Capparos, and R. C. Marcove. 1978. Chemotherapy and thoracotomy for metastatic osteogenic sarcoma: A model for adjuvant chemotherapy and the rationale for the timing of thoracic surgery. Cancer 41:841–849.

Rosen, G., R. C. Marcove, B. Caparros, A. Nirenberg, C. Kosloff, and A. G. Huvos. 1979. Primary osteogenic sarcoma: The rationale for preoperative chemotherapy and delayed surgery. Cancer 43:2163–2177.

Rosen, G., M. L. Murphy, A. G. Huvos, M. Gutierrez, and R. C. Marcove. 1976. Chemotherapy, en bloc resection, and prosthetic bone replacement in the treatment of osteogenic sarcoma. Cancer 37:1–11.

Schullinger, J. N., T. V. Santulli, W. J. Casarella, and R. W. MacMillan. 1977. Wilms' tumor: The role of right heart angiography in the management of selected cases. Ann. Surg. 185:451–455.

Whitmore, W. F., Jr. 1973. Germinal testis tumors in adults, *in* Seventh National Cancer Conference Proceedings. American Cancer Society, New York, pp. 793–801.

Status of the Curability of Childhood Cancers,
edited by J. van Eys and M. P. Sullivan.
Raven Press, New York © 1980.

Optimization of Radiotherapy

Rafael C. Chan, M.D.

*Division of Radiotherapy, The University of Texas Health Science Center at Dallas,
Dallas, Texas*

The optimum care of children with cancer demands the use of multimodal therapy: surgery, irradiation, chemotherapy, and, more recently, immunotherapy when applicable. This approach carried out by experienced physicians in well-staffed and well-equipped medical centers has improved the prognosis of children with cancer many times. The interaction of different treatment modalities requires that one be aware of the impact of one modality on another. The interaction between chemotherapy and radiotherapy can be particularly significant (Table 1) (Chan and Sutow 1979). It is imperative that we anticipate these potential hazards and plan each multimodal treatment program to minimize or circumvent them.

Optimum radiotherapy requires precise treatment planning and accurate dosimetry to ensure that the tumor dose is precisely known and maximized while the dose to normal tissue is kept to a minimum. Optimization would not be possible with only one beam, such as in a cobalt-60 unit or 4-MeV linear accelerator, which have identical beam characteristics. Photon beams of high energy levels and electron beams with different energy levels are essential for an optimally equipped radiotherapy department (Figure 1) (Fletcher et al. 1976).

Table 1. *Major Therapy-Limiting Toxic Effects of Drugs Commonly Used with Radiotherapy*

Complication	VCR*	AMD	CYT	ADR	HD-MTX
Leukopenia	—	+†	++	+++	+++
Thrombocytopenia	—	+++	+	+	++
Neurotoxicity	++	—	—	—	—
Cardiotoxicity	—	—	+	+++	—
Cystitis	—	—	+++	—	—
Mucositis	—	++	—	++	+++
Gastrointestinal toxicity	++	++	++	++	++
Cellulitis (local)	++	++	—	++	—
Erythema	—	++	—	—	+
Hepatotoxicity	—	—	—	—	+++

* VCR = vincristine, AMD = actinomycin D, CYT = cyclophosphamide, ADR = Adriamycin, HD-MTX = high-dose methotrexate.

† Increasing numbers of + indicate increasing severity and frequency of complication.

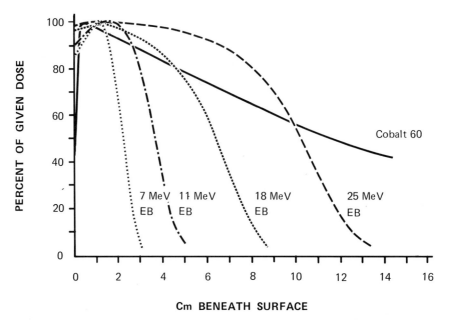

Figure 1. Percent depth dose for various radiation beams. (Adapted with permission from Fletcher, G. H., et al.: Radiotherapy, in the section "Modalities of Cancer Treatment," from *Cancer Patient Care at M. D. Anderson Hospital and Tumor Institute,* edited by R. Lee Clark and Clifton D. Howe. Copyright © 1976 by Year Book Medical Publishers, Inc., Chicago.)

RADIOBIOLOGY

The radiobiological basis of radiation therapy rests upon damaging essential subcelluar structures. Within cells, the critical molecule for radiation damage is DNA, and damage results from breaking one or both of the strands in the DNA (Ward 1975). Single-strand breaks are usually rejoined; this phenomenon forms the basis for radiation repair and sublethal damage. If both strands of DNA are broken and the two breaks are close to each other, neither can be repaired, leading to cell death or loss of reproductive capability. Radiation produces loss of reproductive ability in both malignant and normal cells. While the therapist's objective is to sterilize malignant cells, major complications most frequently result from killing stem cells in self-renewing normal tissues, such as vasculature or skin (Rubin and Casarett 1968). For our purposes, a cell incapable of replicating is a dead cell.

Cell damage, whether lethal or sublethal, is the direct result of ionizing events and thus dose dependent. At low doses single-strand breaks predominate, leading to sublethal damage, while at high doses double-strand breaks leading to cell death predominate. This follows logically from the fact that a single photon or electron track rarely produces a break in both DNA strands; rather, the lethal double-strand lesions occur from two separate ionizing events. The chance of two events occurring in a small volume increases with the total number of events (dose) (Kellerer and Rossi 1972).

These principles provide the rationale for using fractionation schedules in radiotherapy, i.e., certain cells are more or less able to accumulate or repair sublethal damage, depending on their tissue of origin, growth rate, position in the cell cycle, etc. Dose fractionation refers to dividing the prescribed dose of, for example, 5,000 rad into 25 increments of 200 rad each delivered over 5 weeks. Using protocols such as this, local control of the tumor may be achieved with negligible morbidity. Delivery of the same total dose in a single exposure would be devastating. Fractionation of the dose maintains the integrity of normal structures in the following way. A significant portion of a 200-rad dose is registered as sublethal damage in both normal and malignant cells. During the 24-hour interval between dose fractions, most of this damage is repaired. Due to kinetic factors, such as cell cycle position, and probably inherent biochemical repair capabilities, normal cells exhibit slightly greater recovery after each dose fraction. This differential becomes amplified with successive fractions so that a fractionation protocol results in more malignant cell destruction than normal cell damage (Withers 1975).

RADIATION CONSIDERATIONS

The normal tissues in children are actively growing and developing with intensive mitotic activity, so pediatric patients are more likely to suffer adverse effects from irradiation than adults. Irradiation can have several effects on children:

1. Effects on bone growth and development. Irradiation of active centers of bone growth can result in deformity of developing bone. Neuhauser and co-workers (1952) report that doses above 2,000 rad retard bone growth, irrespective of the child's age. Aberrations in bone growth include shortened limbs from epiphyseal damage, scoliosis of the spine, and underdevelopment of various areas. The muscles and soft tissues are often thinner than normal after therapy.

2. Effects on organ function. Effects of irradiation on the lungs and associated clinical syndromes have been well documented. D'Angio (1962) notes that, in the treatment of pulmonary metastases from Wilms' tumor, a dose of 1,200 rad in 10 fractions does not cause clinically evident pulmonary reaction. Irradiation in excess of 1,500 rad to the kidneys is associated with increasing risk of pronounced malfunction, both immediate and late.

3. Effects on the hematopoetic system. Leukopenia and thrombocytopenia can develop, particularly after irradiation of large areas and when cytotoxic agents are being given at the same time. When the white cell count drops below 1,500/mm^3 or the platelets below 100,000/mm^3, careful assessment is needed before continuing therapy.

4. Effects on oncogenesis. Now that pediatric cancer patients are living longer,

the incidence of second primaries is increasing. It is well known that irradiated tissues may develop malignant tumors after a latent period of several years. This phenomenon may be due to a greater tendency for these patients to develop malignant disease or to their exposure to cocarcinogens, either radiation or chemotherapy.

CLINICAL CONSIDERATIONS

Leukemia

Radiotherapy plays a major role in the prevention of meningeal leukemia and in the treatment of extramedullary relapse. Combined modality treatment is now producing long-term disease-free survival in more than half of children with acute lymphocytic leukemia (Simone et al. 1975). The results of preventive central nervous system (CNS) treatment in acute lymphocytic leukemia patients are significantly better than those with treatment instituted after manifestation of CNS disease. Prophylactic treatment for occult CNS disease is usually given as soon as remission is achieved (Figure 2) (Chan and Sutow 1979). A midline tumor dose of 2,400 rad using cobalt-60 or a 4-MeV or 6-MeV linear accelerator is delivered through opposing lateral fields that include the retroorbital space, the anterior edge of the zygomas, and the first two cervical segments. The dose is given over 2½ weeks, and is reduced to 2,000 rad for children 1 to 2 years of age and 1,500 rad for those under 12 months. The same technique is used for patients with overt CNS leukemia, which may occur in a child who

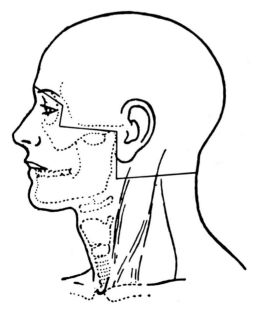

Figure 2. Radiation port in children receiving only cranial irradiation. (Reproduced with permission from Chan, R. C., and W. W. Sutow. 1979. Irradiation and chemotherapy in pediatric tumors. *In* Fletcher, G. H. (ed.): *Textbook of Radiotherapy.* 3rd ed. Lea & Febiger, Philadelphia, in press.)

has been in bone marrow remission for a long time. The combination drug treatment is given prior to the radiation to the cranium.

Neuropsychologic studies fail to demonstrate serious late effects from prophylactic CNS irradiation; however, there have been reports of necrotizing leukoencephalopathy with combination chemotherapy and irradiation to the CNS for leukemia and lymphoma (Rubinstein et al. 1975).

Almost any organ or tissue of the body can be involved in the leukemic process. Radiotherapy can be instituted at the time of diagnosis of an extramedullary infiltrate. The seventh cranial nerve, in contrast to the others, may be the site of leukemic infiltration without demonstrable involvement of meninges or other CNS sites. Initiation of radiotherapy within 24 to 36 hours usually results in restoration of motor function. Parallel opposed fields are used to deliver a dose of 2,500 rad in 2½ weeks. Overt testicular involvement may develop in approximately 10% of boys with leukemia, and following biopsy confirmation of testicular infiltration, radiation therapy is initiated to deliver a dose of 2,500 rad in 10 fractions (Hustu and Aur 1978, Stoffel et al. 1975, Sullivan et al. 1975). Radiotherapy may produce dramatic palliation, with alleviation of severe bone pain. From 1,000 to 1,500 rad are delivered by simple technique in two to three fractions.

Hodgkin's Disease

The 5-year survival rate for stage I and II Hodgkin's disease patients now approaches 90% (Jenkin et al. 1975, Shah et al. 1976, Smith and Rivera 1976). Staging procedures and treatment techniques developed in adults with Hodgkin's disease are, in general, applicable in children. In the latter, in an effort to minimize late effects of therapy, radiotherapy is limited to the involved nodes as far as possible. Fuller et al. (1971) have reported that certain presentations of stage I and II disease are associated with a favorable prognosis when treated by radiotherapy.

Favorable presentations appear to be limited to the following situations:

1. Unilateral disease in the upper third of the neck, lymphocytic predominance, and mixed cellularity;
2. Nodular sclerosing mediastinal disease;
3. Superficial inguinal or femoral nodes of any histologic type.

All other stage I and II presentations are considered unlikely to be cured by radiotherapy alone. For favorable sites, involved areas receive 3,000 rad tumor dose at the rate of 750 to 900 rad per week.

With the development of more effective chemotherapy and the employment of multimodal therapy, survival rates should now improve for patients with unfavorable presentations of Hodgkin's disease. An extended trial of a "sandwich" ACOPP (Adriamycin, Cytoxan, Oncovin, prednisone, and procarbazine)-radiotherapy regimen was developed for unfavorable stage I and II and all stage III presentations of Hodgkin's disease from pilot studies conducted in the Pediatric Department of M. D. Anderson Hospital and Tumor Institute (Sullivan and Fuller 1973). The patients are treated initially with two courses of ACOPP, followed by involved-field radiotherapy and four courses of ACOPP (Figure 3).

Since 1972, 27 children with Hodgkin's disease who were considered unlikely to be cured by irradiation alone were treated with this multimodal therapy (Cullen, Sullivan, Chan, and Butler, manuscript in preparation), including six stage I and II and 21 stage III patients. The complete response rate was 96%. The survival rate is 89%, with a median follow-up of 54+ months. The treatment regimen was well tolerated and highly effective.

Non-Hodgkin's Lymphoma

Information derived from treatment of adults with non-Hodgkin's lymphoma has been of little value in treating children, due to the histologic and biologic differences between the adult and childhood forms of the disease. In children, the lymphoma is so uniformly diffuse that the diagnosis of nodular lymphoma requires confirmation, whereas in adults it may be diffuse or nodular. The types of non-Hodgkin's lymphoma seen in children include diffuse undifferentiated lymphoma, Burkitt's type; diffuse undifferentiated lymphoma, non-Burkitt's type; diffuse poorly differentiated lymphocytic lymphoma, convoluted type; and diffuse histiocytic lymphoma (Sullivan and Butler 1977). Non-Hodgkin's lymphoma in children is characterized by a high incidence of generalized disease at the time of diagnosis, rapid extension of local or regional disease if such spread is present at diagnosis, and a strong tendency for involvement of bone marrow and meninges. For these reasons, radiation therapy is limited to the involved

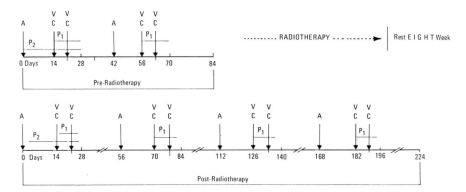

Figure 3. Schema for "sandwich" ACOPP-radiotherapy regimen for Hodgkin's disease in children. (Reproduced with permission from Chan, R. C., and W. W. Sutow. 1979. Irradiation and chemotherapy in pediatric tumors. *In* Fletcher, G. H. (ed.): *Textbook of Radiotherapy.* 3rd ed. Lea & Febiger, Philadelphia, in press.)

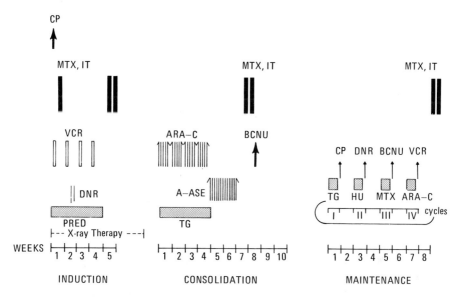

Figure 4. Modified SLA₂L₂ regimen for non-Hodgkin's lymphoma in children (all histologic types except diffuse undifferentiated lymphoma, Burkitt's type). (Adapted with permission from van Eys, J., et al.: Childhood tumors, from *Cancer Patient Care at M. D. Anderson Hospital and Tumor Institute,* edited by R. Lee Clark and Clifton D. Howe. Copyright ©1976 by Year Book Medical Publishers, Inc., Chicago.)

field. Radiotherapy is delivered during the induction phase, before initiation of the consolidation phase, when the patient's marrow is recovering from the myelosuppressive effects of cytotoxic agents. A modification of the SLA₂L₂ regimen for treatment of non-Hodgkin's lymphoma in children developed at Memorial Hospital is currently being used at M. D. Anderson Hospital (Figure 4).

Rhabdomyosarcoma

Rhabdomyosarcoma is the most common soft tissue sarcoma in childhood (Miller 1969). It represents 5–15% of all malignant solid tumors and 4–8% of all malignant disease in children under age 15 (Sutow et al. 1970, Young and Miller 1975). It is now curable in most children whose conditions are diagnosed prior to the development of metastases. The dramatic improvement in survival rates, from less than 20% 15 years ago to approximately 70% at present, is due to a better understanding of the natural history of the disease, careful staging, heightened awareness of histologic features, improved histologic classification, and an effective multimodal approach using surgery, radiation, and chemotherapy (Maurer et al. 1977).

With the activation of the Intergroup Rhabdomyosarcoma Study (IRS) in 1972, a clinical grouping classification that is now widely used was adopted.

Based on extent of disease and completeness of surgical extirpation, four groups were defined (Maurer et al. 1977):

Group I   Localized disease, completely resected. Assessment based on surgical findings, gross inspection of the specimen, and microscopic confirmation of gross resection.

Group II   Grossly resected tumor with microscopic residual disease or regional disease completely resected.

Group III   Incomplete resection or biopsy with gross residual disease locally. No distant metastases.

Group IV   Metastatic disease present at diagnosis.

The radiotherapy techniques recommended vary with the location of the primary tumor. In the current approach, all irradiation for gross or microscopic disease should generously cover the involved mass or compartment. Prophylactic irradiation of adjacent lymph nodes is not recommended. Preliminary evaluation of the relationship between local disease control and radiation therapy dose in IRS patients shows that children 6 years of age and older who received fewer than 4,000 rad had a higher local recurrence rate (32%) than those who received more than 4,000 rad (8–13%) (Tefft et al. 1977). A dose of 5,000 rad in 5 weeks to the primary site is recommended for patients with only microscopic residual disease. For patients with gross residual or metastatic disease or both (Groups III and IV), the dose of radiation to the primary tumor should be 6,000 rad in 6 weeks. In very young children lower doses might be considered because of the increased sensitivity of their normal structures, but no fewer than 4,000 to 4,500 rad in 4 to 5 weeks. Usually parallel opposed fields are used and tumor doses are determined by midplane values along the central axis, with each port being treated every day.

Special measures should be taken for patients with parameningeal lesions (nasopharynx, paranasal sinuses, and middle ear), who are at high risk of developing direct meningeal extensions of disease (Tefft et al. 1978). Diagnostic procedures such as spinal fluid cytology, tomograms of the base of the skull, and computerized axial tomograms of the brain should be done prior to initiation of treatment. If the base of the skull is not involved, no neurologic abnormalities are present, and the cerebrospinal fluid is normal, the radiation field should include a wide margin superiorly to about 2 cm above the base of the skull (Chan and Sutow 1979). However, if there is evidence of meningeal extension, the entire cranial-spinal axis should be irradiated in continuity with the primary site and concomitantly with intrathecal chemotherapy.

Wilms' Tumor

Wilms' tumor is a highly malignant embryonic neoplasm of mixed histologic structure that involves the kidney and occurs primarily in children. The median age of occurrence is 3 years, with the peak incidence between 1 and 3 years.

Ninety percent of cases occur in children age 7 or younger (Sutow 1975). In approximately 5% of the patients, both kidneys are involved (D'Angio et al. 1976).

A collaborative effort of surgeons, pediatricians, radiotherapists, and pathologists led to formation of the National Wilms' Tumor Study Group in 1969. This group helped improve the 2-year survival rate from 20% 3 decades ago to 80% or better within the last 10 years (D'Angio et al. 1976, Ladd 1938, Gross 1953, Farber 1966). The staging scheme formalized by the National Wilms' Tumor Study (NWTS) is widely used currently. The staging is based on clinical, surgical, and pathological considerations and, with the results of NWTS-1 and NWTS-2, has led to the following redefinition of those elements thought to be of prognostic importance (D'Angio et al. 1976):

Group I   Tumor contained within kidney capsule and completely resected.

Group II   Tumor extends locally beyond kidney extension into renal sinus or perirenal soft tissues. Periaortic node involvement. Tumor thrombus in renal vessels completely resected.

Group III   Postsurgically, residual tumor confined to abdomen (biopsy or rupture of tumor, peritoneal implants, involved lymph nodes beyond abdominal periaortic chains, or incomplete resection of tumor).

Group IV   Distant (hematogenous) metastases present.

Group V   Bilateral renal involvement initially or subsequently.

The results of the National Wilms' Tumor Study Therapeutic Trial have been published, along with reports of more specialized aspects of that study (D'Angio 1976, Beckwith and Palmer 1978, Leape et al. 1978, Tefft et al. 1976, Pendergrass 1976). Some of the important conclusions are the following:

1. Postoperative radiation therapy was not necessary in younger patients with early disease. Of Group I patients, 97% of those receiving postoperative irradiation and 92% of those not receiving irradiation were alive after 2 years. All these patients received actinomycin D alone as adjuvant chemotherapy.

2. Double-agent chemotherapy with vincristine and actinomycin D was superior to either agent alone. In patients in Groups II and III, the actuarial projection was 86% alive at 2 years with both drugs.

3. Favorable and unfavorable histologic types were identified. The latter included anaplastic elements and sarcomatous changes. The striking differences in outcome are illustrated in Table 2, which gives 2-year results by histologic type. The differences for relapse-free and overall survival are significant ($p <$ 0.001).

The second National Wilms' Tumor Study's demonstration of the superiority of double-agent chemotherapy in ablating micrometastases led to the use of both agents in Group I children. It was hoped that vincristine could replace

Table 2. *Two-Year Results by Histologic Type*

Type	No. of Patients	Relapse-free Survival Rate (Actuarial)	Overall Survival Rate (Actuarial)
Unfavorable			
Renal sarcoma	22	27%	36%
Diffuse anaplasia	10	10%	20%
Focal anaplasia	14	57%	64%
Favorable	352	79%	91%
Unknown	31	71%	84%

radiotherapy in suppressing microscopic residual disease at the operative site as well as in remote areas such as the lung. The identification of Adriamycin as an effective agent against Wilms' tumor led to a comparison of a three-drug regimen consisting of Adriamycin, actinomycin D, and vincristine to actinomycin D plus vincristine in children with Group II, III, and IV tumors (Bonadonna et al. 1970, Tan et al. 1973).

As increasing success is achieved in the management of children with cancers such as Wilms' tumor, it becomes imperative to refine methods of treatment to the minimum required for success. Determining this minimum is the purpose of the third National Wilms' Tumor Study. Side effects of treatment include disturbances in growth and development, functional impairments, genetic damage, interference with reproductive function, and oncogenesis (Tefft 1977). Both radiation therapy and chemotherapy produce lesions that may remain occult for many years. The currently proposed study will enable us to determine which modes of therapy are required to obtain success with the fewest and mildest late effects.

Radiotherapy techniques for Wilms' tumor depend upon stage, histology, and age. The following are general guidelines:

Stage II, favorable histology. Postoperative radiation therapy is given to the tumor bed, which includes the kidney as outlined on a preoperative excretory urogram, and any associated tumor. Opposing anterior-posterior portals are used, with a dose of 2,000 rad for all patients except those less than 12 months of age, who receive 1,000 rad.

Stage III, favorable histology. Patients who receive radiation therapy are randomized to receive 1,000–2,000 rad, with supplemental doses of up to 1,000 rad to areas of residual bulky disease. The size is adjusted to conform to the extent of disease found at surgery, and fields are similar to those used in stage II patients who have only hilar lymphadenopathy or residual disease confined to the flank. Total abdominal irradiation is given when there is diffuse peritoneal seeding or when there was gross tumor spillage within the abdominal cavity before or during surgery. The remaining kidney is shielded so that the total dose of that organ does not exceed 1,500 rad.

Stage IV, favorable histology. The tumor bed is irradiated postoperatively and the portal used depends on the stage of the primary tumor, with a nominal tumor dose of 2,000 rad and a boost of 1,000 rad to any residual tumor.

Unfavorable histology. All patients with stage I, II, III, or IV disease receive postoperative radiation therapy to the tumor bed. The dose is adjusted on the basis of age of the patient: birth to 12 months, 1,200–1,800 rad; 13 to 18 months, 1,800–2,400; 19 to 30 months, 2,400–3,000; 31 to 40 months, 3,000–3,500; 41 months or more, 3,500–4,000. In patients with pulmonary metastases at the time of diagnosis and a favorable histology, both lungs are treated, regardless of the number and location of metastases. Such patients are given 1,200 rad with a daily fraction of 150 rad using an anterior-posterior field.

Ewing's Sarcoma

Ewing's sarcoma is a primary sarcoma of nonosseous origin involving bone. This highly anaplastic tumor is composed of solidly packed, uniform, small round cells. It occurs primarily in children and young adults, 90% of the patients being under 30 years of age and 70% under 20 years of age. Up to 28% of the patients have metastases at the time of diagnosis. Multimodal approaches have benefited many patients. Especially notable have been studies at St. Jude, Memorial Sloan-Kettering, NCI, and M. D. Anderson, as well as the Intergroup Ewing Sarcoma Study (Hustu et al. 1972, Rosen 1977, Perez et al. 1977, Fernandez et al. 1974, Chan et al. 1979b, Pomeroy and Johnson 1975). Disease-free survival rates as high as 76% have been reported in small series as a result of aggressive therapy (Perez et al. 1977).

With the use of radiation therapy and intensive systemic maintenance chemotherapy, the rate of local control has risen as high as 95% (Fernandez et al. 1974, Chan et al. 1979b). Review of the data from the Intergroup Ewing Sarcoma Study shows that the dose of radiation and the adequacy of the field size influence the local control rate. Local control was achieved in 94% of 34 patients receiving greater than 6,000 rad, 84% of 75 patients receiving 5,000 to 6,000, and 81% of 32 patients receiving 4,000 to 5,000. The local control rate for patients in whom the whole bone was irradiated and who received adequate doses of radiation was 72%. There was a higher rate of local recurrence in patients in whom the field size was confined to a tumor-free margin of less than 5 cm. In addition, the use of Adriamycin appeared to improve control of local recurrences (Perez et al. 1977).

Even in the first 4 to 5 weeks of treatment, fields are drawn to spare as much normal tissue as possible. Shaped fields are employed throughout the treatment and appropriate techniques are used to minimize unintentional irradiation of tissue. Irradiation of the full circumference of the extremity, even in the first portion of treatment, is avoided if possible. If "fall-off" is required on one side of the limb, normal tissues are shielded when possible on the other side to preserve good function in a painfree and nonedematous limb. The anatomical location of the lesion influences the outcome. The Intergroup Ewing Sarcoma

Study showed a relapse rate of about 60% (28/47) for patients with pelvic lesions, 47% (37/79) for those with proximal lesions, 28% (18/64) for those with distal lesions, and 20% (8/41) for those with lesions in other anatomic sites. Because of the high relapse rate for patients with pelvic primaries and sacral disease, a different approach is used to reduce the likelihood of local failure.

REFERENCES

Beckwith, J. B., and N. Palmer. 1978. Histopathology and prognosis of Wilms' tumor: Results of the National Wilms' Tumor Study. Cancer 41:1937–1948.

Bonadonna, G., S. Monfardini, M. Delena, F. Fossati-Bellani, and G. Beretta. 1970. Phase I and preliminary phase II evaluation of Adriamycin. Cancer Res. 30:2572–2582.

Chan, R. C., and W. W. Sutow. 1979. Irradiation and chemotherapy in pediatric tumors, *in* Textbook of Radiotherapy, G. H. Fletcher, ed. 3rd ed. Lea & Febiger, Philadelphia, in press.

Chan, R. C., W. W. Sutow, and R. D. Lindberg. 1979a. Parameningeal rhabdomyosarcoma. Radiology 131:211–214.

Chan, R. C., W. W. Sutow, R. D. Lindberg, M. L. Samuels, J. A. Murray, and D. A. Johnston. 1979b. Management and results of localized Ewing's sarcoma. Cancer 43:215–220.

D'Angio, G. J. 1962. Clinical and biological studies of actinomycin D and roentgen irradiation. Am. J. Roentgenol. 87:100–109.

D'Angio, G. J., A. E. Evans, N. Preslow, J. B. Beckwith, H. Bishop, P. Feigl, W. Goodwin, L. L. Leape, L. F. Sinks, W. Sutow, M. Tefft, and J. Wolff. 1976. The treatment of Wilms' tumor: Results of the National Wilms' Tumor Study. Cancer 38:633–646.

Farber, S. 1966. Chemotherapy in the treatment of leukemia and Wilms' tumor. J.A.M.A. 198:826–836.

Fernandez, C. H., R. D. Lindberg, W. W. Sutow, and M. Samuels. 1974. Localized Ewing's sarcoma: Treatment and results. Cancer 34:143–148.

Fletcher, G. H., H. R. Withers, P. R. Almond, R. D. Lindberg, N. Tapley, D. H. Hussey, and L. D. Delclos. 1976. Radiotherapy, *in* Cancer Patient Care at M. D. Anderson Hospital and Tumor Institute, R. L. Clark and C. D. Howe, eds. Year Book Medical Publishers, Chicago, pp. 14–24.

Fuller, L. M., J. F. Gamble, C. C. Shullenberger, J. J. Butler, and E. A. Gehan. 1971. Prognostic factors in localized Hodgkin's disease treated with regional radiation. Radiology 98:641–654.

Gross, R. E. 1953. Surgery of Infancy and Childhood. W. B. Saunders Co., Philadelphia, 1,000 pp.

Hustu, H. O., and R. J. A. Aur. 1978. Extramedullary leukemia. Clin. Hematol. 7:313–337.

Hustu, H. O., D. Pinkel, and C. B. Pratt. 1972. Treatment of clinically localized Ewing's sarcoma with radiotherapy and combination chemotherapy. Cancer 30:1522–1527.

Jenkin, R. D. T., T. C. Brown, M. V. Peters, and M. J. Sonley. 1975. Hodgkin's disease in children. Cancer 35:979–990.

Kellerer, A. M., and H. H. Rossi. 1972. The theory of dual radiation in action. Curr. Top. Radiat. Res. 8:85–158.

Ladd, W. E. 1938. Embryoma of the kidney (Wilms' tumor). Ann. Surg. 108:885–902.

Leape, L., N. Breslow, and H. C. Bishop. 1978. The surgical treatment of Wilms' tumor: Results of the National Wilms' Tumor Study. Ann. Surg. 187:351–356.

Maurer, H. M., T. Moon, M. Donaldson, C. Fernandez, E. A. Gehan, D. Hammond, D. M. Harp, W. Lawrence, Jr., W. Newton, A. Regab, E. H. Soule, W. W. Sutow, and M. Tefft. 1977. The Intergroup Rhabdomyosarcoma Study: A preliminary report. Cancer 40:2015–2026.

Miller, R. W. 1969. Fifty-two forms of childhood cancer: United States mortality experience, 1960–1966. J. Pediatr. 75:685–689.

Neuhauser, E. B. D., M. H. Wittenborg, C. Z. Berman, and J. Cohen. 1952. Irradiation effects of roentgen therapy on growing spine. Radiology 59:637–650.

Pendergrass, T. W. 1976. Congenital anomalies in children with Wilms' tumor. Cancer 37:403–409.

Perez, C. A., A. Razek, M. Tefft, M. Nesbit, E. O. Borgert, J. Kissane, T. Vietti, and E. A. Gehan. 1977. Analysis of local tumor control in Ewing's sarcoma: Preliminary results of a cooperative intergroup study. Cancer 40:2864–2873.

Pomeroy, T. C., and R. E. Johnson. 1975. Integrated therapy in Ewing's sarcoma. Radiat. Oncol. 10:152–166.

Rosen, G. 1977. Past experiences and future considerations with T-2 chemotherapy in the treatment of Ewing's sarcoma, *in* Management of Primary Bone and Soft Tissue Tumors. Year Book Medical Publishers, Chicago, pp. 187–203.

Rubin, P., and G. W. Casarett. 1968. Clinical Radiation Pathology, Vols. I and II. W. B. Saunders, Philadelphia, 1,057 pp.

Rubinstein, L. J., M. M. Herman, T. F. Long, and J. R. Wilbur. 1975. Disseminated necrotizing leukoencephalopathy: A complication of treated central nervous system leukemia and lymphoma. Cancer 35:291–305.

Shah, N. K., A. I. Freeman, M. Friedman, L. Stutzman, J. Gaeta, A. Ras, and L. F. Sinks. 1976. Hodgkin's disease in children. Med. Pediatr. Oncol. 2:87–98.

Simone, J. V., R. J. A. Aur, H. O. Hustu, and M. Verzosa. 1975. Acute lymphocytic leukemia in children. Cancer 36:770–774.

Smith, K. L., and G. Rivera. 1976. Comparison of the clinical course of Hodgkin's disease in children and adolescents. Med. Pediatr. Oncol. 2:361–370.

Stoffel, T. J., M. E. Nesbit, and S. H. Levitt. 1975. Extramedullary involvement of the testes in childhood leukemia. Cancer 35:1203–1211.

Sullivan, M. P., and J. J. Butler. 1977. Non-Hodgkin's lymphoma of childhood, *in* Clinical Pediatric Oncology, W. W. Sutow, T. J. Vietti, and D. J. Fernbach, eds. 2nd ed. C. V. Mosby Company, St. Louis, 751 pp.

Sullivan, M. P., C. H. Fernandez, C. Perez, and P. Dyment. 1975. Radiotherapy for testicular leukemia, 2500 rads: Local control and relationship to subsequent disease (abstract). Proc. Am. Soc. Clin. Oncol. 16:226.

Sullivan, M. P., and L. M. Fuller. 1973. A chemotherapy-radiotherapy treatment regimen for children with stage III Hodgkin's disease. CA 23:232–241.

Sutow, W. W. 1975. Wilms' tumor. Methods Cancer Res. 13:31–65.

Sutow, W. W., M. P. Sullivan, H. L. Reid, H. G. Taylor, and K. H. Griffith. 1970. Prognosis in childhood rhabdomyosarcoma. Cancer 25:1384–1390.

Tan, C., E. Etcubanas, N. Wollner, G. Rosen, A. Gilladoga, J. Showell, M. Murphy, and I. Krakoff. 1973. Adriamycin: An antitumor antibiotic in the treatment of neoplastic disease. Cancer 32:9–17.

Tefft, M. 1977. Radiation-related toxicities in National Wilms' Tumor Study number 1. Int. J. Radiat. Oncol. Biol. Phys. 2:455–463.

Tefft, M., G. J. D'Angio, and W. Grant. 1976. Postoperative radiation therapy for residual Wilms' tumor: Review of group III patients in National Wilms' Tumor Study. Cancer 37:2768–2772.

Tefft, M., C. H. Fernandez, and T. E. Moon. 1977. Rhabdomyosarcoma: Response with chemotherapy prior to radiation in patients with gross residual disease. Cancer 39:665–670.

Tefft, M., C. Fernandez, M. Donaldson, W. Newton, and T. E. Moon. 1978. Incidence of meningeal involvement of rhabdomyosarcoma of the head and neck in children: A report of the Intergroup Rhabdomyosarcoma Study (IRS). Cancer 42:253–285.

Ward, F. J. 1975. Molecular mechanisms of radiation-induced damage to nucleic acids, *in* Advances in Radiation Biology, Vol. 5, J. T. Lett and H. Adler, eds. Academic Press, New York, pp. 189–239.

Withers, H. R. 1975. The four R's of radiotherapy. Adv. Radiat. Biol. 5:241–271.

Young, J. L., and R. W. Miller. 1975. Incidence of malignant tumors in U.S. children. J. Pediatr. 86:254.

Status of the Curability of Childhood Cancers,
edited by J. van Eys and M. P. Sullivan.
Raven Press, New York © 1980.

Evolution of a Cure for Bone Cancer

Norman Jaffe, M.D.

*Department of Pediatrics, The University of Texas System Cancer Center M. D. Anderson
Hospital and Tumor Institute, Houston, Texas*

Cures for most types of neoplastic disease evolve through a succession of
discoveries. This is particularly true of bone cancer. A major obstacle to cure
was our inability to achieve local control of the primary tumor. An effort was
made to avoid surgical ablation, since most patients appeared destined to die
of their disease. In this context, radiation therapy assumed a dominant role.
With accumulating experience, the limitation of this discipline became apparent
and its role in relation to surgery grew clearer. At the same time it became
obvious that disseminated microscopic disease was present in the majority of
patients at diagnosis. Bone cancer, therefore, was a systemic illness, and any
improvement in survival could only be achieved with therapy directed against
dissemination. This therapy was termed adjuvant treatment. A review of the
events leading to improved cure rates forms the basis of this report. The commonly encountered pediatric malignant bone tumors are used as examples.

SURGICAL TREATMENT OF THE PRIMARY TUMOR

The primary malignant tumor constitutes an uninhibited source of metastases,
so local control is essential for cure. In osteosarcoma, control is usually attempted
with surgery, which, without effective adjuvant therapy, yields an overall
5-year survival rate of approximately 20% (Friedman and Carter 1972). Death
is invariably due to pulmonary metastases, which usually appear within 9 months
of surgery (Jaffe et al. 1974, Marcove et al. 1970, Jeffree et al. 1975). This
experience led to perennial discussions of optimum sites for amputation and
methods of preventing local recurrence and improving survival. These discussions
particularly concerned tumors arising in the distal femur and proximal tibia,
the most common sites of occurrence of osteosarcoma (Sweetnam et al. 1971,
Enneking and Kagan 1975, Lewis and Lotz 1974, Jaffe and Watts 1976, Watts
1979, Parrish 1965).

Several reports documented the incidence of local recurrence as 14–16% (Dahlin and Coventry 1968, Moore et al. 1973, Sweetnam et al. 1971, McKenna et
al. 1966). The risk for developing this complication was felt to be enhanced
by "skip" metastases and unappreciated intramedullary spread of tumor (Ennek-

111

ing and Kagan 1975). As a result, disarticulation, or amputation through the joint proximal to the involved bone, appeared the best method for achieving local control. In contrast, transmedullary amputation improved functional restoration because of the residual stump, but carried an increased risk of local failure.

Review of the literature on results with disarticulation and transmedullary amputation revealed similar cure rates (Lewis and Lotz 1974). This observation and the discovery of effective chemotherapy provided the impetus for adopting transmedullary amputation as a standard procedure in many institutions (Watts 1979, Rosen and Jaffe 1979). The practice was bolstered by advances in diagnostic bone scintigraphy and computerized axial tomography (McNeil et al. 1973, Haynie 1977, Heyman and Treves 1979, de Santos et al. 1979). It was recommended that transection of the tumor-bearing bone be performed 7.0 cm from the lesion as visualized on scintigraphy, and that tumor-free margins be confirmed by frozen section examination and curettage. No adverse effects with this approach were reported (Jaffe and Watts 1976).

En bloc resection and wide local excision are frequently used for removal of parosteal lesions or limb salvage (Jaffe et al. 1974, 1978b, Parrish 1966, Watts 1979, Marcove 1979, McKenna et al. 1966, Wolfel and Carter, 1969). Previously, limited surgery of this nature was invariably complicated by local recurrence. The safety of these procedures, however, particularly for limb salvage, was enhanced by chemotherapy and the advances in diagnostic skill described earlier. Their implementation is predicated on the knowledge that the principles of cancer surgery will not be sacrificed. In all circumstances tumor-free margins must be ensured. Poor cancer surgery may not be excused on the grounds that chemotherapy is an adequate substitute for good surgery.

RADIATION TREATMENT OF THE PRIMARY TUMOR

The development of pulmonary metastases in most patients after surgical ablation and the invariably baleful outcome prompted investigators, beginning in the 1950s, to use radiation therapy for local control (Cade 1955, Lee and MacKenzie 1964, Jenkin et al. 1972). The intent was to spare patients likely to develop pulmonary metastases unnecessary mutilation. Supervoltage treatment with 7,000 to 8,000 rad was administered and ablative surgery was performed 4–6 months later if pulmonary metastases did not appear. Surgery was withheld, however, if metastases were detected or if local control was exceptionally good.

The rationale underlying this approach was based upon the following premises:

1. Radiation therapy might achieve total tumor destruction.
2. Preoperative irradiation might induce a change in cell viability and prevent implantation of tumor cells dislodged during surgery.
3. Preoperative irradiation might alter the character of the tumor and induce an antitumor immune response.

The approach yielded a 5-year survival rate of approximately 20% (Friedman and Carter 1972), comparable to that achieved with surgery alone. The therapeutic strategy, however, was challenged by a number of theoretical and practical considerations:

1. Osteosarcoma is not always radiosensitive (Lee and MacKenzie 1964, Phillips and Sheline 1969, Urtasun et al. 1973).

2. Retention of gross viable tumor is contrary to sound cancer management.

3. Failure of local control with this approach was a perpetual threat. Such failure frequently preceded pulmonary metastases, which initially did not produce major symptoms.

4. Amputation was often required for palliation (Jenkin et al. 1972).

5. Delay in initiation of definitive treatment posed a constant risk of tumor dissemination.

The foregoing considerations eventually prompted investigators to discard radiation therapy as a primary treatment instrument. However, such therapy remains indispensable for treating inoperable tumors (Wilbur et al. 1974, Jaffe 1977). Its efficacy can be enhanced by high-dose methotrexate and Adriamycin (Jaffe et al. 1973, Rosen et al. 1975, Neuberger et al. 1978). Overall, radiotherapy has produced a 5-year survival rate of 12.5% (Friedman and Carter 1972), which probably represents the minimum incidence of local control achievable.

The role of radiation therapy in the treatment of Ewing's sarcoma has been reevaluated in the light of changing concepts about its utility. In several areas its potential still awaits clarification. Its efficacy has been assessed principally in terms of its ability to produce local control, which may also be achieved by chemotherapy.

Radiation therapy administered in the era of single-agent chemotherapy was associated with poor survival rates, varying from 4–5% to 24% (Bhansali and Desai 1963, Falk and Alpert 1967, Phillips and Higinbotham 1967, Pritchard et al. 1975). Local control was apparently achieved in several patients with low-dose radiation, while some recurrences were observed in others treated with higher levels. There did, however, appear to be a slight trend toward increased local control with higher doses (Tefft et al. 1977) (Table 1).

The dismal survival rate achieved in the early chemotherapy period constituted a powerful indictment of ablative surgery. Death from cancer was anticipated for most patients and radiation therapy preferentially was obligated a dominant role (Boyer et al. 1967). In the ensuing years, the techniques of radiotherapy administration improved substantially and multiple-agent chemotherapy received increasing recognition. A new therapeutic era for both disciplines emerged.

Most centers have adopted radiation therapy as the preferred treatment for primary Ewing's sarcoma. Suit (1975) has provided guidelines for achieving local control. He recommends delivery of 4,500 rad in 4½ weeks to the entire affected bone, with generous coverage of all soft tissue likely to be infiltrated by tumor. This is followed by 2,000 rad in 2–2½ weeks to the radiographically

Table 1. *Local Control of Ewing's Sarcoma Primary by Radiation Prior to Intensive Chemotherapy*

Authors	Under 4,000 Rad		Over 4,000 Rad	
	No. of Patients	No. Achieving Local Control	No. of Patients	No. Achieving Local Control
Fernandez et al. (1974)	—	—	40	21
Freeman et al. (1972)	6	2	7	7
Jenkin (1966)	—	—	16	10
Phillips and Higinbotham (1967)	13	10	—	—
Phillips and Sheline (1969)	7	5	11	8
Wang and Schultz (1953)	19	6	13	10
Chabora et al. (1976)	—	—	9	7
Totals	45	23 (51%)	96	62 (65%)

determined area of involvement. The attention of the attending physician is also directed to the biopsy scar, port film localization, and reproducibility of setup. In most instances two fields are treated each day. A cobalt-60 or comparable unit is used, and all affected joints are actively exercised as soon as possible.

With current radiation techniques, local control may be anticipated in over 80% of patients with localized disease (Rosen et al. 1978a, Fernandez et al. 1974, Perez et al. 1977, Jaffe et al. 1976b, Cassady 1979, Hustu et al. 1972). Ewing's sarcoma appears more radiosensitive than osteosarcoma. However, the radiation effect is not complete since the dose response curve after 5,000 rad is not steep (Fernandez et al. 1974).

The efficacy of radiation therapy may be augmented by agents that improve the potential for local control while concurrently ablating disseminated microscopic disease. Reseeding of disease into previously irradiated primary sites may thereby also be avoided. Table 2, adapted from Perez et al. (1977), summarizes data on radiation and chemotherapy dosages used and incidences of local control reported by different institutions.

Radiation therapy has been associated with early and delayed complications, including fractures of the irradiated bone, contractures of the irradiated limb, and the development of second malignant neoplasms (Lewis et al. 1977, Li et al. 1975, Strong et al. 1979). This association has prompted recommendations for surgery in selected cases (Rosen et al. 1978a, Perez et al. 1977). Surgical removal may be preferable for lesions of the rib, metatarsal, metacarpal, fibula, or foot (Cassady 1979). These procedures may result in limited impairment and permanent local control. Similarly, primary amputation and early rehabilitation may be preferable for children under 6 years of age with tumors in weight-bearing bones.

The potential benefit of initial cytoreduction with chemotherapy followed by surgical debulking in Ewing's sarcoma is under investigation (Rosen et al. 1978a, Perez et al. 1977). This approach may permit delivery of lower conven-

Table 2. *Local Control of Ewing's Sarcoma Primary by Radiation and Intensive Chemotherapy**

Investigators	Radiation Dose (Rad)	Local Control (%)
University of San Francisco	4,000–4,500	71–73
Intergroup Ewing's Sarcoma	4,000–5,000	83
Intergroup Ewing's Sarcoma	5,000–6,000	86
M. D. Anderson Hospital	6,000–7,400	67
Memorial Hospital	6,000–8,000	75–88
St. Jude Children's Research Institute	4,700–6,300	93
Pooled data (130 patients)	4,000–8,000 (5,000–6,000 average)	89 (105 patients)

* Chemotherapy included two or more of the following agents: vincristine, actinomycin D, cyclophosphamide, and Adriamycin.
From Perez et al. (1977).

tional doses of radiation. The approach is being investigated particularly in Ewing's sarcoma of the pelvis, which is characterized by a high incidence of local failure (Tefft et al. 1978).

SYSTEMIC TREATMENT OF MALIGNANT BONE TUMORS

Three major disciplines have contributed toward systemic treatment of malignant bone tumors: radiation therapy, chemotherapy, and immunotherapy.

Radiation Therapy

Since the lungs are the initial site for the development of metastases, the utility of prophylactic pulmonary irradiation in osteosarcoma was investigated. Contradictory results were obtained. Two studies reported failure to prevent pulmonary metastases with 1,500 rad and actinomycin D (Rab et al. 1976, Jenkin et al. 1972). In contrast, similar studies by others, including a cooperative group, suggested that pulmonary irradiation was effective (Lougheed et al. 1967, Bruer et al. 1978). Further investigations appear warranted.

The efficacy of prophylatic pulmonary irradiation in Ewing's sarcoma is also undetermined. In the Intergroup Ewing's Sarcoma Study, preliminary results suggested that such irradiation may decrease the incidence of pulmonary metastases. The effect was similar to that achieved with the addition of Adriamycin to the combination of vincristine, actinomycin D, and cyclophosphamide (VAC) (Perez et al. 1977). A single case report also suggested that prophylactic pulmonary irradiation was beneficial (Mintz et al. 1976).

Total body irradiation with chemotherapy was administered to Ewing's sarcoma patients in an effort to destroy disseminated metastases. Stepwise improvements in disease-free survival were noted (Jenkin 1970, Millburn et al. 1968). However, the procedure has not been universally adopted, since it is associated with severe morbidity and pancytopenia, preventing delivery of effective combination chemotherapy.

Central nervous system irradiation has been advocated by some for patients with Ewing's sarcoma on the grounds that meningeal involvement similar to that with leukemia occurs (Marsa and Johnson 1971, Johnson and Pomeroy 1975). The concept and therapeutic program, however, have been rejected by others (Rosen et al. 1974, Rosen et al. 1978a, Jaffe et al. 1976b).

Chemotherapy

A major advance in the treatment of bone cancer occurred with the discovery of chemotherapeutic agents that were effective against the disease. This effectiveness was initially demonstrated against overt metastases. The use of these agents as adjuvant therapy was a logical next step. The strategy is based on the assumption that chemotherapy is more effective against microscopic disease than against bulk tumor. Clinical and experimental evidence for this assumption has been presented (Schabel 1975, Farber 1966).

Osteosarcoma

In the 1960s the chemotherapeutic agents used to treat osteosarcoma produced inconsistent and mediocre results. The agents included phenylalanine mustard (Sullivan et al. 1963), mitomycin C (Sutow 1971), cyclophosphamide (Finkelstein et al. 1969, Haggard 1967, Pinkel 1962, Sutow 1971), and 5-fluorouracil (Groesbeck and Cudmore 1963).

During the past decade, therapeutic research has revealed that osteosarcoma need no longer be considered chemoresistant. Response rates in patients with overt disease of 35–45% were achieved with high-dose methotrexate with citrovorum factor "rescue" (MTX-CF) (Jaffe 1976, Jaffe et al. 1973, 1980, Rosen et al. 1975), Adriamycin (Cortes et al. 1974), and cis-dichlorodiammineplatinum II (Ochs et al. 1978). In several instances the responses were complete and long-term. Four general types of adjuvant programs are currently in use: MTX-CF, Compadri regimens, Adriamycin, and cis-dichlorodiammineplatinum II.

The results obtained with the adjuvant programs are outlined in Table 3. When compared to results with historical control patients, they reveal an improved survival. Over a 3–5-year follow-up, they show an escalation in the cure rate from 20% to as high as 90%.

A major criticism of osteosarcoma investigations has been the use of historical controls. This was buffered by a recent report from the Mayo Clinic describing a substantial improvement in the disease-free interval and a 40–50% 3–5-year actuarial survival in patients treated without adjuvant chemotherapy (Taylor et al. 1978). This report prompted several investigators to reevaluate previous

Table 3. *Adjuvant Therapy for Osteosarcoma*

Authors	Other Agents	Actuarial 3–5-Year Disease-free Survival (%)
	High-Dose Methotrexate Regimens	
Jaffe et al. (1980)	Adriamycin, vincristine	40–80
Rooon ot al. (1070)	Adriamyoin, oyolophoophamido, vincriotinc	65–90
Pratt et al. (1977)	Adriamycin, cyclophosphamide, vincristine	50
Eilber et al. (1978)	Adriamycin	60
Etcubanas and Wilbur (1978)	Adriamycin, cyclophosphamide, vincristine	40
	Compadri Regimens (I–III)	
Sutow et al. (1976)	L-Phenylalanine mustard, cyclophosphamide, vincristine	35–55
	Adriamycin	
Cortes et al. (1979)		45–50
	Cis-dichlorodiammineplatinum (II)	
L. J. Ettinger et al. (in preparation)	Adriamycin	90

studies. The 20% 3–5-year actuarial survival in historical control patients was confirmed (Gehan et al. 1978, Miké and Marcove 1978, Jaffe et al. 1974).

Limb Salvage

Enthusiasm generated by the results achieved with chemotherapy provided the impetus to investigate the possibility of limb salvage with functional restoration in osteosarcoma patients. In the initial studies, the efficacy of chemotherapy alone or in combination with radiation therapy was assessed (Rosen et al. 1976, Jaffe et al. 1978b). The chemotherapy with or without radiotherapy was administered preoperatively and was followed by en bloc local resection and insertion of an internal prosthesis.

In 41 of 61 cases reported in the literature (67%), tumor destruction of 40% to 100% was achieved (Jaffe et al. 1978b, Rosen et al. 1976, Eilber et al. 1979). Although isolated instances of poor wound healing and sepsis were encountered, most patients acquired useful, functioning limbs. Recently, similar tumor destruction was achieved by intra-arterial infusions of cis-platinum and transcatheter occlusion (Chuang et al. 1979). Limb salvage in one such patient is illustrated in Figures 1–4.

Preoperative chemotherapy in limb salvage may be only partially effective. This has generated concern that the delay before definitive surgery could increase the incidence of pulmonary metastases. The magnitude of the risk is unknown, since destruction of microscopic disease and destruction of bulk tumor are not necessarily mutually exclusive. Different factors may obtain in each circum-

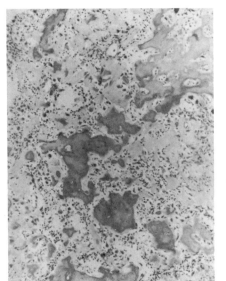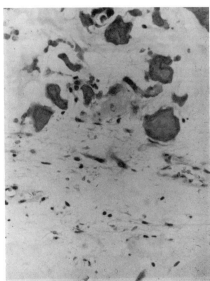

Figure 1. Left, Biopsy specimen from an osteosarcoma of the right distal femur. Intramedullary osteoid tissue and malignant cells are present. The tumor also has a predominantly cartilaginous component. Right, Posttreatment section. Intramedullary residual osteoid and chondroid tissue is apparent. Intervening tissue is poorly cellular, with rare atypical cells.

stance, including degree of oxygenation, pH level, metabolic products generated, and adequacy of arterial supply. Current investigations in limb salvage center on determining the risks and benefits of surgery with and without preoperative chemotherapy (Rosen and Jaffe 1979).

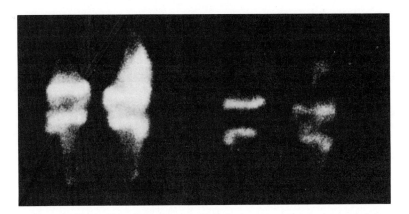

Figure 2. Left, Pretreatment arteriogram of lesion shown in Figure 1. A densely vascular, undifferentiated tumor of the distal diaphysis and metaphysis is noted. There is a large soft tissue component. Right, Posttreatment angiogram. Tumor vascularity and size have dramatically diminished.

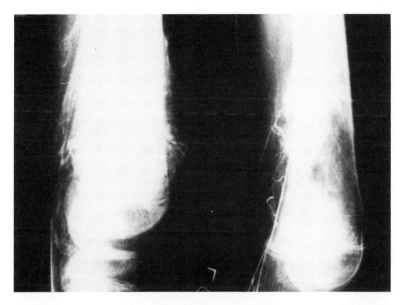

Figure 3. Left, Radionuclide bone scan of same tumor prior to initiation of treatment. There is a marked increase in isotope uptake at the distal femur. Right, Repeat radionuclide bone scan on completion of treatment. Marked decrease in isotope uptake has occurred. The post-treatment angiogram and radionuclide findings were accompanied by complete disappearance of pain.

Ewing's Sarcoma

Investigations in Ewing's sarcoma over the past 2 decades have demonstrated tumor regression and improved survival with vincristine (Sutow 1968), cyclophosphamide (Samuels and Howe 1967), actinomycin D (Senyszen et al. 1970), Adriamycin (Tan et al. 1973), BCNU (Palma et al. 1972), and mithramycin (Kofman et al. 1971). Chemotherapy regimens use combinations of these agents with different mechanisms of action and minimal overlapping toxicity.

Actinomycin D and Adriamycin enhance the efficacy and toxicity of radiation therapy (Cassady et al. 1975, D'Angio 1962). To improve treatment and prevent complications, chemotherapy and radiation therapy should be skillfully integrated.

With current methods of treatment, 3–5-year actuarial survival in patients with localized Ewing's sarcoma has improved from 8–24% to approximately 40–95% (Table 4). The results represent a major advance, but contrast sharply with those obtained in patients with metastatic disease. The results for the latter are uniformly poor, with a cure rate of probably less than 20%. Treatment of patients in this category represents a major challenge.

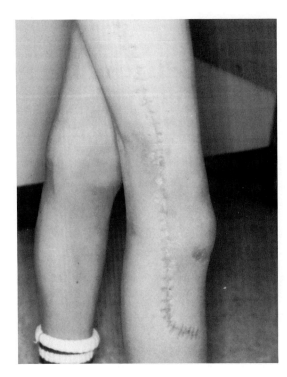

Figure 4. Right leg following en bloc local resection and insertion of an internal prosthesis.

IMMUNOTHERAPY

A clinical trial using interferon as adjuvant therapy was initiated in Stockholm in 1971 (Strander et al. 1973). A recent report reveals that 24 osteosarcoma patients have been treated (Strander 1977). To date, 60% have failed to develop metastases, compared to 15% of historical controls and 25% of concurrent controls. The results are promising, but the number of cases is too small to permit meaningful statistical analysis.

Table 4. *Actuarial Disease-free Survival in Localized Ewing's Sarcoma*

Authors	3–5-Year Survival Rate (%)
Fernandez et al. (1974)	25
Pomeroy and Johnson (1975)	55
Jaffe et al. (1976b)	65
Rosen et al. (1978a)	75
Chan et al. (1979)	55
Cassady (1979)	70

Transfer factor was administered to five patients who were clinically free of metastases at initiation of treatment (Levin et al. 1975). They had remained tumor free for 12–24 months after diagnosis at the time of the report. The number of cases is once again too small to permit meaningful interpretation.

Adoptive immunotherapy in a small number of patients did not produce statistically significant differences between disease-free survival for this group and for a control group (Neff and Enneking 1975).

TREATMENT OF ESTABLISHED METASTATIC DISEASE

Pulmonary metastases in osteosarcoma may appear at diagnosis or during adjuvant therapy. Late metastases after discontinuation of therapy have also been reported (Sutow 1976, Jaffe et al. 1976b, Eilber et al. 1978). The latter are usually treated with a coordinated multidisciplinary approach integrating surgery, radiation therapy, and chemotherapy. The conceptual development and clinical application of this approach were accelerated by the observation of a change in metastatic patterns induced by chemotherapy (Eilber et al. 1979, Pratt et al. 1977, Jaffe et al. 1978a). Metastases appeared to be reduced in number and delayed in appearance. They were frequently detected through pulmonary tomography or computerized axial tomography. Approximately 30–60% of patients with such metastases have been rendered free of disease (Table 5).

DIAGNOSTIC TECHNIQUES

The development of the interdisciplinary approaches described earlier was undoubtedly accelerated by advances in diagnostic techniques, particularly computerized axial tomography, radionuclear scanning, and angiography. These innovative procedures contributed to improvements in operative techniques and earlier detection and eradication of metastases. Occasionally computerized axial tomography was employed to ensure precision of radiation ports and monitor response to therapy. Angiography was also used to therapeutic advantage. Thus,

Table 5. *Results with Treatment of Pulmonary Metastases from Osteosarcoma*

Authors	No. of Patients Treated	3–5-Year Survival Rate (%)
Jaffe et al. (1976a)	41	34
Rosen et al. (1978a)	45	60
Rosenberg et al. (1979)	18	61
Sutow et al. (1979)	44	40
Giritsky et al. (1978)	12	53
Huang et al. (1978)	13	30
Telander et al. (1978)	28	55

intra-arterial chemotherapy was administered for osteosarcoma and transcatheter occlusion was performed to eradicate giant cell tumors (Chuang et al. 1979, Jaffe 1977, Wallace et al. 1979). Undoubtedly, additional discoveries will also prove beneficial.

SUMMARY

This review has outlined obstacles to the cure of bone cancer and attempts to overcome them. Such attempts have included the skillful and judicious application of the three major disciplines, which have been integrated over the past decade. Advances in diagnostic skills have also been contributory. Major advances in survival rates have been produced, but additional progress is still required. This will probably depend upon the acquisition of new knowledge and therapeutic discoveries.

REFERENCES

Bhansali, S. K., and P. B. Desai. 1963. Ewing's sarcoma: Observations on 107 cases. J. Bone Joint Surg. 45A:541–553.

Boyer, C. W., Jr., T. J. Brickner, Jr., and R. H. Perry. 1967. Ewing's sarcoma: Case against surgery. Cancer 20:1602–1606.

Bruer, K., P. Cohen, V. Schweisguth, and A. M. M. Hart. 1978. Irradiation of the lung as an adjuvant therapy in the treatment of osteosarcoma of the limbs: An E.O.R.T.C. randomized study. Eur. J. Cancer 14:461–471.

Cade, S. 1955. Osteogenic sarcoma: A study based on 113 patients. J. R. Coll. Surg. Edinb. 1:79–111.

Cassady, J. R. 1979. Radiation therapy in Ewing's sarcoma, in Bone Tumors in Children, N. Jaffe, ed. P. S. G. Publishing Co., Littleton, Mass., pp. 191–204.

Cassady, J. R., M. P. Richter, A. J. Piro, and N. Jaffe. 1975. Radiation-Adriamycin interactions: Preliminary clinical observations. Cancer 36:946–949.

Chabora, B. M., C. Rosen, W. Cham, G. J. D'Angio, and M. Tefft. 1976. Radiotherapy of Ewing's sarcoma. Radiology 120:667–671.

Chan, R. C., W. W. Sutow, R. D. Lindberg, M. L. Samuels, J. A. Murray, and D. A. Johnston. 1979. Management and results of localized Ewing's sarcoma. Cancer 43:1001–1006.

Chuang, V. P., S. Wallace, R. S. Benjamin, and N. Jaffe. 1979. Therapeutic intra-arterial infusion of cis-platinum in the management of malignant bone tumors: A preliminary report (Abstract), in Proceedings of the 27th Annual Meeting of the Association of University Radiologists, May 6–10, 1979, Rochester, N.Y.

Cortes, E. P., J. F. Holland, J. J. Wang, L. F. Sinks, J. B. Blom, H. Senn, A. Bank, and O. Glidewell. 1974. Amputation and Adriamycin in primary osteosarcoma. N. Engl. J. Med. 291:998–1000.

Cortes, E. P., T. F. Necheles, J. F. Holland, and O. Glidewell. 1979. Adriamycin (ADR) alone versus ADM and high dose methotrexate citrovorum factor rescue (HDMTX-CF) as adjuvant to operable primary osteosarcoma (OS): A randomized study by cancer and leukemia group B (CALGB) (Abstract). Proc. Am. Assoc. Cancer Res. 20:412.

Dahlin, D. C., and M. B. Coventry. 1968. Osteogenic sarcoma: A study of six hundred cases. J. Bone Joint Surg. 49A:101–110.

Dahlin, D. C., M. B. Coventry, and P. W. Scanlon. 1961. Ewing's sarcoma: A critical analysis of 165 cases. J. Bone Joint Surg. 43A:185–192.

D'Angio, G. J. 1962. Clinical and biologic studies of actinomycin D and roentgen irradiation. Am. J. Roentgenol. 87:100–109.

de Santos, L. A., M. E. Bernadino, and J. A. Murray. 1979. Computed tomography in the evaluation of osteosarcoma: Experience with 25 cases. Am J. Roentgenol. 132:535–560.

Eilber, F. R., T. Grant, and D. L. Morton. 1978. Adjuvant therapy for osteosarcoma: Preoperative and postoperative treatment. Cancer Treat. Rep. 62:213–216.

Eilber, F. R., D. L. Morton, and T. T. Grant. 1979. En bloc resection and allograft replacement for osteosarcoma of the extremity, *in* Bone Tumors in Children, N. Jaffe, ed. P. S. G. Publishing Co., Littleton, Mass., pp. 159–167.

Enneking, W. F., and A. Kagan. 1975. "Skip" metastases in osteosarcoma. Cancer 36:2192–2205.

Etcubanas, E., and J. R. Wilbur. 1978. Adjuvant chemotherapy for osteogenic sarcoma. Cancer Treat. Rep. 62:283–287.

Falk, S., and M. Alpert. 1967. Five year survival of patients with Ewing's sarcoma. Surg. Gynecol. Obstet. 124:319–324.

Farber, S. 1966. Chemotherapy in the treatment of leukemia and Wilms' tumor. JAMA 198:826–836.

Fernandez, C. H., R. D. Lindberg, W. W. Sutow, and M. L. Samuels. 1974. Localized Ewing's sarcoma: Treatment and results. Cancer 34:143–148.

Finkelstein, J., R. E. Hittle, and U. D. Hammond. 1969. Evaluation of a high dose cyclophosphamide regimen in childhood tumors. Cancer 23:1239–1244.

Freeman, A. I., C. Satchatello, J. Gatta, N. K. Shah, J. J. Wang, and L. F. Sinks. 1972. An analysis of Ewing's tumor in children at Roswell Park Memorial Institute. Cancer 29:1563–1569.

Friedman, M. A., and S. K. Carter. 1972. The therapy of osteogenic sarcoma: Current status and thoughts for the future. J. Surg. Oncol. 4:482–510.

Gehan, E. A., W. W. Sutow, T. Uribe-Botero, M. Romsdahl, and T. L. Smith. 1978. Osteosarcoma: The M. D. Anderson experience 1950–1974, *in* Immunotherapy of Cancer: Present Status of Trials in Man, W. E. Terry and D. Windhorst, eds. Raven Press, New York, pp. 271–282.

Giritsky, A. S. E., Etcubanas, and F. B. D. Mark. 1978. Pulmonary resection in children with metastatic osteogenic sarcoma. J. Thorac. Cardiovasc. Surg. 73:354–362.

Groesbeck, H. P., and J. T. P. Cudmore. 1963. Evaluation of 5-fluorouracil (5-Fu) in surgical practice. Am. Surg. 29:638–691.

Haggard, M. 1967. Cyclophosphamide (NSC-26271) in the treatment of children with malignant neoplasms. Cancer Chemother. Rep. 51:403–405.

Haynie, T. P., III. 1977. Radionuclide bone imaging in primary bone tumors, *in* Management of Primary Bone and Soft Tissue Tumors (Proceedings of The University of Texas System Cancer Center M. D. Anderson Hospital and Tumor Institute 21st Annual Clinical Conference on Cancer). Year Book Medical Publishers, Inc., Chicago, pp. 97–105.

Heyman, S., and S. Trever. 1979. Scintigraphy in pediatric bone tumors, *in* Bone Tumors in Children, N. Jaffe, ed. P. S. G. Publishing Co., Littleton, Mass., pp. 79–96.

Huang, M. N., H. Takita, and H. O. Douglas. 1978. Lung resection for metastatic osteogenic sarcoma. J. Surg. Oncol. 10:179–182.

Hustu, H. O., D. Pinkel, and C. B. Pratt. 1972. Treatment of clinically localized Ewing's sarcoma with radiotherapy and combination chemotherapy. Cancer 30:1522–1526.

Jaffe, N. 1977. Current concepts in the management of disseminated malignant bone disease in childhood. Can. J. Surg. 20:537–539.

Jaffe, N. 1976. Osteogenic sarcoma: State of the art with high-dose methotrexate treatment. J. Clin. Orthopaed. 120:95–102.

Jaffe, N., S. Farber, D. Traggis, C. Geiser, B. S. Kim, L. Das, A. Frauenberger, I. Djerassi, and J. R. Cassady. 1973. Favorable response of metastatic osteogenic sarcoma to pulse high-dose methotrexate with citrovorum rescue and radiation therapy. Cancer 31:1367–1373.

Jaffe, N., E. Frei III, E. Smith, J. R. Cassady, R. M. Fuller, and M. Zelen. 1978a. A hypothesis for the pattern of pulmonary metastases in osteogenic sarcoma: Impact of adjuvant therapy (Abstract). Proc. Am. Assoc. Cancer Res. 19:488.

Jaffe, N., E. Frei III, D. Traggis, and Y. Bishop. 1974. Adjuvant methotrexate citrovorum factor treatment of osteogenic sarcoma. N. Engl. J. Med. 291:996–997.

Jaffe, N., M. Link, D. Traggis, E. Frei, H. Watts, P. Beardsley, D. Cohen, and H. Abelson. 1980. The role of high-dose methotrexate in osteogenic sarcoma. J. Natl. Cancer Inst. (in press).

Jaffe, N., D. Traggis, J. R. Cassady, R. M. Fuller, H. Watts, and E. Frei. 1976a. Multidisciplinary treatment for micrometastatic osteogenic sarcoma. Br. Med. J. 2:1039–1041.

Jaffe, N., D. Traggis, S. Sallan, and J. R. Cassady. 1976b. Improved outlook for Ewing's sarcoma with combination chemotherapy (vincristine, Adriamycin and cyclophosphamide) and radiation therapy. Cancer 38:1925–1930.

Jaffe, N., and H. Watts, 1976. Multidrug chemotherapy in primary treatment of osteosarcoma. J. Bone Joint Surg. 58A:634–635.

Jaffe, N., H. Watts, K. E. Fellows, and C. Vawler. 1978b. Local en bloc resection for limb preservation. Cancer Treat. Rep. 62:217–223.

Jeffree, C. M., C. H. G. Price, and H. A. Sessons. 1975. The metastatic patterns of osteosarcoma. Br. J. Cancer 32:87–107.

Jenkin, R. D. T. 1970. Ewing's sarcoma: A trial of adjuvant total body irradiation. Radiology 96:151–155.

Jenkin, R. D. T. 1966. Ewing's sarcoma: Study of treatment methods. Clin. Radiol. 17:97–106.

Jenkin, R. D. T., W. E. C. Allt, and P. J. Fitzpatrick. 1972. Osteosarcoma: An assessment of management with particular reference to primary irradiation and selective delayed amputation. Cancer 30:393–400.

Johnson, R. E., and T. C. Pomeroy. 1975. Evaluation of therapeutic results in Ewing's sarcoma. Am J. Roentgenol. 123:583–587.

Kofman, S., C. P. Perlia, and S. G. Economou. 1971. Mithramycin in the treatment of Ewing's sarcoma with radiation therapy and adjuvant chemotherapy. Cancer 27:1051–1054.

Lee, E. S., and D. H. MacKenzie. 1964. Osteosarcoma: A study of the value of preoperative megavoltage radiotherapy. Br. J. Surg. 51:252–274.

Levin, A. S., V. S. Beyer, H. H. Fudenberg, J. Wybran, A. J. Hackett, J. O. Johnston, and L. E. Spitler. 1975. Osteogenic sarcoma: Immunotherapy with tumor-specific transfer factor. J. Clin. Invest. 55:487–499.

Lewis, R. J., and M. P. Lotz. 1974. Medullary extension of osteosarcoma: Implications for rational therapy. Cancer 33:371–375.

Lewis, R. J., R. C. Marcove, and C. Rosen. 1977. Ewing's sarcoma: Functional effects of radiation therapy. J. Bone Joint Surg. 59A:325–331.

Li, F. P., J. R. Cassady, and N. Jaffe. 1975. Risk of second tumors in survivors of childhood cancer. Cancer 35:1230–1235.

Lougheed, M. N., J. D. Palmer, I. Henderson, and J. M. McIntyre. 1967. Radiation and regional chemotherapy in osteogenic sarcoma, *in* Excerpta Medica International Congress Series No. 105, Progress in Radiology. Excerpta Medica Foundation, Amsterdam, pp. 1124–1128.

Marcove, R. 1979. En bloc resection and prosthetic replacement in osteosarcoma, *in* Bone Tumors in Children, N. Jaffe, ed. P. S. G. Publishing Co., Littleton, Mass., pp. 143–158.

Marcove, R. C., V. Miké, J. V. Hajek, A. G. Levin, and R. V. P. Hutter. 1970. Osteogenic sarcoma under the age of twenty-one: A review of one hundred forty-five operative cases. J. Bone Joint Surg. 52A:611–623.

Marsa, G. W., and R. E. Johnson. 1971. Altered pattern of metastases following treatment of Ewing's sarcoma with radiotherapy and adjuvant chemotherapy. Cancer 27:1051–1054.

McKenna, R. J., C. P. Schwinn, K. Y. Soong, and N. C. Higinbotham. 1966. Sarcomata of the osteogenic series (osteosarcoma, fibrosarcoma, chondrosarcoma, periosteal osteogenic sarcoma, and sarcomata arising in abnormal bone): An analysis of 552 cases. J. Bone Joint Surg. 48A:1–26.

McNeil, B. J., J. R. Cassady, C. F. Geiser, N. Jaffe, D. Traggis, and S. Treves. 1973. Fluorine-18 bone scintigraphy in children with osteosarcoma or Ewing's sarcoma. Radiology 109:627–631.

Miké, V., and R. C. Marcove. 1978. Osteogenic sarcoma under the age of 21: Experiences at Memorial Sloan-Kettering Cancer Center, *in* Immunotherapy of Cancer: Present Status of Trials in Man, W. D. Terry and D. Windhorst, eds. Raven Press, New York, pp. 283–292.

Millburn, L. F., L. O'Grady, and F. R. Hendrickson. 1968. Radical radiation therapy and total body irradiation in the treatment of Ewing's sarcoma. Cancer 22:919–925.

Mintz, U., Z. Keinan, and B. Wainrach. 1976. Prophylactic irradiation of the lung in Ewing's sarcoma. Chest 70:393–395.

Moore, G. E., R. E. Gerner, and A. Brugarolas. 1973. Osteogenic sarcoma. Surg. Gynecol. Obstet. 136:359–366.

Neff, J. R., and W. E. Enneking. 1975. Adoptive immunotherapy in primary osteosarcoma. J. Bone Joint Surg. 57A:145–148.

Neuberger, P. E., J. R. Cassady, and N. Jaffe. 1978. Esophagitis due to Adriamycin and radiation therapy for childhood malignancy. Cancer 42:417–423.

Ochs, J. J., A. I. Freeman, H. O. Douglass, Jr., D. J. Higby, E. R. Mindell, and T. Sinks. 1978. Cis-dichloro-diammine platinum (II) in advanced osteogenic sarcoma. Cancer Treat. Rep. 62:239–245.

Palma, J., S. Gartani, A. Freeman, L. Sinks, and J. F. Holland. 1972. Treatment of metastatic Ewing's sarcoma with BCNU. Cancer 30:909–913.

Parrish, F. F. 1966. Treatment of bone tumors by total excision and replacement with massive autologous and homologous grafts of bone. J. Bone Joint Surg. 68A:968–990.

Perez, C., J. Herson, J. Kimball, and W. W. Sutow. 1978. Prognosis after metastasis in osteosarcoma. Cancer Clin. Trials 1:315–320.

Perez, C. A., A. Razek, M. Tefft, M. Nesbit, O. Burgert, J. Kissane, T. Vietti, and E. A. Gehan. 1977. Analysis of local tumor control in Ewing's sarcoma. Cancer 40:2864–2873.

Phillips, R. F., and N. L. Higinbotham. 1967. The curability of Ewing's endothelioma of bone in children. J. Pediatr. 70:391–397.

Phillips, T. L., and C. E. Sheline. 1969. Radiation therapy of malignant bone tumors. Radiology 92:1537–1545.

Pinkel, D. 1962. Cyclophosphamide in children with cancer. Cancer 15:42–69.

Pomeroy, T. C., and R. E. Johnson. 1975. Combined modality therapy for survival in Ewing's sarcoma. Cancer 35:36–47.

Pratt, C., E. Shanks, O. Hustu, C. Rivera, J. Smith, and P. M. Kumar. 1977. Adjuvant multiple drug chemotherapy for osteosarcoma of the extremity. Cancer 39:51–57.

Pritchard, D. J., D. Dahlin, R. Dauphine, W. Taylor, and J. Beabout. 1975. Ewing's sarcoma. J. Bone Joint Surg. 57A:10–16.

Rab, C. T., J. C. Ivins, D. S. Childs, R. E. Capps, and D. J. Pritchard. 1976. Elective whole lung irradiation in the treatment of osteogenic sarcoma. Cancer 38:939–942.

Rosen, G., B. Caparros, C. Mosende, B. McCormick, A. G. Huvos, and R. C. Marcove. 1978a. Curability of Ewing's sarcoma and considerations for future therapeutic trials. Cancer 41:888–899.

Rosen, G., A. G. Huvos, C. Mosende, E. J. Beattie, Jr., P. R. Exelby, and R. C. Marcove. 1978b. Chemotherapy and thoracotomy for metastatic osteogenic sarcoma: A model for adjuvant chemotherapy and the rationale for the timing of thoracic surgery. Cancer 41:841–849.

Rosen, G., and N. Jaffe. 1979. Chemotherapy for malignant spindle cell tumors of bone, *in* Bone Tumors in Children, N. Jaffe, ed. P. S. G. Publishing Co., Littleton, Mass., pp. 107–130.

Rosen, G., M. L. Murphy, A. G. Huvos, M. Gutierrez, and R. C. Marcove. 1976. Chemotherapy, en bloc resection, and prosthetic bone replacement in the treatment of osteogenic sarcoma. Cancer 37:1–11.

Rosen, G., A. Nirenberg, H. Juergens, B. Kosloff, B. M. Mehta, R. C. Marcove, and A. G. Huvos. 1979. Osteogenic sarcoma: Three year disease free survival in excess of 80% with combination chemotherapy including effective high dose methotrexate with citrovorum factor rescue. J. Natl. Cancer Inst. (in press).

Rosen, G., C. Tan, A. Sanmaneechai, E. J. Beattie, Jr., R. Marcove, and M. L. Murphy. 1975. The rationale for multiple drug chemotherapy in the treatment of osteogenic sarcoma. Cancer 35:936–945.

Rosen, G., N. Wollner, C. Tan, J. Wu, S. I. Haydn, G. Chem, G. J. D'Angio, and M. L. Murphy. 1974. Disease-free survival in children with Ewing's sarcoma treated with radiation therapy and adjuvant four-drug sequential chemotherapy. Cancer 33:386–393.

Rosenberg, S. A., M. W. Flye, D. Conkle, C. A. Seipp, A. S. Levine, and R. M. Simon. 1979. Treatment of osteogenic sarcoma: Aggressive resection of pulmonary metastases. Cancer Treat. Rep. 63:753–756.

Samuels, M. L., and C. D. Howe. 1967. Cyclophosphamide in the management of Ewing's sarcoma. Cancer 20:961–966.

Schabel, F. M., Jr. 1975. Concepts for systemic treatment of micrometastases. Cancer 35:15–24.

Senyszen, J. J., R. E. Johnson, and R. E. Curran. 1970. Treatment of metastatic Ewing's sarcoma with Adriamycin (NSC-3053). Cancer Chemother. Rep. 54:103–107.

Strander, H. 1977. Antitumor effects of interferon and its possible use as an antineoplastic agent in man. Tex. Rep. Biol. Med. 35:629–635.

Strander, H., K. Cantell, C. Carlstrom, and P. A. Jakobsson. 1973. Clinical and laboratory investigations on man: Systemic administration of potent interferon to man. J. Natl. Cancer Inst. 51:733–742.

Strong, L. C., J. Herson, B. M. Osborne, and W. W. Sutow. 1979. Risk of radiation-related subsequent malignant tumors in survivors of Ewing's sarcoma. J. Natl. Cancer Inst. 62:1401–1406.

Suit, H. D. 1975. Role of therapeutic radiology in cancer of bone. Cancer 35:930–935.

Sullivan, M. P., W. W. Sutow, and G. Taylor. 1963. L-phenylalanine mustard as a treatment for metastatic osteogenic sarcoma in children. J. Pediatr. 63:227–237.

Sutow, W. W. 1968. Vincristine (NSC-GF574) therapy for malignant solid tumors in children (except Wilms' tumor). Cancer Chemother. Rep. 52:485–487.

Sutow, W. W. 1971. Evaluation of dosage schedules of mitomycin C (NSC-26980) in children. Cancer Chemother. Rep. 55:285–289.

Sutow, W. W. 1976. Late metastases in osteosarcoma. Lancet 1:856.

Sutow, W. W., E. A. Gehan, T. J. Vietti, A. E. Frias, and P. G. Dyment. 1976. Multidrug chemotherapy in primary treatment of osteosarcoma. J. Bone Joint Surg. 58A:629–633.

Sutow, W. W., J. Herson, and C. Perez. 1979. Survival after metastases in osteosarcoma. J. Natl. Cancer Inst. (in press).

Sweetnan, R., J. Knowleden, and H. Sneddon. 1971. Bone sarcoma treatment by irradiation, amputation or a combination of the two. Br. Med. J. 2:263–267.

Tan, C., E. Etcubanas, N. Wollner, C. Rosen, A. Gilladoga, P. Showel, M. L. Murphy, and I. H. Krakoff. 1973. Adriamycin and antiumor antibiotic in the treatment of neoplastic disease. Cancer 32:9–17.

Taylor, W. F., J. G. Ivins, D. C. Dahlin, and O. J. Pritchard. 1978. Osteogenic sarcoma experience at the Mayo Clinic 1963–1974, *in* Immunotherapy of Cancer: Present Status of Trials in Man, W. E. Terry and D. Windhorst, eds. Raven Press, New York, pp. 257–269.

Tefft, M., B. Chabora, and C. Rosen. 1977. Radiation in bone sarcomas: A re-evaluation in the era of intensive systemic chemotherapy. Cancer 39:806–816.

Tefft, M., A. Rozck, C. Perez, O. Bugert, E. A. Gehan, P. Griffin, J. Kissane, T. Vietti, and M. Nesbit. 1978. Local control and survival related to radiation dose and volume and to chemotherapy in non-metastatic Ewing's sarcoma of pelvic bones. J. Radiat. Oncol. Biol. Phys. 4:367–372.

Telander, R. L., P. C. Pairolero, D. J. Prichard, F. H. Sim, and G. S. Gilchrist. 1978. Resection of pulmonary metastatic osteogenic sarcoma in children. Surgery 84:335–341.

Urtasun, R. C., P. McGonnachie, and T. Merz. 1973. Radiation damage to the periphery and center of human osteogenic sarcoma. Cancer 31:1354–1358.

Wallace, S., M. Granmayeh, L. A. de Santos, J. A. Murray, M. M. Romsdahl, R. B. Bracken, and K. Jonsson. 1979. Arterial occlusion of pelvic bone tumors. Cancer 43:322–328.

Wang, C. C., and M. D. Schultz. 1953. Ewing's sarcoma. N. Engl. J. Med. 248:571–576.

Watts, H. G. 1979. Surgical management of malignant bone tumors in children, *in* Bone Tumors in Children, N. Jaffe, ed. P. S. G. Publishing Co., Littleton, Mass., pp. 131–142.

Wilbur, J. R., E. Etcubanas, T. Long, E. Glatstein, and T. Leavitt. 1974. Four drug therapy and irradiation on primary and metastatic osteogenic sarcoma (Abstract). Proc. Am. Assoc. Cancer Res. 15:816.

Wolfel, D. A., and P. R. Carter. 1969. Parosteal osteosarcoma. Am. J. Roentgenol. 105:142–146.

Status of the Curability of Childhood Cancers,
edited by J. van Eys and M. P. Sullivan.
Raven Press, New York © 1980.

Osteosarcoma: The Pathological Study of Specimens from En Bloc Resection in Patients Receiving Preoperative Chemotherapy

Alberto G. Ayala, M.D., Bruce Mackay, M.D., Ph.D., Norman Jaffe, M.D.,* W. W. Sutow, M.D.,* Robert Benjamin, M.D.,† and John A. Murray, M.D.‡

Departments of Pathology, *Pediatrics, †Developmental Therapeutics, and ‡Surgery, The University of Texas System Cancer Center M. D. Anderson Hospital and Tumor Institute, Houston, Texas

Preoperative chemotherapy (and occasionally radiation therapy) is being used with increasing frequency in limited salvage procedures (Jaffe et al. 1978). The degree to which it produces tumor destruction may serve as an indication for postoperative administration of adjuvant chemotherapy. The purpose of this communication is to establish and describe the pathological features of chemotherapy-induced effects in five patients who were treated at M. D. Anderson Hospital and Tumor Institute.

MATERIALS AND METHODS

At M. D. Anderson Hospital and Tumor Institute, patients suspected of having a bone tumor usually undergo a needle biopsy. The specimens obtained are fixed in 10% buffered formalin for a minimum of 3 hours and decalcified overnight in dilute formic acid. The next morning the tissue is processed through the Ultratechnicon (a 4-hour procedure), embedded in paraffin, and stained with hematoxylin and eosin. The entire procedure takes approximately 24 hours. Open biopsies may require a longer time for fixation and decalcification, depending on the amount of bone present. A 3-mm-thick fragment of tissue is routinely taken and fixed in gluteraldehyde for ultrastructural studies.

In segmentally resected bone lesions, the length and diameter of the bone fragment are measured, and the outer surface is carefully inspected for gross tumor permeation. After the bone is sectioned longitudinally by a band saw, the cut surface, cortex, and margins are examined. The bone is photographed, radiographed, and, in patients who have received tetracycline, examined by ultraviolet light. By means of an Isomet low-speed diamond saw, a 3-mm-thick slice of the entire cut surface is taken and blocked into multiple squares, each of which is numbered (Figures 1 and 2). In this manner the epicenter and

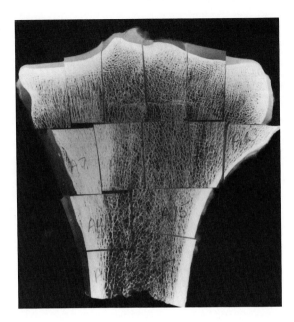

Figure 1. Specimen radiograph of 3-mm-thick slice of proximal tibia. Each block is labeled and then submitted for decalcification and routine sectioning.

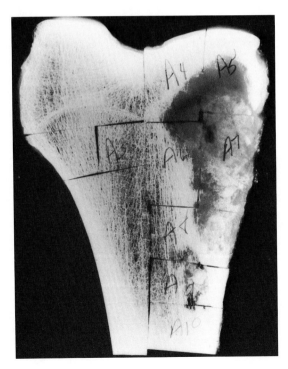

Figure 2. Specimen radiograph from Case 2. Epicenter, periphery, and normal bone are included for study.

Table 1. *Categories of Response (Therapeutic Effect)*

I. No effect or doubtful effect
  A. No effect
    Most of tumor viable
    Necrosis in up to 30%
  B. Doubtful effect
    Most of tumor viable
    Necrosis in up to 40%
    May be minimal evidence of fibrovascular regeneration
II. Partial tumor effect
  A. 40–50% tumor destruction
    Definite evidence of fibrovascular regeneration
  B. 50–60% tumor destruction
    Fibrovascular regeneration
III. Definite tumor effect
  A. 60–90% tumor destruction
    Viable tumor may be present
    Frank evidence of fibrovascular regenerative activity
  B. Complete tumor effect
    No viable or minimally viable tumor
    Major fibrovascular regeneration

periphery of the lesion in one plane are studied. Additional sections can be taken as needed.

The objectives of the biopsy are to confirm the diagnosis of osteosarcoma, recognize the variants, and subclassify the lesion as osteoblastic, chondroblastic, or fibroblastic. Histologic examination of the resected specimen helps in evaluating the effect of chemotherapy on tumor tissue. A quantitative estimation is made of necrosis, degree of fibrosis with regeneration, and tumor viability, and the category of response, or chemotherapeutic effect (Table 1), is determined.

CASE 1

A 15-year-old boy was referred to M. D. Anderson Hospital with a radiologic diagnosis of osteosarcoma of the right proximal tibia. Findings from a needle biopsy were felt to be equivocal, but an open biopsy confirmed the diagnosis. The patient was treated with high-dose methotrexate administered as 7.5 g/m² at 7–10-day intervals for a total of eight courses. In January 1979 he underwent local resection of the proximal tibia.

Initial Biopsy

An open biopsy of the right tibia provided, in aggregate, a sample of tumor tissue 4 cm in diameter. The tumor was an osteoblastic osteosarcoma with irregular depositions of osteoid and numerous small, hyperchromatic malignant cells (Figure 3). Areas of the tumor consisted mainly of sclerotic bone.

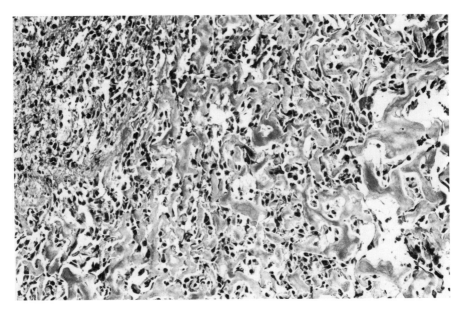

Figure 6. Case 2. Pretherapy biopsy shows osteoblastic osteosarcoma. Note delicate osteoid and hyperchromatic sarcomatous stroma; reduced from ×150.

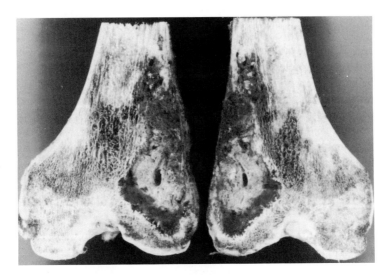

Figure 7. Case 2. Distal femur. Large metaphyseal-epiphyseal tumor is present. Periphery shows 3–4-mm-thick osteosclerotic rim, inside of which is area of edematous, gelatinous tissue, seen in illustration as dark tissue. Tumor was grossly necrotic.

Initial Biopsy

A few cylindrical fragments of bone disclosed abundant lace-like osteoid depositions with a hyperchromatic sarcomatous stroma (Figure 6). Areas of the tumor consisted of relatively acellular, solid, irregular bone. The diagnosis was osteoblastic osteosarcoma.

Resection of the Distal Femur after Therapy

An 11-cm-long segment of distal femur was resected. The outer surface showed a small amount of fibroadipose tissue and skeletal muscle. Longitudinal sections disclosed a large, irregular lesion predominantly involving the lateral condyle (Figure 7) and occupying the metaphysis and epiphysis. The tumor measured 9 cm long and 6 cm at the widest point. At the periphery of the lesion was a 3–4-mm-thick, sclerotic rim of fibro-osseous tissue. Immediately within the lesion was a zone of gelatinous, translucent tissue, while the central portion of the tumor was grayish and contained sclerotic bone. The cortex was irregular, but was not penetrated. Ultraviolet examination of the specimen disclosed fluorescence of the sclerotic rim at the periphery of the tumor.

Microscopic Examination

Examination of multiple sections revealed no evidence of viable tumor. The periphery of the lesion was made up of reactive fibro-osseous tissue. The cystic

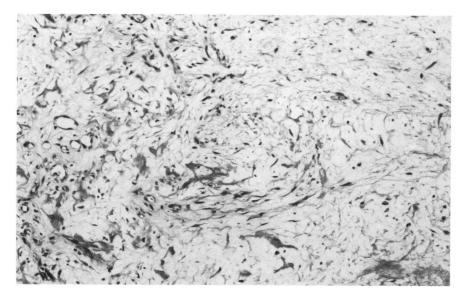

Figure 8. Case 2. Periphery of lesion. Note loose connective tissue with fibroblasts and capillaries. There is no evidence of osteosarcoma; reduced from ×100.

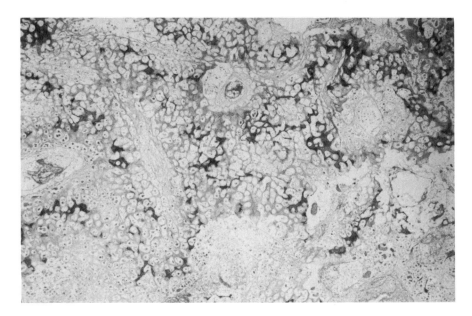

Figure 9. Case 2. Center of lesion. Note irregular osteoid and partially calcified bone. Rare "ghost" cells are seen, but no viable tumor is present; reduced from ×150.

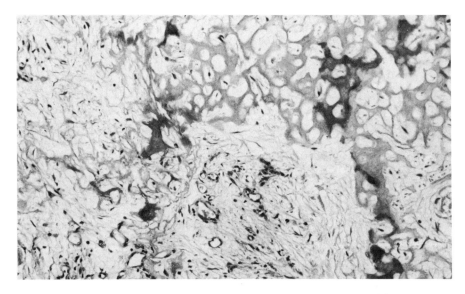

Figure 10. Case 2. Higher magnification demonstrates framework of osteoid is present, but without viable cells. Note active fibrovascular proliferation; reduced from ×220.

tissue adjacent to this rim consisted of loose myxoid connective tissue without tumor (Figure 8). The central portion contained focally calcified, irregular osteoid, but there was no evidence of malignant cells (Figure 9). Throughout the lesion was an active fibrovascular proliferation indicative of a regenerative process (Figure 10). This was also considered to be an example of complete tumor destruction, response category IIIB.

CASE 3

A 16-year-old girl was referred to M. D. Anderson Hospital with a lump in the knee associated with minimal pain. Radiographs showed a mixed lytic and blastic lesion of the proximal tibia, and the diagnosis on needle biopsy was chondroblastic osteosarcoma. The patient received four courses of high-dose methotrexate (7.5 g/m² at 7–10-day intervals). There was an initial response, but after the fourth course the tumor appeared to escape control. Two additional courses failed to control the disease. The therapy was then changed to intra-arterial cis-platinum. The patient received two courses (150 mg/m²), after which she underwent an en bloc resection with insertion of an internal prosthesis.

Initial Biopsy

The biopsy demonstrated islands of malignant cartilage between spicules of normal bone. Dense sclerotic abnormal bone was also present. The diagnosis was chondroblastic osteosarcoma (Figure 11).

Resection of Proximal Right Tibia after Therapy

The respected specimen consisted of the proximal right tibia, measuring 10.5 cm long. The outer surface was covered by fibroconnective tissue. Examination of a longitudinal section revealed a metaphyseal-epiphyseal tumor that was well circumscribed and measured 6.7×6.0×5.0 cm (Figure 12). In the epiphysis the lesion approached the articular cartilage, although the latter was not penetrated. The cortex was permeated, allowing the tumor to extend beyond the bone, but the periosteum limited and separated the tumor from the adjacent soft tissue. The tumor bulge was approximately 3 cm thick. The cut surface showed a gray-white discoloration with sclerosis, which fluoresced under ultraviolet light. A 2-cm-wide margin of normal bone was present at the distal site of resection.

Microscopic examination disclosed some viable tumor with approximately 60–70% tumor necrosis (Figure 13) and evidence of fibroblastic and vascular proliferation. The rim of sclerosis consisted of reactive bone, rather than the healed edge of the tumor. A response category of IIIA was assigned.

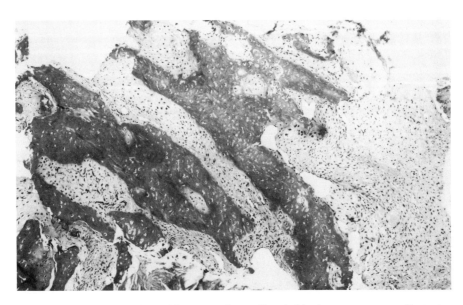

Figure 11. Case 3. Pretherapy biopsy specimen. Chondroblastic osteosarcoma. Illustration shows spindle-shaped, somewhat sarcomatous proliferation growing between normal bone spicules; reduced from ×100.

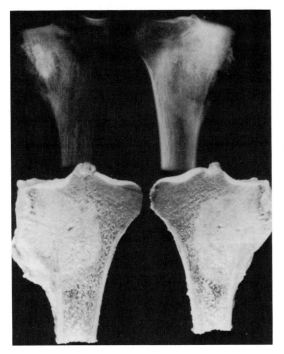

Figure 12. Case 3. Specimen radiograph (top) and bisected tibia (bottom). Tumor is well demarcated from surrounding normal bone. Destruction of cortex produces a nodular bulge outside bone. Tumor is still limited by periosteum.

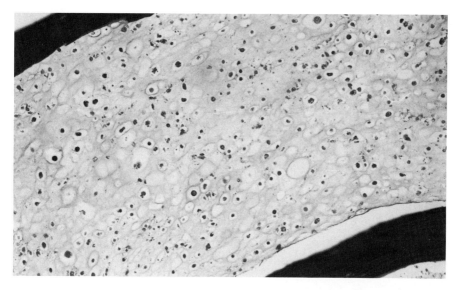

Figure 13. Case 3. Post-therapy. Illustration demonstrates pyknosis and disintegration of nuclei. No viable tumor cells are present; reduced from ×200.

CASE 4

A 19-year-old man was referred to M. D. Anderson Hospital in November 1978 with a diagnosis of a bone tumor involving the right radius. A needle biopsy confirmed the diagnosis of osteosarcoma. The patient received three intra-arterial infusions of cis-platinum (120 mg/m^2) and on February 7, 1979, underwent resection of the right distal radius with reconstruction by means of Steinman pins and poly-methylmethacrylate.

Initial Biopsy

A needle biopsy of the right distal radius provided three cylindrical fragments of bony tissue measuring, in aggregate, 1 cm long and 0.2 cm in diameter. Histologically, there was a predominantly cartilaginous proliferation with osteoid depositions. The specimen was interpreted as chondroblastic osteosarcoma.

Resection of Distal Radius after Therapy

The resected specimen was a 5-cm-long segment of the distal radius. Covering the specimen was a thin layer of skeletal muscle and fibroconnective tissue. When the specimen was bisected, the cut surface revealed obliteration of the

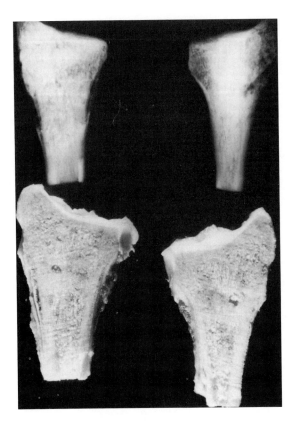

Figure 14. Case 4. Radiograph (top) shows irregular calcification, while specimen (bottom) displays disarray of normal bony trabeculae, which are replaced by granular tissue.

medullary cavity by dense sclerotic tissue. This could be better appreciated on the radiograph of the specimen (Figure 14). The patient had received tetracycline prior to undergoing resection, so the specimen was examined under ultraviolet light. Scattered foci of fluorescence indicative of new bone or osteoid formation were disclosed. The entire surface was cut in multiple blocks for histologic examination.

Microscopically, there was abundant bone and cartilage material with relatively few cells. The cartilaginous areas contained many necrotic nuclei, although there were areas with viable cells. These areas alternated with zones of bone and osteoid deposition in which the stroma was no longer malignant, but was replaced by a loose, myxoid fibroblastic proliferation and numerous capillaries.

The tumor was confined to the medullary cavity, except for one area in which the cortex was penetrated with microscopic extension into the adjacent skeletal muscle. This area was still covered by muscle, however, and the resection margin was free of tumor. The estimated tumor destruction was 75–80%. Definite tumor effect was documented; the response category was considered to be IIIA.

CASE 5

A 21-year-old woman was referred to M. D. Anderson Hospital in April 1979 with a biopsy-confirmed diagnosis of osteosarcoma of the left distal femur. She received three courses of intra-arterial cis-platinum (90 mg/m²) in about 2 months. In June 1979 the patient underwent an en bloc resection of the distal femur with the insertion of a customized prosthetic replacement.

Initial Biopsy

An open biopsy of the femur disclosed a few fragments of a malignant cartilaginous tumor, which had spindle cells at the periphery of the chondroid lobules and some depositions of osteoid. This lesion was initially interpreted as a chondroblastic osteosarcoma.

Resection of the Left Femur after Therapy

The resected specimen was a 10.8-cm-long segment of distal femur. The outer surface was covered by fibroconnective tissue and muscle that did not contain tumor. Examination of the longitudinal section disclosed a metaphyseal-epiphyseal lesion involving both condyles (Figure 15). The periosteum on the medial condyle was elevated. The cut surface had irregular areas of sclerosis alternating with focal hemorrhage. A 1.5-cm-wide margin of normal bone was present. Although there was some evidence of cartilage in the sections, the predominant component was osteoid with bone, indicating an osteoblastic osteosarcoma. The tumor was extremely anaplastic, with large bizarre cells and abnormal mitosis. The major portion was viable and only 30–40% of the lesion showed necrosis. There was only focal fibroblastic proliferation (Figure 16). The tumor effect was considered to be doubtful; a response category of IB was assigned.

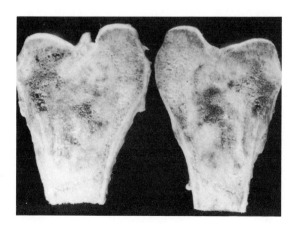

Figure 15. Case 5. Distal end of femur. Irregular metaphyseal lesion shows ill-defined, blastic tumor that is permeating cortex.

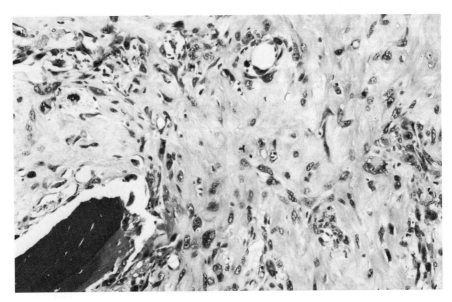

Figure 16. Case 5. Viable osteosarcoma with numerous bizarre cells.

RESULTS

Table 2 summarizes the salient features of these five cases. The osteoblastic osteosarcomas from the proximal tibia and distal femur (Cases 1 and 2) were essentially similar in morphology and demonstrated rather sclerotic patterns, with lace-like depositions of osteoid and stroma composed of small to medium-sized, round to oval sarcomatous cells. The responses to chemotherapy were also similar, with coagulative necrosis of the tumor cells and reparative fibrovascular proliferation.

The two chondroblastic osteosarcomas (Cases 3 and 4) also showed coagulative necrosis, but the stromal responses were minimal and limited to the periphery of the lesions. Although the extent of necrosis exceeded 60%, viable cells were present in both cases.

In Case 5, a pleomorphic osteosarcoma, predominantly osteoblastic, showed approximately 40% necrosis, but the major portion of the tumor was viable. There were, however, some areas of fibrovascular regeneration.

Ultraviolet light was used to evaluate the tumor margins and to demonstrate skip metastases. Cases 2 and 3 showed a partial rim of fibro-osseous tissue surrounding the lesion that was evidently reactive, suggesting some limiting of tumor growth. Skip metastases were not found.

COMMENT

Osteosarcoma is the most common primary malignant tumor of bone, occurring most often in children and young adults. It is defined as a malignant tumor

Table 2. Assessment of Post-Chemotherapy Changes in Primary Osteosarcoma Lesions

Patient Age/Sex	Cell Type	Site of Primary Tumor	Preoperative Chemotherapy		Category of Histopathologic Response
			High-Dose Methotrexate	Intra-arterial Cis-platinum	
15/M	Osteoblastic	Proximal tibia	Yes	No	IIIB
17/M	Osteoblastic	Distal femur	No	Yes	IIIB
16/F	Chondroblastic	Proximal tibia	Yes	Yes	IIIA
19/M	Chondroblastic	Distal radius	No	Yes	IIIB
21/F	Osteoblastic	Distal femur	No	Yes	IB

composed of a sarcomatous stroma that produces osteoid or bone. However, the diagnosis actually comprises several distinct clinicopathological osteosarcoma variants, including medullary (conventional) osteosarcoma, telangiectatic osteosarcoma, periosteal osteosarcoma, parosteal osteosarcoma, well-differentiated intraosseous osteosarcoma, osteosarcoma of jawbone, Paget's osteosarcoma, and postirradiation osteosarcoma. These variants (Dahlin and Unni 1977) differ from the medullary or conventional osteosarcoma in their biologic behavior and must be recognized in order to assess the effectiveness of chemotherapeutic modalities. Thus, telangiectatic osteosarcoma, a predominately lytic tumor, carries a poorer prognosis than the conventional osteosarcoma and has a high tendency to recur in the stump (Matsuno et al. 1976).The intra-osseous, well-differentiated osteosarcoma, like its surface counterpart, the parosteal osteosarcoma, is relatively benign and is characterized by an innocuous-appearing, fibro-osseous morphology, multiple recurrences, and late metastases (Unni et al. 1977). Periosteal osteosarcoma (Unni et al. 1976, Spjut et al. 1977) (juxtacortical chondrosarcoma by the World Health Organization classification, Schajowicz 1977), also a surface lesion, differs from parosteal osteosarcoma by having a poorly differentiated histology with large amounts of cartilaginous tissue; its prognosis appears to be worse than that of parosteal osteosarcoma, but better than that of conventional osteosarcoma. Osteosarcomas occurring in the jawbones, those associated with Paget's disease, and those developing in irradiated bones are well-known variants.

The most common osteosarcoma is the central medullary, or conventional, osteosarcoma (Dahlin et al. 1977). This lesion arises in the metaphysis of long bones, especially the distal femur and proximal tibia and humerus, and rarely in the diaphysis or in a flat bone. It can be subdivided into three histologic categories: osteoblastic, chondroblastic, and fibroblastic. The first type demonstrates abundant osteoid, which may be calcified or noncalcified, and radiologically the lesion appears sclerotic. Chondroblastic osteosarcoma contains an anaplastic cartilaginous proliferation with depositions of osteoid. Absence of cartilage or significant amounts of osteoid characterizes a fibroblastic osteosarcoma. In the past, these subtypes were only of academic interest, since differences in survival were statistically insignificant. Dahlin and Coventry in 1967 reported a 5-year survival rate of 17% for patients with osteoblastic lesions, 22% for chondroblastic, and 25% for fibroblastic. With the advent of chemotherapy, subtyping may be of future value.

Needle biopsies of bone can be adequately processed within 24 hours, but this requires close collaboration between the radiologist performing the biopsy and the pathologist. We have described our successful experience at M. D. Anderson Hospital (de Santos et al. 1979). Occasionally it is not possible to make a definitive diagnosis on the basis of the needle biopsy; in such cases an open biopsy is required. This was true in Case 1, involving an osteoblastic osteosarcoma. The needle biopsy specimen was representative of the lesion since it contained irregular osteoid and ossified material distinct from the normal bony spicules, but the tissue was inadequate because no malignant cells were seen. In such cases, we are conservative in our interpretation. The tissue obtained by needle biopsy may indicate the subtype of osteosarcoma, but the interpretation should be correlated with that provided by the radiologic examination. Nevertheless, one should be cautious in reaching a conclusion, since scanty material may not be representative of the overall lesion. In an open biopsy, subtyping is more feasible.

The main purpose of the histopathologic examination of a previously treated osteosarcoma is to assess the chemotherapeutic effect. High-dose methotrexate and cis-platinum have shown definite tumor effects against osteosarcoma, but the response varies and some patients show no response. Our findings of complete tumor destruction in one patient with osteoblastic osteosarcoma treated with high-dose methotrexate and another treated with intra-arterial cis-platinum and definite tumor effect in two patients with chondroblastic osteosarcomas treated with intra-arterial cis-platinum raise the possibility of a specific tumor effect. In one chondroblastic osteosarcoma patient, the initial treatment with high-dose methotrexate failed but the tumor responded to intra-arterial cis-platinum.

Tumor effect on chondroblastic osteosarcomas is difficult to evaluate since the cartilaginous component in tumors of untreated patients often shows patchy necrosis. In our two patients, the major area of necrosis was in the epicenter of the lesions, while the periphery appeared to contain viable cells.

The pathological findings indicating the response of an osteosarcoma to preoperative chemotherapy should serve as a guide in the selection of drugs and dosages for adjuvant chemotherapy. A tumor showing a category II response probably needs additional chemotherapeutic agents for optimal results, while altogether different drugs would be indicated for those with a category I response. Those with a category III response should receive the same treatment as was previously administered.

CONCLUSIONS

The guidelines presented for assessing response to preoperative chemotherapy appear practical, but further experience is required to establish their reliability. For example, tumor response may be influenced by many different cell type elements. Therefore, cooperation between the pathologist and clinical oncologist is of major importance, and studies should be continued.

REFERENCES

Dahlin, D. C., and M. B. Coventry. 1967. Osteogenic sarcoma: A study of 600 cases. J. Bone Joint Surg. 49A:101–110.

Dahlin, D. C., and K. K. Unni. 1977. Osteosarcoma of bone and its important recognizable varieties. Am. J. Surg. Pathol. 1:61–72.

de Santos, L. A., J. A. Murray, and A. G. Ayala. 1979. The value of percutaneous needle biopsy in the management of primary bone tumors. Cancer 43:735–744.

Jaffe, M., M. Watts, K. E. Fellows, and G. Vawle. 1978. Local en bloc resection for limb preservation. Cancer Treat. Rep. 62:217–223.

Matsuno, T., K. K. Unni, R. A. McLeod, and D. C. Dahlin. 1976. Telangiectatic osteosarcoma. Cancer 38:2538–2547.

Schajowicz, F. 1977. Juxtacortical chondrosarcoma. J. Bone Joint Surg. 59B:473–480.

Spjut, H. J., A. G. Ayala, L. de Santos, and J. A. Murray. 1977. Periosteal osteosarcoma, *in* Management of Primary Bone and Soft Tissue Tumors (The University of Texas System Cancer Center 21st Annual Clinical Conference, 1976). Year Book Medical Publishers, Inc., Chicago, pp. 79–95.

Unni, K. K., D. C. Dahlin, and J. W. Beabout. 1976. Periosteal osteogenic osteosarcoma. Cancer 37:2466–2475.

Unni, K. K., D. C. Dahlin, R. A. McLeod, and D. J. Pritchard. 1977. Intra-osseous well-differentiated osteosarcoma. Cancer 40:1337–1347.

Status of the Curability of Childhood Cancers,
edited by J. van Eys and M. P. Sullivan.
Raven Press, New York © 1980.

The Persistent Challenge of Neuroblastoma

P. A. Voûte, A. Vos, J. F. M. Delemarre, J. de Kraker, J. M. V.
Burgers, and O. A. van Dobbenburgh

*Werkgroep Kindertumoren Emma Kinderziekenhuis and Antoni van Leeuwenhoek
Ziekenhuis, The Netherlands Cancer Institute, Amsterdam, The Netherlands*

To appreciate the challenge in neuroblastoma, one must understand the embryology and anatomy of the sympathetic nervous system, as well as the clinical signs of neuroblastoma and catecholamine metabolism. Only against this background can therapeutic problems be properly understood and eventually solved.

EMBRYOLOGY

After a fertilized ovum has gone through the morula and blastula stages, the first signs of the development of the central nervous system appear in the gastrula stage. The neural plate, which consists of ectodermal cells, forms in what is referred to as the neurula stage. The margins of the neural plate are elevated to create the neural folds, which are separated by a midline neural groove. With further growth, progressive fusion between the folds takes place. In this way the neural tube is formed, and the connection with the ectoderm disappears. During separation of the neural tube, a chain of cells appears on either side in the angle between the tube and the remaining ectoderm. These two longitudinal columns form the neural crest. From the distal part of the neural crest cells begin to migrate. The dorsally migrating cells are partially responsible for formation of the melanoblasts. The ventrally migrating cells develop into the spinal ganglia, the ganglia of the sympathetic side chain, the prevertebral ganglia, the paraganglia, and the chromaffin bodies. The cells migrating from the neural crest, which form the sympathetic nervous system, are called sympathetic neuroblasts, primitive sympathetic cells, or sympathogonia. The sympathogonia migrate further to the adrenal medulla and the paraganglion of Zuckerkandl at the bifurcation of the aorta. A great number of paraganglia are formed in the retroperitoneal space along the aorta.

The sympathogonia are still pluripotential cells at this stage and differentiate into chromaffin cells, neurofibrous cells, and sympathetic ganglion cells. The differentiation starts in the fetus of 10 weeks (Coupland 1965) and continues long after birth in the adrenal medulla, even to adulthood.

Apart from the sympathetic side chain, which forms at an early stage of development, sympathetic plexuses such as the plexus celiacus, mesentericus, and renalis are formed. In adults these consist of ganglion cells and sporadic chromaffin cells. In the fetus and newborn a large variety in cell morphology is found. Chromaffin cells are formed in great numbers in the side chain and the plexuses. The paraganglia are also important at this age, both anatomically and endocrinologically. About the age of 2 to 3 years the paraganglia regress. The adrenal medulla is then the most important organ left, and could be considered the suprarenal paraganglion. In a fetus or newborn child one finds the typical rosette formation in the sympathogonia in the side chain, plexuses, paraganglia, and adrenal medulla. In the development of a sympathogonium into a ganglion cell, pheochromocyte, or neurofibrous tissue, there is great variation. This variation can create diagnostic difficulties when a tumor arises in the sympathetic system. A clear-cut ganglioneuroma or pheochromocytoma is not difficult to diagnose, but one may also find all the developmental stages in between. This has caused great variation in the nomenclature of tumors of the sympathetic system in children: neurocytoma, embryonal sympathoma, sympathetic blastoma, sympathicogonioma, gangliosympathicoblastoma, ganglioneuroblastoma, pheochromoblastoma, pheochromoneuroblastoma, and others. It is not clear why the name neuroblastoma is most often used, since sympathicoblastoma is a much better name.

Before going further, it is necessary to define some tumor types: A *pheochromocytoma* is a tumor consisting of pheochromocytes, i.e., cells that produce, store, and secrete pressor amines. A *ganglioneuroma* consists of ganglion cells and nerve fibers without any detectable metabolic products. A *neuroblastoma* is a tumor consisting of sympathogonia that multiply, much as they do during the embryonic period. They attain partial differentiation into rosettes and ganglion cells, as well as into immature chromaffin cells, and may produce normal and abnormal products. Ganglioneuromas and pheochromocytomas can develop as the result of maturation of a neuroblastoma. The normal sympathogonia will develop into ganglion cells or chromaffin cells. The same is true for a neuroblastoma.

Beckwith and Perrin (1963) performed microscopic examinations on the adrenals of stillborn infants and found 40% more neuroblastomas than expected on the basis of known clinical frequency. According to their observation, many more children than are diagnosed at some time have subclinical neuroblastomas. Most of these tumors are apparently controlled by the normal regulation mechanisms of the body and regress spontaneously. Children with clinically manifest tumors may be "just the tip of the iceberg."

PATHOLOGY

The undifferentiated tumor consists of small, spheroidal cells devoid of arrangement or differentiation, and often no more specific diagnosis is possible than undifferentiated round cell malignant tumor, compatible with neuroblastoma. The cells resemble the migratory neural crest cells of early embryos. The first sign of differentiation is the formation of rosettelike structures consisting of cells surrounding a central tangle of fine fibers exactly like the structure of developing sympathetic ganglia in the embryo. In the maturing neuroblastoma, transition into ganglioneuroma can be found. The tumor may have abundant nerve fiber material forming large areas bounded by small neuroblasts. Large cells with prominent nucleoli, similar to ganglion cells, are usually present as well. The fully differentiated ganglioneuroma consists entirely of mature ganglion cells. Typical pheochromocytes can also be found in neuroblastomas. A correct classification is impossible. As long as immature cells are found, one usually speaks of a neuroblastoma. The term "ganglioneuroblastoma" gives a false feeling of security because this is a highly malignant tumor.

FAMILIAL OCCURRENCE OF NEUROBLASTOMA AND OTHER DISTURBANCES OF NEURAL CREST ORIGIN

Familial neuroblastoma has been reported only sporadically (Zucker 1974, Chatten and Voorhess 1967) because very few patients reach reproductive age. Neuroblastoma and pheochromocytoma in one family have been reported by Donath et al. (1965). Pheochromocytomas and ganglioneuromas with neurofibromatosis of Recklinghausen are found too often for the association to be accidental, but neuroblastomas have also been found with von Recklinghausen's disease (Witzleben and Landy 1974). Hirschsprung's disease with aganglionic colon appears to be basically a disturbance of a neural crest development and has been reported with neuroblastoma in one patient. Heterochromia is found with cervical neuroblastomas; the pigment of the iris is of neural crest origin.

AGE INCIDENCE

Neuroblastomas are seldom seen in persons over the age of 14. Seventy-five percent of the patients are younger than 4 years and 50% younger than 2 years. Neuroblastomas can be found immediately after birth, with metastases in the placenta (Strauss and Driscoll 1964). As they are truly embryonic tumors arising in early life, their occasional appearance in adolescents and adults is probably due to an exacerbation of growth in a tumor that had been clinically dormant since childhood. As might be expected, ganglioneuromas and pheochromocytomas manifest themselves clinically later in life than neuroblastomas.

LOCALIZATION

Neuroblastomas can be found wherever sympathetic nervous system tissue is present (Figure 1), such as in the sympathetic side chain, visceral ganglia, paraganglia, adrenal medulla, bladder, and inner genitalia. Because of the often rapid growth of the tumor, it is difficult to pinpoint the exact place of origin.

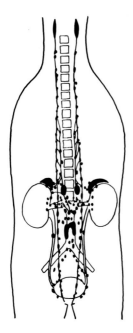

Figure 1. Schematic illustration showing where sympathetic nervous tissue is present.

Seventy percent of the tumors arise in the abdomen, half of these in the adrenals, the other half in the paraganglia, visceral ganglia, and abdominal side chain. The remaining 30% originate in the cervical, thoracic, and pelvic side chains (Figure 2).

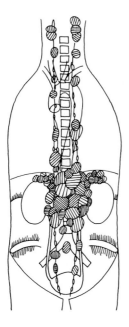

Figure 2. Schematic illustration showing where neuroblastomas may be found.

CLINICAL SYMPTOMS

By and large, the site of the tumor can explain the clinical symptoms of both the primary tumor and the metastases. These symptoms can be outlined as follows:

I. Clinical symptoms of the primary tumor
   A. Anatomic
      Head and neck: palpable mass and Horner's syndrome.
      Chest: upper thoracic localization can give rise to dyspnea and dysphagia, lower thoracic localization seldom produces symptoms.
      Abdomen: palpable mass, with or without tenderness.
      Pelvis: defecation and urination problems.
      For all these sites the possibility exists that the tumor arising from the side chain has extended into the spinal canal. In such cases, depending on the area of extension, various neurological symptoms of cord depression may be found. Such tumors are called "hourglass" or "dumbbell" tumors.
   B. Metabolic
      Hypertension, flushing, periods of excessive sweating, and irritability, due to excessive production and excretion of catecholamines. Also, watery diarrhea with atonic bowel and profound loss of potassium. The exact mechanism causing this diarrhea is not known. Some attribute it to dopamine excretion, but prostaglandins are also thought to be a cause. Diarrhea occurs with neuroblastomas, especially those that show signs of maturation to ganglioneuromas.
   C. Neurologic
      Opsomyoclonus and cerebellar ataxia. Several hypotheses have been proposed to explain the etiology of these signs. Catecholamines cannot be the cause because only 2% of patients with neuroblastomas have these symptoms. One hypothesis is that the tumor produces another, unidentified tumoral mediator that affects the cerebellum. Another explanation is that the host immune response to the tumor cross-reacts with brain cells. This better fits with the observation that children with opsomyoclonus have a favorable prognosis due to their more mature tumor (Roberts and Freeman 1975).

II. Clinical symptoms of metastases
   A. Metastatic signs in patients under 1 year were first described by Pepper (1901). Diffuse liver metastases can give rise to an enormously enlarged liver with prolonged jaundice and circulatory problems. Subcutaneous metastases can also be found. This subcutaneous and liver metastatic spread is due to the fetal circulation, as described by Wieberdink (1957).
   B. Skeletal and bone marrow sites of metastases, as described first by Hutchison (1907), are predominant in patients over 1 year. This metastatic spread can cause bone pain and signs resembling those of rheumatic fever or leukemia. One type of skeletal metastasis,

the orbital metastasis, causes protrusion of the eye. Skeletal metastases can be difficult to differentiate from Ewing's sarcoma. Further metastatic spread can occur in the lymph nodes. Some organs are never the site of metastases, including the brain, spinal cord, heart, and lungs. Pulmonary metastases, however, are possible in far-advanced cases by extensive lymphatic spread or direct ingrowth through the diaphragm (Zucker 1974).

CATECHOLAMINE METABOLISM

One of the most striking characteristics of neuroblastomas is the excessive production of catecholamines, which can be found as tumor markers in the urine. It is not strange that catecholamines are produced, because in normal sympathetic tissue dopamine and the epinephrines play an important role in the function of the sympathetic nervous system. The enzyme phenylalanine hydroxylase produces tyrosine out of phenylalanine. Both tyrosine and phenylalanine are extracellular amino acids. In the sympathetic cells intracellular 3,4-dihydroxyphenylalanine (dopa) is produced by the enzyme tyrosine hydroxylase. The total amount of tyrosine in the body is high in comparison to that of dopa. Decarboxylation by dopa decarboxylase produces the first catecholamine, dihydroxyphenylamine (dopamine). Norepinephrine is formed by dopamine-β-oxidase, after which phenylethanolamine-N-methyl transferase forms epinephrine. In the normal sympathetic tissue these intracellular substances are stored and used, epinephrine in the adrenal glands, norepinephrine and dopamine in the sympathic nerve ends and ganglion cells.

Two enzymes are responsible for the metabolism of the catecholamines, catechol-O-methyl transferase (COMT) and monoamine oxidase (MAO). The former exists in high concentrations in liver and kidney, and the latter is present in the mitochondria of the sympathetic cells. Most excreted catecholamines are O-methylated by COMT in the body. This is the most important metabolic pathway. The structure of the catecholamines is as follows:

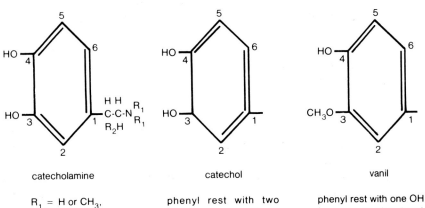

catecholamine

R_1 = H or CH_3,
R_2 = H or OH

catechol

phenyl rest with two OH groups on positions 3 and 4

vanil

phenyl rest with one OH group on position 4 and OCH_3 group on position 3

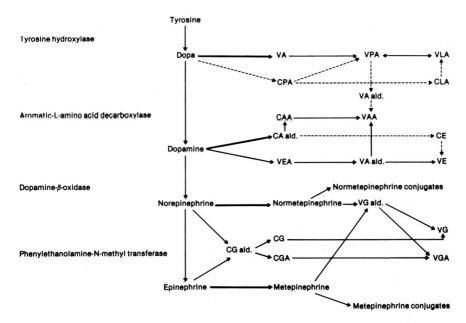

Figure 3. Metabolic pathways of the intracellular amino acid dopa and the catecholamines dopamine, norepinephrine, and epinephrine.

As shown in Figure 3, the metabolic process is quite complicated. Excretion of VGA (VMA)[1] and VAA (HVA) can be measured for diagnostic purposes, but this is of limited value because the quantity excreted depends largely on which enzyme is used.

In neuroblastoma patients many of the above-mentioned metabolites can be found in abnormal quantities. There are two reasons for this:

1. Higher production of dopa and dopamine, with a relative insufficiency of the next enzyme in the synthesis of the epinephrines.

2. Higher production of dopa and dopamine because of more producing cells. In a certain number of cells a deficient enzyme system exists because of the chaotic reproduction of enzyme-producing cells. The produced dopa and dopamine must be metabolized along alternative pathways and their metabolites appear in the urine.

In chaotic sympathetic tumor cells the enzyme concentrations are not syn-

---

[1] Abbreviations: VA = vanil alanine, VPA = vanil pyruvic acid, VLA = vanil lactic acid, CPA = catechol pyruvic acid, CLA = catechol lactic acid, CA ald. = catechol acetic aldehyde, CAA = catechol acetic acid, CE = catechol ethanol (DHPE), VAA = vanil acetic acid (homovanillic acid, HVA), VE = vanil ethanol, VA ald. = vanil acetic aldehyde, VEA = vanil ethylamine, VG = vanil glycol (HMPG), VG ald. = vanil glycol aldehyde, VGA = vanil glycolic acid (vanilmandelic acid, VMA), CG ald. = catechol glycol aldehyde, CG = catechol glycol, CGA = catechol glycolic acid.

chronized. Synthesis becomes deregulated and metabolism can follow secondary pathways (Figure 4).

Much of the dopa is decarboxylated to dopamine, which is then hydroxylated to norepinephrine. This last step occurs only when enough dopamine-β-oxidase is present. When this is not the case, dopamine is a good substrate for MAO in the cells, forming CAA and thereafter VAA and eventually VE. In still less differentiated cells, dopamine is not formed because of the deficient aromatic-L-amino acid decarboxylase. Dopa accumulates and forms a good substrate for COMT. Vanil alanine is formed, which is not a suitable substrate for decarboxylating, but can be transaminated to VPA and reduced to VLA. In a still more anaplastic neuroblastoma, tyrosine hydroxylase may not be present and dopa cannot be formed in such a case. No abnormal excretion products are formed.

Finally, cystathionine and homoserine are found in the urine of patients with neuroblastomas. Both occur in nervous tissue as well as in the liver. It is very possible that these abnormal amino acids are caused by liver function disturbances due to metastases.

A previous study by Voûte (1968) demonstrated the value of determining the presence and level of the metabolites. In that study, the clinical status, pathologic diagnosis, and excretory patterns of 30 patients were extensively studied. Twelve had symptoms of neuroblastoma before the age of 1 year, three of whom died. Of the remaining 18, 13 died. In 28 of the patients the pathologic diagnosis of neuroblastoma or ganglioneuroblastoma was made. These patients had similar clinical pictures. Two had distinct ganglioneuromas with neuroblastoma excretory patterns. The excretory pattern of the urine of these patients was very different. The amounts of VGA, VG, VAA, and VLA were determined in milligrams per gram of creatinine, and the presence of CAA and VE was

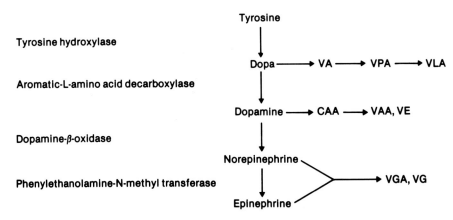

Figure 4. Degradation of dopa and the catecholamines when normal synthesis is blocked by tumorous deregulation.

Table 1. *Ratio of VGA + VG to VAA in Healthy Persons**

Age (yrs)/ No. Persons	VGA + VG (μmol/g creatinine), Mean Value	VAA (μmol/g creatinine), Mean Value	$\dfrac{VGA + VG}{VAA}$
0–1/6	81	82	1:0.99
1–2/5	37	37	1:1
2–6/6	37	36	1:1.03
6–13/5	24	24	1:1
>13/10	19	19	1:1

* Mol. weight VGA = 198, VG = 184, VAA = 182.

noted. Four patients had normal or slightly increased levels of excretion of VGA and VG, while VAA was markedly elevated. One patient excreted markedly more VG and VGA (555 mg/g creatinine and 833 mg/g creatinine, respectively). Three patients excreted a small amount of VE. Ten patients excreted CAA and VLA at the beginning of their disease, and five more excreted CAA and VLA later in the course of their disease. One patient did not excrete any metabolites. Excretion can also be expressed as micromoles per gram of creatinine. In this manner, one can get an idea of the amount of epinephrines and dopamine produced. The sum of VGA and VG levels gives information about the production of epinephrines, as does the VAA level about dopamine. Calculation of the ratio of VGA and VG to VAA makes it easy to compare the two production lines as long as no VLA or CAA is found in the urine. In 32 normal persons of different ages, this ratio was calculated (Table 1). In 26 cases the ratio was between 1:0.8 and 1:1.2, in 32 between 1:0.6 and 1:1.3.

Marked differences were found among the patients. Observation of the excretion patterns of patients who were cured shows that their ratios of VGA + VG to VAA were higher than those in normal persons (Table 2). Patients older than 1½ years showed lower ratios. When CAA or VLA is excreted, its value should be added to VAA, but CAA was not quantitatively determined in these patients (Table 3). In cured patients the ratio returned to near normal. Patients who excreted VE, CAA, or VLA at any stage of their disease had a very bad prognosis. The only exception occurred when the primary tumor could be extirpated completely and no metastases were present, as was the case in the last three patients in Table 2.

The following diagnoses were made: neuroblastoma in 18 patients, ganglioneuroblastoma in eight, and ganglioneuroma in two. There was no difference between the clinical behavior of the neuroblastomas and that of the ganglioneuroblastomas. Thus, there seems to be no reason why the differentiation between neuroblastoma and ganglioneuroblastoma should be maintained.

On the basis of this study, the following conclusion concerning prognosis

Table 2. *Ratio of VGA + VG to VAA in Cured Patients*

VGA + VG (μmol/g creatinine)	VAA (μmol/g creatinine)	VLA	CAA	VGA +VG / VAA
7,300	2,200	–	–	1:0.30
4,300	1,500	–	–	1:0.35
460	290	–	–	1:0.65
250	260	–	–	1:1.05
3,000	1,900	–	–	1:0.65
270	160	–	–	1:0.60
1,300	420	–	–	1:0.30
960	760	–	–	1:0.80
390	410	–	–	1:1.05
89	120	–	–	1:1.35
330	510	++	+	1:1.55
54	170	–	–	1:3.15
360	1,100	–	++	1:3.05

Table 3. *Ratio of VGA + VG to VAA in Patients Who Died*

VGA + VG (μmol/g creatinine)	VAA (μmol/g creatinine)	VLA	CAA	VGA + VG / VAA
210	360	–	–	1:1.70
540	1,500	–	–	1:2.75
220	520	–	–	1:2.35
110	280	–	–	1:2.55
450	970	–	–	1:2.15
100	310	–	–	1:3.10
2,200	1,900	+	+++	1:0.85
36	38	–	–	1:1.05
980	1,000	–	+	1:1.00
10,900	7,300	++	++	1:0.65
110	1,700	++	++	1:15.45
320	520	+	–	1:1.60
180	840	+	–	1:4.65
2,400	1,600	–	++	1:0.65
2,400	1,800	–	++	1:0.75

was drawn: Urinanalysis provides the most important information regarding the prognosis of the patient with neuroblastoma. Absence of excretion or excretion of CAA, VLA, and VE is prognostically unfavorable. The possibility of cure exists with total resection. The ratio of VGA + VG to VAA has prognostic value as long as CAA, VE, and VLA are not excreted. An elevated ratio indicates a favorable prognosis, but the prognosis is also influenced by the age of the patient. In general, the younger the child, the better the prognosis.

TREATMENT PROGRAM

Following the clinical staging system of Evans et al. (1971) (Table 4), we used the following treatment regimen, which takes into account clinical findings and metabolite excretion:

Stage I
- A. Complete removal of tumor, no further therapy if excretion of metabolites returns to normal. If not, search for second primary tumor or metastases and restaging.
- B. Incomplete removal of tumor.
    1. Favorable excretion, radiotherapy.
    2. Unfavorable excretion, radiotherapy and chemotherapy.

Stage II
- A. Extirpation of tumor and affected lymph nodes when feasible.
    1. Normal excretion of metabolites, no further therapy.
    2. Increased excretion of metabolites, chemotherapy.
- B. Extirpation of tumor and lymph nodes impossible or incomplete, radiotherapy followed by chemotherapy, eventually reexploration.

Stage III
Treatment nearly always same as that for stage IIB, chemotherapy after radiotherapy.

Stage IV
Chemotherapy only feasible treatment, extirpation of tumor if possible and radiotherapy.

Stage IV-S
Consists of infants with metastases primarily in liver and subcutaneous tissue. Extirpation of primary tumor at beginning of treatment or if necessary. Low-dose irradiation of liver and low-dose short-term chemotherapy stimulate regression and may induce seemingly spontaneous cure.

Table 4. *Clinical Staging System of Evans et al. (1971)*

Stage	Description
I	Tumor confined to organ or structure of origin.
II	Tumor extending in continuity beyond organ or structure of origin, but not crossing midline. Homolateral lymph nodes may be involved.
III	Tumor extending in continuity beyond the midline. Bilateral regional lymph nodes may be involved.
IV	Dissemination with metastases in skeleton, organs, soft tissue, distant lymph nodes, etc.
IV-S	Same as stage I or II, but also dissemination in liver, spleen, or bone marrow, without radiographic evidence of bone metastases.

Surgical Treatment

Total removal of a tumor still gives the best chance of cure. Whether efforts should be made to extirpate large parts of a tumor when there is no hope of total removal is very much open for discussion. Surgery should also be considered after improvement following radiotherapy and chemotherapy.

Radiotherapy

A major radiotherapeutic attack is a good approach for tumors that cannot be treated surgically. A dose of 3,000 rad in 3–4 weeks is usually prescribed. In certain circumstances a higher dose can be given to a reduced volume. In patients with IV-S disease, radiotherapy should be used to induce regression of the tumor. In our experience, 500–600 rad in two sessions to the entire liver brings about the desired result.

Chemotherapy

An evaluation of chemotherapeutic treatment in children with neuroblastoma poses a number of difficult problems because, when treating patients with a favorable prognosis, one must take into consideration the likelihood of spontaneous regression and differentiation. Chemotherapy is combined with surgery and radiotherapy. We use chemotherapy differently in patients with favorable excretion patterns and those with unfavorable. In the former, usually IV-S patients, we use:

Prednisolone, 20 mg/m²/day,
Cyclophosphamide, 20 mg/m²/day.

This therapy is continued for 2 months after normal excretion of metabolites is achieved. In the unfavorable excretion group, usually older patients, combination chemotherapy (OPEL) is used:

Oncovin (vincristine), 2 mg/m²/1×14 days i.v.,
Prednisolone, 20 mg/m²/day p.o. for 2 months and then halved,
Endoxan (cyclophosphamide), 50 mg/m²/day p.o. for 14 days, 14 days' rest, and repeat,
Ledertrexate (methotrexate), 2.5 mg/m²/day p.o. for 14 days, 14 days' rest, and repeat.

If a recurrence or no response is found, we use:

Prednisolone, 20 mg/m²/day p.o. for 2 months, then halved,
Adriamycin, 60 mg/m²/1×3 wk i.v.,
Cytosine arabinoside, 100 mg/m²/day s.c.,
Vincristine, 1 mg/m²/1×3 wk i.v.

Many other chemotherapy programs are currently being used. Cyclophosphamide, dimethyl triazeno imidazole carboxamide, and vincristine alone or combined with Adriamycin (Finkelstein et al. 1979) and vincristine, Adriamycin, nitrogen mustard, and dimethyl triazeno imidazole carboxamide (Jaffe 1976).

TREATMENT RESULTS

A total of 105 patients were treated according to the treatment outlined and 29 (28%) have been cured (Table 5). Nine patients had stage IV-S disease, five of whom have been cured. Three had received low-dose irradiation of the liver because of liver enlargement; none had more than 2 months of chemotherapy. Four patients died, two during an operative procedure undertaken to alleviate severe compression of the lung and trachea. Two patients died after complete remissions of 6 and 8 months; when disease recurred, after the age of 12 months, they behaved the same as the unfavorable group. All nine patients had favorable excretion patterns.

The 24 other cured patients were divided as follows:

Fifteen patients had stage I disease. One had three primary tumors (left adrenal, abdominal, and thoracic side chain). Two needed radiotherapy because of incomplete tumor removal. Twelve were treated only surgically. Nine had unfavorable excretion patterns. Three had "hourglass" tumors, which had to be extirpated in two sessions.

All seven stage II patients needed radiotherapy, after which excretion patterns returned to normal. Two received chemotherapy until their excretion patterns were normal. All had originally had unfavorable excretion patterns.

Both stage IV patients were treated with chemotherapy, radiotherapy, and surgery. They are doing well 4 and 6 years after treatment. One still has an elevated excretion level without anatomically detectable tumor or metastases.

The treatment results for the 76 patients who died can be summarized as follows:

One of two stage I patients died of surgical complications; the other died 9 months later of sudden generalized disease. The second patient had a pathologic diagnosis of ganglioneuroma. Both had unfavorable excretion patterns.

Table 5. *Results in 105 Patients Treated for Neuroblastoma*

Stage	No. Patients	No. Cured	No. Who Died
I	17	15	2
II	9	7	2
III	6		6
IV	64	2	62
IV-S	9	5	4
Total	105	29	76

Both stage II patients were treated with surgery, radiotherapy, and chemotherapy. Both had unfavorable excretion patterns and died of generalized disease.

All six stage III patients were treated as stage II patients and died of generalized disease.

All 62 stage IV patients had unfavorable excretion patterns (six did not excrete tumor metabolites early in their disease), and 51 had bone marrow metastases. All were first treated with chemotherapy, and their bone marrow was cleared of metastases very easily. Radiotherapy was given to the primary tumor, after which surgery was performed on the primary tumor. In only nine patients could a complete excision of the primary tumor be performed. Fifty-eight patients had remissions of 2 to 16 months, with a median duration of 7½ months.

The primary tumor and osseous and lymph node metastases could be influenced by chemotherapy, but not as much as bone marrow metastases. Bone marrow recurrences were found during treatment, but only after obvious recurrence of the primary tumor or lymph node and bone metastases.

In this series of patients, no metastases were found in the central nervous system or lung. Metastases in the dura never penetrated into the brain.

THE CHALLENGE

The challenge in treating children with neuroblastoma is great. This is the most common solid tumor of childhood, but it has not shown the dramatic improvement in treatment results found in other childhood malignant diseases. The only progress that has been made is that we can identify the 25% of patients who do not need any therapy beyond surgery. This lack of progress is quite striking in comparison with results with nephroblastoma, for which treatment has improved so rapidly that now we have to find the 30% of patients with nephroblastoma who can be cured with surgery alone out of the 90% of patients who are cured.

Important questions remain, however.

Why do some tumors spontaneously regress or mature into benign ganglioneuromas?

Why do spontaneous remissions mostly occur in younger patients and why do younger patients do better?

Why are other neural crest disorders often found in combination with neuroblastomas?

Why is an "hourglass" neuroblastoma more mature or completely mature within the spinal canal and immature outside?

Why does a neuroblastoma metastasize to the dura, but then limit its growth to the outside and leave the dura adjacent to the brain intact?

Why do strange neurologic signs, such as opsomyoclonus and cerebellar atrophy, occur in older children with more differentiated tumors?

Why are metastases never found in the central nervous system, heart, and lung?

Why is it easy to induce remissions in bone marrow metastases and not in the primary tumor and lymph node and bone metastases?

Answers to these questions cannot be provided as yet, but we can construct hypotheses that may stimulate further investigations. If neuroblastomas are more common in stillborns, as Beckwith and Perrin (1963) report, children must have a strong tendency to differentiate unripe sympathetic tissue. Children under 1 year of age with clinically manifest tumors apparently lack this tendency and for some reason the sympathogonia migrate in the wrong direction. It is possible that an intrauterine factor, such as a viral infection, gives rise to this behavior. The virus that most affects nervous tissue, especially the side chain, is the herpes virus. It is known to be teratogenic, oncogenic, and neurotropic. Investigations in this field are being performed; the cytomegalovirus, for instance, has received attention (Wertheim and Voûte 1976). But as in all oncoviral research, one must demonstrate that viral DNA or parts of it can be found in the DNA of the tumor cells. The finding of chromosomal aberrations in tumor cells but not host cells can help demonstrate this.

It seems that neuroblastomas usually arise from aberrant localization of sympathetic tissue. Perhaps this tissue is more susceptible to oncogenic factors because it lacks normal environmental control. Teratogenic factors could also account for the other aberrations from the neural crest.

Neuroblastomas in younger patients seem to possess a more or less differentiated enzyme system, according to the patients' excretory patterns. The younger patients can be treated so as to stimulate the tumor's potential for spontaneous regression. It seems possible that brief courses of low-dose irradiation or treatment with corticosteroids alone or combined with cyclophosphamide can regulate the organism. The clinical findings that primary neuroblastomas or their metastases are not likely to occur adjacent to normal nervous tissue and that no metastases occur in the central nervous system suggest that a substance must be present that stimulates differentiation. Perhaps this substance is the nerve growth factor (Levi-Montalcini and Calissano 1979). As has been shown, however, it is the immediate contact of embryonic nervous tissue with nerve growth factor for a long period that causes differentiation. Nerve growth factor does not seem to be a useful treatment tool when it must be given parenterally.

Cerebellar ataxia with opsoclonus-myoclonus is usually found with differentiated neuroblastomas. Does this represent an overreaction of the patient's defense mechanism? Could it be that an immunological defense mechanism is trying to destroy the tumor but, as with autoimmune disease, is also directed at the cerebellum? The good response of such patients to ACTH treatment supports this theory (Nicherson and Hutter 1979).

Obviously, current chemotherapy schedules do not cure all children with bone and lymph node metastases, so other schedules must be used. Neuroblastoma is sensitive to chemotherapy, as shown by the fact that bone marrow metastases can be treated easily. But the levels of chemotherapy reached in the primary tumor, lymph nodes, and bone are not high enough. Higher levels of chemotherapy must be used, causing higher toxicity to the bone marrow. Autologous bone marrow transplantation could be helpful. The fact that bone marrow can be cleared of metastases makes bone marrow transplantations feasible. If some metastases are transplanted this way, it is not serious while the lung is the first filter for circulating tumor cells. Metastases do not seem to find the lung a suitable site for development. Our current treatment program, based on the experimental work of Millar et al. (1978) and Hedley et al. (1978), is promising. Using high-dose phenylalanine mustard, we have destroyed the entire tumor burden in five patients. Bone marrow toxicity can be overcome by autologous transplantation. The problem with this treatment is the intestinal tract, where, as in the bone marrow, the entire fast-dividing mucosa is destroyed. Our five patients died of this problem because intractable bleeding occurred. It is hoped that, in due time, this problem will be solved.

There is a future in treatment for the 70% of patients with neuroblastoma who cannot be cured by current chemotherapy schedules. Neuroblastoma is sensitive to chemotherapy; we have to use that chemotherapy in a different way with good supporting care. The problem of prophylaxis is equally important. Additional investigations will perhaps solve this problem. Science cannot be stopped. One would like to have the knowledge of tomorrow to save the patients of today.

REFERENCES

Beckwith, J. B., and E. V. Perrin. 1963. In situ neuroblastomas: A contribution to the natural history of neural crest tumors. Am. J. Pathol. 43:1089–1104.

Chatten, J., and M. L. Voorhess. 1967. Familial neuroblastoma. N. Engl. J. Med. 277:1230–1236.

Coupland, R. E. 1965. The Natural History of the Chromaffin Cell. Longmans, London.

Donath, A., H. Käser, B. Roos, W. Ziegler, O. Oetliker, J. P. Colombo, and M. Bettex. 1965. Le phéochromocytome familial. Helv. Paediatr. Acta 20:1–18.

Evans, A. E., G. J. D'Angio, and J. Randolph. 1971. A proposed staging for children with neuroblastoma. Cancer 27:374–378.

Finkelstein, J. Z., M. R. Klemperer, A. Evans, I. Bernstein, S. Leikin, S. McCreadie, J. Grosfeld, R. Hittle, J. Weiner, H. Sather, and D. Hammond. 1979. Multiagent chemotherapy for children with metastatic neuroblastoma: A report from the Children's Cancer Study Group. Med. Pediatr. Oncol. 6:179–188.

Hedley, D. W., J. L. Millar, T. J. McElwain, and M. Y. Gordon. 1978. Acceleration of bone-marrow recovery by pre-treatment with cyclophosphamide in patients receiving high-dose melphalan. Lancet 2:966–967.

Hutchison, R. 1907. On suprarenal sarcoma in children with metastases in the skull. Q. J. Med. 1:33–41.

Jaffe, N. 1976. Neuroblastoma. Cancer Treat. Rev. 3:61–82.

Levi-Montalcini, R., and P. Calissano. 1979. The nerve-growth factor. Sci. Am. 240:44–53.

Millar, J. L., B. N. Hudspith, T. J. McElwain, and T. A. Phelps. 1978. Effect of high dose melphalan on marrow and intestinal epithelium in mice pretreated with cyclophosphamide. Br. J. Cancer 38:137–142.

Nicherson, B. G., and J. J. Hutter. 1979. Opsomyoclonus and neuroblastoma. Clin. Pediatr. (Phila.) 18:446–448.

Pepper, W. A. 1901. A study of congenital sarcoma of the liver and suprarenal. Am. J. Med. Sci. 121:287–299.

Roberts, K. B., and J. M. Freeman. 1975. Cerebellar ataxia and occult neuroblastoma, without opsoclonus. Pediatrics 56:464–465.

Strauss, L., and S. G. Driscoll. 1964. Congenital neuroblastoma involving the placenta. Pediatrics 34:23–31.

Wertheim, P., and P. A. Voûte. 1976. Neuroblastoma, Wilms' tumor and cytomegalovirus. J. Natl. Cancer Inst. 57:701–703.

Wieberdink, J. 1957. Foetal haemic metastases: An explanation of the Pepper type of metastases in adrenal neuroblastoma. Br. J. Cancer 11:378–383.

Witzleben, C. L., and R. A. Landy. 1974. Disseminated neuroblastoma in a child with von Recklinghausen's disease. Cancer 34:786–790.

Voûte, P. A. 1968. Neuroblastoom, Ganglioneuroom, Phaeochromocytoom: Een Klinische, Biochemische en Pathologisch Anatomische Studie over Drie Tumoren van Het Sympathisch Zenuwstelsel (thesis). Oosthoek, Utrecht.

Zucker, J. M. 1974. Retrospective study of 426 neuroblastomas treated between 1950 and 1970. Maandschr. Kindergeneesk. 42:369–385.

Status of the Curability of Childhood Cancers,
edited by J. van Eys and M. P. Sullivan.
Raven Press, New York © 1980.

Brain Tumors: The New Frontier

Ayten Cangir, M.D., and Jan van Eys, Ph.D., M.D.

*Department of Pediatrics, The University of Texas System Cancer Center M. D. Anderson
Hospital and Tumor Institute, Houston, Texas*

Central nervous system (CNS) tumors are the second most common malignant tumors in children (Young et al. 1975). The incidence is about 24 per million per year in both whites and blacks. In a recently reported series, about 4.5% of all CNS tumors were intraspinal and about 95% were intracranial (Farwell et al. 1977).

About 70% of intracranial tumors are gliomas, which include astrocytomas, glioblastomas, oligodendrogliomas, ependymomas, and medulloblastomas. Medulloblastomas and astrocytomas occur with about the same frequency (Bloom and Walsh 1975). The remaining intracranial tumors comprise meningiomas, neurinomas, pituitary adenomas, craniopharyngiomas, choroid plexus tumors, papillomas, pinealomas, hemangiomas, epidermoidomas, teratomas, sarcomas, and metastases. The gliomas are a heterogeneous group of interrelated entities derived from astrocytes, oligodendroglias, and the ependyma (Vogel 1977). Traditionally, gliomas have been classified by histologic criteria (Bailey and Cushing 1926, Earle et al. 1957, Rubinstein 1972, Zülch and Wechsler 1968).

Of the intracranial tumors, craniopharyngiomas carry an excellent prognosis. With conservative surgery and postoperative irradiation, the 10-year control rate reaches about 90% (Kramer 1976, Bloom 1978). The glioblastomas (grade IV astrocytomas) and anaplastic astrocytomas (grade III) carry the worst prognosis. With conventional therapy, which includes a biopsy or partial resection of the tumor followed by irradiation, the median survival is about 9 months in patients with glioblastomas and about 12 months in those with medulloblastomas and ependymomas. The 5-year survival rate is less than 5% for patients with glioblastomas, about 20% for those with medulloblastomas and ependymomas (Farwell et al. 1977).

Although the prognosis of children with most types of brain tumors has been poor, the introduction of chemotherapy has been delayed by fear of using antineoplastic agents in brain tumors because of the "blood-brain barrier," and by difficulties in evaluating response to chemotherapy in children with permanent neurologic damage. Nonetheless, along with improvements in diagnostic capability with the introduction of computerized tomography and sophisticated new surgical and radiotherapeutic advances, trials of new chemotherapeutic agents have produced an armamentarium of drugs effective against CNS tumors. These drugs include vincristine (VCR), procarbazine hydrochloride, BCNU (1,3-bis(2-chloroethyl)-1-nitrosourea), CCNU (1-(2-chloroethyl)-3-cyclohexyl-1-nitrosourea), and methotrexate (MTX) (Lampkin et al. 1967, Lassman et al. 1969, Rosenstock et al. 1976, Kumar et al. 1974, Walker and Hurwitz 1970, Wilson et al. 1970, Hoogstraten et al. 1973, Rosen et al. 1977, Sumer et al. 1978, Shapiro 1977).

The purpose of this paper is to review our experience with chemotherapeutic agents in the management of patients with CNS tumors in the past 5 years.

DIAGNOSTIC PROCEDURES AND EVALUATION OF RESPONSE

A physical examination, including complete neurologic testing, with documentation of abnormal signs at the time of diagnosis and during the follow-up period is essential for accurate evaluation. The most valuable laboratory study is the computerized tomography (CT) scan. Radionuclide scanning and examination of cerebrospinal fluid (CSF) for cytologic type and tumor markers are also indicated. Myelography is still valuable for anatomic localization of spinal cord tumors. The use of pneumoencephalography and angiography may also be helpful in some cases, but these studies are not used as frequently as they used to be because much of the information can be obtained by CT scans. Cerebrospinal fluid cytology is informative in tumors with meningeal spread, such as medulloblastomas and ependymomas. Cerebrospinal fluid polyamines have been shown to be significantly increased in patients with medulloblastomas. The concentration of these markers in the CSF declines with the regression of medulloblastomas and increases with the recurrence of these tumors. Accordingly, the CSF polyamine assay is a valuable tool in monitoring patients with medulloblastomas (Marton et al. 1979).

Endocrine Function Studies

Recent studies have demonstrated a decrease in hypothalamic-pituitary functions in patients who receive radiation to the hypothalamic-pituitary axis (Richards et al. 1976, Samaan et al. 1975, Shalet et al. 1976, Wara et al. 1977). It is our policy to obtain baseline hormone levels in patients about to undergo irradiation. Thereafter, an endocrine evaluation is done at yearly intervals. Appropriate hormonal replacement therapy is instituted in patients with hormonal deficits.

Evaluation of Response to Chemotherapeutic Agents

Evaluation of response to chemotherapeutic agents in patients with brain tumors has been very difficult. Conventional criteria are not applicable in patients with CNS tumors, as even patients with complete tumor regression may have a neurologic deficit. Accordingly, we have adopted more appropriate criteria in defining responses to chemotherapy in children with brain tumors:

1. *Unequivocal response (UR),* unequivocal improvement in neurologic status and the radionuclide or CT scan and decreased steroid dependence for 3 months or more.

2. *Probable or partial response (PR),* improvement in neurologic status with stability of the radionuclide or CT scan, or vice versa, or stability of neurologic function and scan and a nonescalating steroid dose for 3 months or more.

3. *No response (NR),* progression of signs or symptoms and continued steroid dependence, or a response for less than 3 months.

COMBINATION CHEMOTHERAPY FOR RECURRENT BRAIN TUMORS

Experience with CCNU, VCR, and Intrathecal MTX

Normally the brain is protected by the "blood-brain barrier," which selectively permits drug penetration. It is generally believed that lipid-soluble substances accumulate better in the brain. For this reason, lipid-soluble nitrosoureas were developed to treat intracranial neoplasms. Because of the established effectiveness of CCNU, a combination chemotherapy regimen including this nitrosourea, vincristine, and intrathecally administered methotrexate was developed for children with recurrent brain tumors in 1974. Of the 12 children treated on this regimen, four each had UR, PR, and NR. The overall response rate was 66% (van Eys 1975). The dosage schedule for this regimen is shown in Table 1. Although the response rate was good, the toxicity of CCNU was cumulative.

Experience with Combination Chemotherapy Including Nitrogen Mustard, Vincristine, Procarbazine, and Prednisone (MOPP)

The MOPP chemotherapy regimen was implemented in 1975, and it was based on the following rationale: (1) the agents included had been shown to be effective against brain tumors as single agents; (2) nitrogen mustard is lipid

Table 1. *Combination Chemotherapy with CCNU, VCR, and MTX in Children with Recurrent Brain Tumors*

Drug	Dosage
CCNU	130 mg/m² p.o. on day 1
VCR	1.5 mg/m² i.v. on days 1, 8, and 15
MTX	12 mg/m² i.t. on days 1, 8, and 15
Restart cycle on day 43	

Table 2. *Dosage Regimen for MOPP Chemotherapy*

Drug	Dosage
Nitrogen mustard	6 mg/m² i.v. on days 1 and 8
Vincristine sulfate	1.4 mg/m² i.v. (not more than 2 mg per dose) on days 1 and 8
Procarbazine	50 mg/m² p.o. on day 1, 100 mg/m² p.o. on day 2, and 100 mg/m² p.o. on days 3 through 10
Prednisone	40 mg/m²/day p.o. on days 1 through 10, tapering off over the following 3 days
	Restart cycle on day 29

soluble; and (3) this combination had been used to treat children with Hodgkin's disease and its toxicity was very well documented (Young et al. 1973). The dosage regimen for MOPP is given in Table 2. Initially this treatment was given at M. D. Anderson Hospital and Tumor Institute; later, three other member institutions of the Southwest Oncology Group collaborated in the study. The earlier results of that study have previously been published (Cangir et al. 1978).

Twenty-three children with primary CNS tumors were treated with this combination chemotherapy. All but one had had progressive or recurrent tumors following surgery and irradiation; in addition, nine had received prior chemotherapy. Seventeen of 20 patients (85%) responded to MOPP chemotherapy, including seven who had received prior chemotherapy with single or multiple agents such as VCR, the nitrosoureas, intrathecal MTX, and VM-26. Three comatose patients who were being kept on Decadron without benefit recovered from their comas. The median survival of responders was 11 months, while nonresponders survived only 2 months.

Updated information on a group of patients treated with MOPP for recurrent brain tumors indicates that six of 17 responders are still alive 31–54 months from the initiation of MOPP chemotherapy. Four of these patients are off therapy and surviving with no evidence of disease. Characteristics of these four patients are summarized in Table 3. Two of six surviving patients experienced recurrences and are now under different treatment regimens. One of these patients experienced a recurrence 3 months after cessation of MOPP chemotherapy.

Results with MOPP chemotherapy demonstrate that this treatment regimen is effective against recurrent brain tumors in children, that medulloblastomas and other gliomas are equally sensitive to chemotherapy, and that patients who fail on one chemotherapy regimen can respond to another.

To evaluate the value of nitrogen mustard in the MOPP schedule, a randomized trial comparing MOPP and OPP (no nitrogen mustard) was begun in 1976 by the Southwest Oncology Group. Preliminary results of this study suggest that MOPP chemotherapy is superior to OPP in children with recurrent medul-

Table 3. Characteristics of Four Responders Who Survived More Than 3 Years Following MOPP Chemotherapy

Patient No.	Age (years)/ Sex	Histologic Type of Tumor	Previous Therapy	Pre-MOPP Evaluation	Post-MOPP Evaluation	Duration of Response (months)	Duration of Survival (months)
1	14/M	Not biopsied. Initially CT scan and pneumoencephalograms suggested a brain stem tumor; this was confirmed at surgical exploration	XRT	Bedridden, positive CT scans	Fully functional, complete normalization of CT scans	46+	46+
2	14/M	Astrocytoma	Surgery, XRT	Major paralysis, positive CT scans	Fully functional, normalization of CT scans	49+	49+
3	7½/F	Astrocytoma	Biopsy only	Major paralysis, complete block on myelogram	Fully functional, no neurologic evidence of block (myelograms unsuccessful)	39+	39+
4	9/M	Medulloblastoma	Surgery, XRT, VCR + MTX	Bedridden, major paralysis, abnormal vertebral angiograms or scintograms	Fully functional in self-skills, negative CT scans	54+	54+

loblastomas. However, the number of patients is too small to draw a definite conclusion.

CHEMOTHERAPY AS A PRIMARY APPROACH

A study of 488 children suggests that the median age for the occurrence of CNS tumors is 6 years. This means 50% of children with CNS tumors are under 6 years of age. The peak incidence occurs at age 3 (Farwell et al. 1977). Medulloblastomas and poorly differentiated ependymomas spread along the meninges. To eradicate the disease by radiation therapy, the whole brain and spinal cord must be treated. However, it is preferable to defer or completely avoid irradiation in young children, if possible, for the following reasons:

1. Radiation therapy causes retardation of growth.
2. Hypothalamic-pituitary deficiency can occur following irradiation.
3. Second malignant neoplasms of the brain have been reported following irradiation (Bachman and Ostrow 1978, Modan et al. 1974, Foley et al. 1975, Noetzli and Malamud 1962).
4. Necrosis of the brain is a rare but possible complication of irradiation.

For these reasons, we administered chemotherapy to six children under 2 years of age with brain tumors. Histologic diagnoses included three medulloblastomas, two astrocytomas (both in the spinal cord), and one ependymoma. Because of the encouraging experience with MOPP chemotherapy in recurrent brain tumors, this treatment regimen was selected as primary therapy in five of these infants, while the sixth received radiotherapy to the area of the primary tumor. The main toxic effect has been myelosuppression, which has necessitated dosage adjustments in four patients. However, there has not been a major complication. Response to chemotherapy in these infants has been encouraging, and all are surviving without evidence of progression of disease for 2 to 35 months, with a median of 6 months (Table 4).

In addition to these six infants, a 3-year-, 9-month-old boy with medulloblastoma who presented in an extremely debilitated state with tumor cells in the CSF received MOPP therapy as primary treatment. The relatively slow process of cranial-spinal axis irradiation seemed undesirable. The child received two courses of MOPP without incident. His spinal fluid cleared of tumor cells, and his neurologic status improved. There was no need for maintenance steroids. Following two courses of chemotherapy, cranial-spinal axis irradiation was again administered without difficulty. Four additional courses of MOPP were given, with some adjustment of doses necessary, but without myelosuppression. The patient is currently able to walk and learn again. This experience demonstrates that MOPP chemotherapy can be given in a "sandwich" style with radiation therapy without major complications.

Table 4. MOPP as Primary Therapy in Children with Brain Tumors Under 4 Years of Age*

Patient No.	Age at Start of Therapy	Diagnosis	No. of MOPP Courses	Survival Status	Toxic Effect
1	6 mo.	Medulloblastoma	1	Alive, disease free, 2+ months	—
2	1 yr./6 mo.	Medulloblastoma	4	Alive, disease free, 6+ months	Myelosuppression,† irritability
3	1 yr./5 mo.	Astrocytoma grade I, spinal cord	4	Alive, with disease, 6+ months	Myelosuppression, irritability
4	3 yr./9 mo.	Medulloblastoma	6	Alive, disease free, 6+ months	Myelosuppression†
5	6 mo.	Ependymoma	6	Alive, disease free, 7+ months	Myelosuppression, rritability
6	6 mo.	Astrocytoma grade II, spinal cord	22	Alive, disease free, 35+ months	Myelosuppression†

* As of October 5, 1979.
† Dosage adjustments were made according to the guidelines usually used for administering MOPP to Hodgkir's disease patients.

ADJUNCTIVE CHEMOTHERAPY

Five-year survival of children with glioblastomas, medulloblastomas, and ependymomas is very poor. Since chemotherapy has been effective in patients with recurrent brain tumors, trials of adjunctive chemotherapy for children with these tumors are justified. Such trials require cooperative group studies to obtain conclusive data. Several such cooperative group studies have been undertaken.

The Brain Tumor Study Group evaluated the use of BCNU, radiotherapy, or both, in the treatment of patients who were operated upon and had histologic evidence of anaplastic glioma. This study demonstrated no significant improvement in survival for patients receiving BCNU in addition to radiation therapy over that for patients receiving radiation therapy alone.

The Children's Cancer Study Group initiated a study in 1975 to examine the treatment of medulloblastomas and ependymomas in children. Patients were randomized to radiation therapy alone or radiation therapy plus chemotherapy with VCR, CCNU, and prednisone. Preliminary results of this study show no significant difference in survival between these two groups (Evans et al. 1979).

The International Society of Pediatrics designed a study of the treatment of medulloblastomas and ependymomas. Patients were randomized to radiation therapy alone or radiation therapy plus chemotherapy with VCR and CCNU. Thirty institutions, mostly in Europe, contributed 131 patients. In the radiotherapy group, eight of 66 have developed tumor recurrence and six have died. Of 65 in the radiotherapy plus chemotherapy group, five have experienced recurrence and three have died (Bloom and Walsh 1975).

The Southwest Oncology Group's study was initiated in 1974. Patients with medulloblastomas and ependymomas were randomized to receive treatment with radiation therapy alone or radiation therapy plus chemotherapy including VCR, intrathecal methotrexate, and intrathecal hydrocortisone. The most recent evaluation on this study demonstrated no significant difference in survival between the two groups of patients.

SUMMARY

Chemotherapy has been proven effective in recurrent brain tumors in children. In particular, MOPP chemotherapy provides palliation in up to 70% of children with recurrent brain tumors. This treatment regimen has shown equal effectiveness against medulloblastomas and other gliomas. Four of 17 responders to MOPP chemotherapy are surviving without evidence of disease from 36 to 54 months. This demonstrates that long-term control of brain tumors is possible with chemotherapy even after recurrence. Preliminary results of a SWOG study demonstrate that MOPP chemotherapy is superior to OPP chemotherapy in children with medulloblastomas.

As primary treatment, MOPP chemotherapy has been tolerated well without major complications in five infants. These children are surviving without evidence of progression of disease for 2–36 months. One boy tolerated a treatment regimen with MOPP–radiation therapy–MOPP with unequivocal response. Although the number of patients in this trial is small, it represents an initial step into a new area in the management of young children with CNS tumors.

Cooperative group trials of adjuvant chemotherapy have been unsuccessful in improving the survival rate of patients with brain tumors. Since chemotherapy is effective against recurrent brain tumors, adjunctive chemotherapy should theoretically increase the poor survival rate of patients with medulloblastomas, ependymomas, and glioblastomas. It is most probable that selection of antineoplastic agents, dosage regimens, and timing of these regimens play very important roles in the outcome of adjunctive chemotherapy. Accordingly, future trials should be designed to further explore these areas.

REFERENCES

Bachman, D. S., and P. T. Ostrow. 1978. Fatal long-term sequelae following radiation "cure" for ependymoma. Ann. Neurol. 4:319–321.

Bailey, P., and H. Cushing. 1926. A Classification of the Tumors of the Gloma Group on a Histogenetic Basis with a Correlated Study of Prognosis. Lippincott, Philadelphia, 175 pp.

Bloom, H. J. 1978. Management of some intracranial tumors in children and adults, *in* Recent Advances in Clinical Oncology. Alan R. Liss, Inc., New York, pp. 55–84.

Bloom, H. J. G., and L. S. Walsh. 1975. Tumours of the central nervous system, *in* Cancer in Children: Clinical Management, H. J. G. Bloom, J. Lemerle, M. K. Neidhardt, and P. A. Voûte, eds. Springer-Verlag, Berlin, pp. 93–119.

Cangir, A., J. van Eys, D. H. Berry, E. Hvizdala, and S. K. Morgan. 1978. Combination chemotherapy with MOPP in children with recurrent brain tumors. Med. Pediatr. Oncol. 4:253–261.

Earle, K. M., E. H. Rentschler, and S. R. Snodgrass. 1957. Primary intracranial neoplasms: Prognosis and classification of 513 verified cases. J. Neuropathol. Exp. Neurol. 16:321–331.

Evans, A. E., R. D. Jenkin, I. Ertel, and C. Wilson. 1979. Adjuvant chemotherapy for medulloblastoma, interim report from CCG 942, *in* Proceedings of the Fifteenth Annual Meeting of the American Society of Clinical Oncology, Abstract C-556. Waverly Press, Baltimore, p. 425.

Farwell, J. R., G. J. Dohrmann, and J. T. Flannery. 1977. Central nervous system tumors in children. Cancer 40:3123–3132.

Foley, K. M., J. M. Woodruff, and J. B. Posner. 1975. Radiation-induced malignant schwannomas (Abstract). Neurology 25:354.

Hoogstraten, B., J. A. Gottlieb, E. Caoili, W. G. Tucker, R.-W. Talley, and A. Haut. 1973. CCNU (1-(2-chloroethyl)-3-cyclohexyl-1-nitrosourea) (NSC-79037) in the treatment of cancer. Cancer 32:38–43.

Kramer, S. 1976. Craniopharyngioma: The best treatment is conservative surgery and postoperative radiation therapy, *in* Current Controversies in Neurosurgery, T. P. Morley, ed. W. B. Saunders, Philadelphia, pp. 336–343.

Kumar, A. R. V., J. Renaudin, C. B. Wilson, E. B. Boldrey, K. J. Enot, and V. A. Levin. 1974. Procarbazine hydrochloride in the treatment of brain tumors, Phase II study. J. Neurosurg. 40:365–371.

Lampkin, B. C., A. M. Mauer, and B. H. McBride. 1967. Response of medulloblastoma to vincristine sulfate: A case report. Pediatrics 39:761–763.

Lassman, L. P., G. W. Pearce, J. Banna, and R. D. Jones. 1969. Vincristine sulfate in the treatment of skeletal metastases from cerebellar medulloblastoma. J. Neurosurg. 30:42–49.

Marton, L. J., M. S. Edwards, V. A. Levin, W. P. Lubich, and C. B. Wilson. 1979. Predictive value of cerebrospinal fluid polyamines in medulloblastoma. Cancer Res. 39:993–997.

Modan, B., H. Mart, D. Baidatz, R. Steinitz, and S. G. Levin. 1974. Radiation-induced head and neck tumors. Lancet 1:277–279.

Noetzli, M., and N. Malamud. 1962. Postirradiation fibrosarcoma of the brain. Cancer 15:617–622.

Richards, G. E., W. M. Wara, M. M. Grumbach, S. L. Kaplan, G. E. Sheline, and F. A. Conte. 1976. Delayed onset of hypopituitarism: Sequelae of therapeutic irradiation of central nervous system, eye, and middle ear tumors. J. Pediatr. 89:553–559.

Rosen, G., F. Ghavimi, A. Nirenberg, C. Mosende, and B. M. Metha. 1977. High-dose methotrexate with citrovorum factor rescue for the treatment of central nervous system tumors in children. Cancer Treat. Rep. 61:681–690.

Rubinstein, L. J. 1972. Atlas of Tumor Pathology. 2nd series, Fasc. 6. Tumors of the Central Nervous System. Armed Forces Institute of Pathology, Washington, D.C.

Samaan, S. A., M. M. Bakdash, J. B. Caderao, A. Cangir, R. H. Jesse, and A. J. Ballantine. 1975. Hypopituitarism after external radiation: Evidence for both hypothalamic and pituitary origin. Ann. Intern. Med. 83:771–777.

Shalet, S. M., C. G. Beardswell, P. Morris-Jones, F. M. Bamford, G. G. Ribero, and D. Pearson. 1976. Growth hormone deficiency in children with brain tumors. Cancer 37:1144–1148.

Shapiro, W. R. 1977. High-dose methotrexate in malignant gliomas. Cancer Treat. Rep. 61:753–756.

Sumer, T., A. I. Freeman, M. Cohen, A. M. Bremer, P. R. Thomas, and L. F. Sinks. 1978. Chemotherapy in recurrent noncystic low-grade astrocytomas of the cerebrum in children. J. Surg. Oncol. 10:45–54.

van Eys, J. 1975. Chemotherapy for gliomas in children. Cancer Bull. 27:16–19.

Vogel, F. S. 1977. Nomenclature for gliomas. Natl. Cancer Inst. Monogr. 46:51–60.

Walker, M. D., and B. S. Hurwitz. 1970. BCNU (1,3-bis(2-chloroethyl)-1-nitrosourea) (NSC-409962) in the treatment of malignant brain tumors. Cancer Chemother. Rep. 54:263–271.

Wara, W. M., G. E. Richards, M. M. Grumbach, S. I. Kaplan, G. E. Sheline, and F. A. Conte. 1977. Hypopituitarism after irradiation in children. Int. J. Radiat. Oncol. Biol. Phys. 2:549–552.

Wilson, C. B., E. B. Boldrey, and K. J. Enot. 1970. 1,3-bis(2-chloroethyl)-1-nitrosourea (NSC-409962) in the treatment of brain tumors. Cancer Chemother. Rep. 54:273–281.

Young, J. L., Jr., and R. W. Miller. 1975. Incidence of malignant tumors in U.S. children. J. Pediatr. 86:254–258.

Young, R. C., V. T. DeVita, and R. E. Johnson. 1973. Hodgkin's disease in childhood. Blood 42:163–179.

Zülch, K. J., and W. Wechsler. 1968. Pathology and classification of gliomas. Prog. Neurol. Surg. 2:1–84.

STATUS OF THE CURABILITY OF HEMOPOIETIC MALIGNANT DISEASES

Status of the Curability of Childhood Cancers,
edited by J. van Eys and M. P. Sullivan.
Raven Press, New York © 1980.

Status of the Curability of Hemopoietic Malignant Diseases

Jan van Eys, Ph.D., M.D.

Department of Pediatrics, The University of Texas System Cancer Center M. D. Anderson Hospital and Tumor Institute, Houston, Texas

The progress in the management of childhood lymphoid diseases has been phenomenal. Modern chemotherapy was born in the treatment of childhood lymphocytic leukemia. All of our current structure of cooperative study groups originated in the first investigations into this childhood malignant disease. Definitions of phase I, II, or III studies, definitions of responses, and agreements on end results reporting all contributed to setting cure as the end point for these investigations. Figure 1 shows the steady progress in prolonged survival that has been accomplished through these studies. But eventually there was a plateau. For a period of time, no major improvements occurred.

To be able to cure a disease, you need to know what the disease is. The

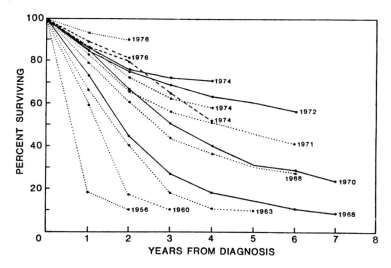

Figure 1. Survival rates for children with acute lymphocytic and acute undifferentiated leukemia, based on data generated for a report of a cooperative group effort to the Board of Scientific Counselors of the Division of Cancer Treatment, National Cancer Institute, and supplied by Dr. D. Hammond. The years indicate when each study was begun.

fact is that until recently we did not know how to define leukemia in a scientific way. The following definition is found in a leading textbook on pediatric oncology:

> Leukemia is a protean group of diseases of unknown cause that have in common a high fatality rate due to complications of bone marrow failure or infiltration of tissues because of a generalized proliferation of immature or abnormal leukocytes or both (Fernbach 1977).

We were playing a game that was no different from the television diversion introduced by Steve Allen and perpetuated by Johnny Carson—"the question man." Here is the answer, what was the question; we can now cure, what are we curing?

The fact that we got as far as we did proves that intuitively we did recognize a common denominator in various forms of leukemia, even if our scientific definitions did not allow reproducible criteria for study. This is now rapidly changing. The current nosology shows a very intriguing pattern of leukemia subsets that are beginning to generate insights into normal cellular ontology and phylogeny. We now think we have a new set of questions again, so that answers can be devised that make sense. We will hear much about such new concepts in leukemia and lymphoma.

These new concepts do not negate the possibility of a single common etiology of cancer, however. The same stimulus may have very different results in different specialized cells, or in cells with different degrees of differentiation. In addition, therapy, which basically is still selective cell kill, may need to be very different in different malignant diseases, even though the basic defect is the same. It is highly likely that we will formulate many further questions on the basis of our current insights.

To be able to conquer leukemia, we need to define what the malignant cell is. To be able to prevent cancer, we need to understand its etiology. That will be our next question. Curability is an answer to leukemia, but if we try to imagine what the question is we may draw a laugh—the question eventually ought to be more basic than that.

In the meantime, however, we are approaching cures, to the benefit of our current patients.

REFERENCE

Fernbach, D. J. 1977. Natural history of acute leukemia, *in* Clinical Pediatric Oncology, 2nd ed., W. W. Sutow, T. J. Vietti, and D. J. Fernbach, eds. C. V. Mosby Co., St. Louis, pp. 291–333.

Status of the Curability of Childhood Cancers,
edited by J. van Eys and M. P. Sullivan.
Raven Press, New York © 1980.

Impact of the New Nosology on Acute Lymphocytic Leukemia

Ellen R. Richie, Ph.D., and Lawrence S. Frankel, M.D.

Department of Pediatrics, The University of Texas System Cancer Center M. D. Anderson Hospital and Tumor Institute, Houston, Texas

The application of nosology to hematopoietic malignant disease has had a profound impact, particularly on the treatment of childhood acute lymphocytic leukemia (ALL). Classification schemes for ALL based on immunologic markers have established several subtypes of this disease, which require different treatment protocols to achieve optimal therapy. Although it is now firmly established that ALL is a heterogeneous disease with respect to the origin of the malignant cells, the number of possible subtypes and their associated prognoses are still under investigation. The immunologic classification of ALL is based in large part on identification of membrane constituents that are characteristic components of thymus-derived (T) and bone marrow–derived (B) lymphocyte populations. The underlying concept supporting this scheme is that each type of lymphocytic leukemia, presumed to be a clonal proliferation of transformed lymphocytes, has a normal lymphocytic counterpart that can be identified by cell membrane characteristics. It is conceivable that every stage of antigen-independent or -dependent normal lymphocyte differentiation can undergo neoplastic transformation. The fact that leukemias with immature surface phenotypes predominate in number may reflect a difference in pathogenesis or the relative susceptibility of primitive lymphoid cells to neoplastic transformation, perhaps due to expression of appropriate transformation-sensitive molecules on immature cell membranes.

Nevertheless, immunologic assessment of leukemic cells from different patients has revealed that the clinical entity termed ALL includes lymphoid precursors as well as subsets of T and B lymphocytes, and that the cellular origin of the leukemic cells profoundly affects clinical responsiveness. Although this discussion will focus on the contribution of immunologic markers to the nosology of ALL, other parameters, including morphology, cytochemistry, cytogenetics, and biochemical markers, provide additional relevant information to the overall scheme.

Before assigning leukemic cells to the T or B cell series, it is necessary to define the surface markers that distinguish the two major normal lymphocyte populations. A large number of membrane receptors and antigens (both of which

Table 1. *Surface Membrane Receptors and Antigens on Human T and B Lymphocytes*

Marker	T	B
Sheep erythrocyte receptor*	+	−
T antigens	+	−
Surface membrane immunoglobulin	−	+
Mouse erythrocyte receptor	−	+
Epstein-Barr virus receptor	−	+
B differentiation antigen	−	+
Ia antigen*·†	±	+
C3 receptor*·†	±	+
Fcγ receptor*·†	±	+
Fcμ receptor	±	+
Fcα receptor	±	−
Fcε receptor	±	±

* Expressed on third-population lymphocytes.
† Expressed on nonlymphoid cells.
+ Expressed on a majority of cells.
− Not detectable.
± Expressed as a subpopulation.

have been thoroughly discussed in recent reviews) have been identified on T and B lymphocyte surfaces (Table 1) (Ross 1979, Chess and Schlossman 1977, Siegal 1978). In addition, although the idea is still controversial, several investigators have proposed the existence of a heterogeneous third lymphocyte population, termed "null" lymphocytes, which bear high-affinity Fc receptors but lack other markers characteristic of T and B lymphocytes (Horowitz and Garrett 1976, Winfield et al. 1977). Included in this third lymphocyte population are K cells, which mediate antibody-dependent cytotoxicity, and natural killer cells, which are cytotoxic to a variety of targets in the absence of antibody.

Several points concerning surface membrane receptors deserve comment. First, certain surface receptors are found on subsets of T and B lymphocytes, as well as on null lymphocytes and nonlymphoid cells. For example, the complement receptor (C3R) originally considered to be a characteristic B cell surface receptor is expressed on null lymphocytes and monocytes, and recently has been found on a subpopulation of normal T lymphocytes in peripheral blood and thoracic duct lymph (MacDermott et al. 1975, Shore et al. 1979). Second, the phenotypic expression of surface membrane components may vary qualitatively or quantitatively, depending on the differentiation status of a given cell. In the T cell series, the characteristic sheep erythrocyte receptor (ER) is expressed on less than 10% of fetal thymocytes at 8–10 weeks' gestation, while 80% of the cells express C3R (Gatien et al. 1975). With increasing gestational age the proportions of thymocytes positive for ER and C3R are gradually reversed, so that at birth the majority of thymocytes are ER positive (ER+) and C3R negative (C3R−). In the B cell series, immature lymphocytes express a low level of surface membrane immunoglobulin (SmIg), which increases as the cell differentiates into a functional B lymphocyte and diminishes again after the antigen triggers further differentiation to the plasma cell stage (Perkins et al. 1972, Raff et al. 1976). Qualitative as well as quantitative changes in surface marker expression occur during B lymphocyte maturation. Data obtained from investigations of murine and human B cell ontogeny are integrated in Table 2 into a theoretical scheme of membrane markers expressed during antigen-independent B lymphocyte differentiation (Owen et al. 1977, Kearney et al. 1977, Gelfand et al. 1974, Rosenberg and Parish 1977, Hämmerling et al. 1976). This scheme probably masks the heterogeneity of B cell subsets. For example, SmIg+, C3R− lymphocytes may be precursors of SmIg+, C3R+ lymphocytes, or these two membrane phenotypes may occur on distinct B cell subpopulations.

A final point concerning lymphocyte surface receptors is that particular receptors define functionally distinct lymphocyte subsets. In this regard, T lymphocytes with $Fc\mu$ receptors function as helper cells for mitogen-induced B cell differentiation, while T lymphocytes bearing $Fc\gamma$ receptors have suppressor activity in this system (Moretta et al. 1977b).

In addition to surface receptors, cell membrane antigens distinguish between T and B lymphocytes, as well as among their respective subsets. Ia-like or DR (D locus–related) antigens are encoded by genes within or closely associated with the HLA-D region of the major histocompatibility complex. These antigens not only are expressed throughout B cell maturation (Table 2), but have been found on stem cells, monocytes, myeloblasts, and T and null lymphocytes, as well as on various types of leukemic lymphocytes, including ALL, and chronic lymphocytic and acute myelogenous leukemia (Chess and Schlossman 1977, Chess et al. 1976, Vogler et al. 1978, Schlossman et al. 1976). B differentiation antigen (BDA) is also present at all stages of B cell maturation but, unlike the Ia antigens, is not expressed on other cell types (Balch et al. 1978).

Normal T lymphocyte subsets can be identified by the presence of differentiation antigens, which are expressed, often transiently, during ontogeny or, in the adult, as precursor cells mature to functional lymphocytes. In the mouse,

Table 2. *Theoretical Sequence of Surface Marker Expression During Antigen-Independent B Lymphocyte Differentiation*

Lymphocyte Marker	Hypothetical Differentiation Stages			
	1*	2	3	4†
Cytoplasmic Ig	+	−	−	−
SmIg	−	+	+	+
Fc receptor	−	−	+	+
C3R	−	−	−	+
Ia antigen	+	+	+	+
B differentiation antigen	+	+	+	+

* Pre-B cell.
† Mature B cell.

expression of T cell surface antigens is a reliable index of cellular differentiation. The capacity to induce T-specific antigens on a subpopulation of bone marrow cells by in vitro exposure to thymic hormones supports the concept of a prothymocyte population already committed to differentiate along the T cell axis (Scheid et al. 1975). Within the thymus, the prothymocyte acquires thymus leukemia (TL) antigen, high-density theta antigen, and Ly 123 differentiation antigens (Touraine et al. 1977). As differentiation proceeds, TL is lost and theta density diminishes with a concomitant increase in H2 density. Peripheral T cells express Ly 123+, Ly 1+23−, or Ly 1−23+ phenotypes, each of which is associated with particular functional potentials (Cantor and Boyse 1977). For example, Ly 1+23− T cells function as helper cells in the antibody response to thymus-dependent antigens, whereas Ly 1−23+ cells have a cytotoxic effector or suppressor function (Cantor and Boyse 1977).

As in the murine system, expression of T lymphocyte antigen has been induced on a subpopulation of human bone marrow cells after in vitro incubation with thymosin (Touraine et al. 1977). Although many of the heteroantisera produced against normal or malignant human T cells react with both immature and mature T lymphocytes, certain antisera, after multiple absorptions, detect discrete T cell subsets. Heteroantisera have been produced against T-specific antigens that are present on thymocytes but undetectable on peripheral T cells (Chess and Schlossman 1977, Mohanakumar and Metzgar 1974). In addition, heteroantisera have been prepared against functionally distinct peripheral T cell subsets. For example, two human peripheral blood T cell populations have been termed TH_2+ and $TH_2−$ (Evans et al. 1978). The TH_2+ subset, which accounts for approximately 20% of circulating T cells, proliferates poorly to soluble antigens and contains cells with cytotoxic effector and suppressor functions (Evans et al. 1978, Reinherz and Schlossman 1979). The $TH_2−$ subset proliferates optimally to soluble antigens and provides helper function in several systems (Evans et al. 1978). In another approach, antimonkey thymocyte antiserum that has been absorbed with Molt-4, a T lymphoblastoid cell line, has been shown to detect antigens on a T cell subpopulation that suppresses mitogen-induced B cell differentiation (Balch and Ades 1979).

Although heteroantisera are valuable reagents, the antibody specificities elicited by a given immunization protocol are often variable, and multiple absorptions are necessary to render a given antiserum T cell or subset specific. Recently, these problems have been circumvented by employing the hybridoma technique to raise monoclonal antibodies that are specific for functional T cell subsets (Reinherz et al. 1979a, Kung et al. 1979). These antibodies have obvious relevance for the classification of lymphoid malignant diseases.

The various immunologic surface receptors and antigens have been applied to the classification of ALL. Individual leukemic cells arising from clonal proliferation of an initially transformed lymphocyte may differ in maturation status and corresponding surface marker phenotype. Furthermore, it is likely that surface membrane and functional properties are not stable traits of all members of a leukemic clone (Nowell 1976). Indeed, chromosomal instability, emergence of drug-resistant subclones, and changes in morphology and surface markers have been reported at relapse in ALL patients (Zuelzer et al. 1976, Borella et al. 1979, Goldstone et al. 1979). Nevertheless, considerable progress has been made in sorting out clinically relevant subgroups in ALL on the basis of immunologic markers present on leukemic cells at diagnosis.

Three distinct subgroups of ALL exist: the T cell, the B cell, and the non–T, non–B cell. We can now correlate clinical presentation, laboratory immunologic criteria, and therapeutic response patterns. A disease that had been considered a single entity has begun to unravel.

Relatively few patients ($< 10\%$) have SmIg+ leukemic blasts. Most of these patients show unusual clinical or cytologic features that appear to be rare presentations of Burkitt's lymphoma or poorly differentiated lymphoma and may be associated with a poor prognosis (Brouet et al. 1976, Flandrin et al. 1975).

T cell leukemia accounts for approximately 20% of ALL cases and is associated with several poor prognostic factors, including older age, high white blood cell count, and mediastinal involvement. This subgroup, in which males predominate, was initially identified in the laboratory by the E rosetting capacity of the leukemic cells (Tsukimoto et al. 1976, Sen and Borella 1975). A laboratory parameter was then available to identify a group of patients with a distinct therapeutic response pattern. Since standard therapy was associated with a poor outcome in these patients, a new approach to treatment was required. Preliminary trials using the same combination chemotherapy that was successful against convoluted cell lymphoma demonstrated an improved response rate in T cell leukemia patients (Sullivan and Frias 1977). Since 1976, patients with T cell leukemia have been treated in a Southwest Oncology Group (SWOG) study headed by Dr. Margaret Sullivan with an aggressive chemotherapeutic approach and have experienced significant improvement in therapeutic response. In a current SWOG study group, 49 patients were established as having T cell leukemia, based on greater than 20% ER+ blasts on bone marrow examination. Of these patients, 88% attained complete remission. Of the 43 patients in remission, 65% have maintained remission up to 33 months after initiation of treatment. This experience proves that appropriate therapy can change the clinical response pattern and improve the therapeutic outcome in an otherwise poor-risk group.

As additional immunologic markers are used to characterize leukemic cells, it becomes apparent that T cell ALL is itself heterogeneous with regard to surface membrane phenotype and perhaps prognosis. Although most leukemic T cells are ER+, several investigators have reported patients whose leukemic cells expressed T antigens even though they were not capable of forming E rosettes, a surface phenotype consistent with a primitive stage of normal T cell development (Brouet and Seligmann 1978, Greaves and Janossy 1978, Kaplan et al. 1977, Anderson et al. 1979). A group of SWOG investigators have identified a significant subgroup of these patients (approximately 5%) who are currently receiving standard ALL therapy without a significant difference in the response pattern compared to that of T antigen–negative patients. However, additional follow-up time is necessary to determine whether distinctive therapeutic responses will be observed.

Surface membrane receptors that may be expressed in various combinations on the surface of leukemic T cells include, but are not limited to, thermolabile and thermostabile ERs, C3Rs, Fcγ, Fcμ, and TH$_2$ antigen. The E rosette–forming capacity of leukemic T cell populations from various patients may differ with respect to the thermostability of the E rosette–forming cells. Many, but not all, leukemic T cell populations form E rosettes at both 4°C and 37°C, as do normal human thymocytes or activated peripheral blood T cells (Galili and Schlesinger 1975, Richie and Patchen 1978). Another characteristic common to early fetal thymocytes and leukemic T cells from some patients is C3R expression. On leukemic T cells, C3Rs are often expressed concomitantly with ERs (Stein et al. 1976, Lin and Hsu 1976). However, C3R expression may also occur on T antigen+, ER− leukemic cells (Richie et al. 1980). Finally, ER+ leukemic cells may express Fcμ or Fcγ receptors, or both (Moretta et al. 1977a).

T leukemia cells express antigens detected by anti-human thymocyte sera, as well as antigens detected by antisera with broad specificity for both immature thymocytes and mature peripheral T cells (Schlossman et al. 1976, Greaves and Janossy 1978, Kaplan et al. 1977, Anderson et al. 1979, Mills et al. 1975). Although the leukemic cells from most patients with T cell ALL do not express Ia antigen, a patient with Ia-positive leukemic T cells has been reported (Greaves and Janossy 1978). The Ia+, T antigen+, ER+ phenotype has been found on a subset of normal peripheral T cells (Greaves and Janossy 1978).

Recently, subset derivation of T cell ALL has been achieved using heteroantisera specific for the TH$_2$ antigen present on approximately 20% of normal peripheral blood T cells (Evans et al. 1978). Leukemic cells from 25 patients (including seven adults) were either TH$_2$+ or TH$_2$−, while no patient had both TH$_2$+ and TH$_2$− leukemic subclones (Reinherz et al. 1979b). All five patients with TH$_2$+ leukemic cells were less than 21 years of age and only two presented with a mediastinal mass, whereas 11 of the 13 children with TH$_2$− leukemic cells presented with a mediastinal mass. The fact that overall survival was greater for the TH$_2$+ group suggests that subset antigenic characterization of T cell leukemias relates to prognosis within this ALL subgroup (Reinherz et al. 1979b).

Since antigenic phenotype correlates with functional activity of normal T cell subsets, it will be of interest to determine if the TH$_2$+ T cell leukemias have cytotoxic effector or suppressor function. Indeed, leukemic T cells from a child with ALL and hypogammaglobulinemia suppressed immunoglobulin production in vitro when mixed with normal T and B cells (Broder et al. 1978).

The third major subgroup of ALL (representing approximately 70% of all cases) is termed non-T, non-B ALL because the leukemic blasts fail to express immunologic markers unique to either the T or B cell series. These patients have the most favorable prognosis in terms of therapeutic response. In the non-

T, non-B subgroup, as defined by leukemic cells that are ER−, SmIg−, and common ALL antigen+, a complete continuous remission rate in excess of 70% may be possible. Ia-like antigen expression on these leukemic cells has prompted the suggestion that these cells are of pre-B cellular origin. Although Ia antigens are present on pre-B leukemic cells, Ia antigens are also expressed on null ALL cells, which do not contain cytoplasmic immunoglobulin, and, as previously mentioned, Ia antigens are present on a variety of other leukemic and normal cells, including stem cells.

The finding that the blast cells from most patients with non-T, non-B ALL contain terminal deoxynucleotidyl transferase (TdT), which is found in immature thymocytes and not in peripheral T cells, suggests a pre-T cellular origin (McCaffrey et al. 1975). However, this enzyme has been found in pre-B leukemic cells, as well as in a small percentage of normal bone marrow cells (possibly lymphoid progenitors) (Vogler et al. 1978, Janossy et al. 1979). As previously mentioned, several investigators have reported ER− leukemic blasts that express T antigen. It seems likely, then, that non-T, non-B ALL includes very early progenitors of the lymphoid series that may not be committed to the T or B cell pathways of differentiation. This is supported by the recent finding that lymphoblastic crisis in some cases of chronic myelogenous leukemia (CML) involves cells containing both cytoplasmic IgM and the Philadelphia chromosome (Tucker et al. 1979).

If the non-T, non-B ALL subgroup indeed represents neoplastic expansion of a primitive lymphoid progenitor, one might expect to find characteristic cell surface entities shared by leukemic cells and their normal counterparts. Greaves and colleagues (1975) have developed an anti-ALL antiserum by injecting rabbits with ALL blasts that were preincubated in vitro with anti-human lymphocyte antigens. After appropriate absorption, the antiserum distinguished an antigen or antigen complex on non-T, non-B ALL, some cases of CML in blast crisis, as well as certain undifferentiated acute leukemias and lymphomas (Roberts et al. 1978). The antigen-positive blasts in common ALL (cALL) are also Ia+, but ER−, HuTLA (T antigen)−, and SmIg−.

Further work has supported the interpretation that the cALL antigen is not a leukemic-specific antigen, but a differentiation antigen occurring on normal lymphoid progenitor cells. In fetal, neonatal, and regenerating marrow, non-T, non-B type cells that resemble small lymphocytes and are TdT+ show weak reactivity for the cALL antigen (Greaves and Janossy 1978, Janossy et al. 1979). Although there is no formal evidence as yet, these cells are considered to be lymphoid precursors. Therefore, the cALL antigen most likely is not unique to leukemia cells, but rather is a normal differentiation antigen present transiently during the early stages of lymphoid cell maturation.

Approximately 10% of patients with T antigen+, E+ leukemia showed weak but definite expression of the cALL antigen on the leukemic T cells. These results were interpreted to indicate the existence of an infrequent subgroup of ALL with a phenotype intermediate between that of the common form of non-T, non-B ALL and the T cell subgroup (Greaves and Janossy 1978). It is not yet known whether the prognosis of patients with the infrequent cALL+, T antigen+ subgroup will correspond to that of patients with the major non-T, non-B or the T cell subgroup of ALL.

In another subgroup of patients previously classified in the non-T, non-B series, the leukemic cells are SmIg− but contain small amounts of cytoplasmic IgM indicative of a pre-B cell origin (Vogler et al. 1978). Pre-B leukemic cells may express Fc or C3 receptors, or both, in contrast to normal pre-B cells. Identification of these patients in the SWOG studies has revealed that clinical findings at diagnosis and laboratory parameters do not differ from those for non-T, non-B patients. The remission induction rate and maintenance of remission appear to be similar to those for patients with non-T, non-B cell leukemia (Crist et al. 1979). This subgroup will have to be followed for several years to determine if pre-B ALL represents a distinct clinical entity.

Experimental evidence to date shows that the leukemic blasts of patients in the major ALL subgroup have the surface phenotype of SmIg−, ER−, T antigen−, cALL antigen+, Ia+. It is imperative to search for additional parameters of variability, for while the outlook is generally favorable for patients in this subgroup, there is still an undefined subgroup of patients who relapse during or after completion of therapy. One approach to identifying this subgroup is to define additional immunologic receptors or antigens not expressed on leukemic cells of all non-T, non-B ALL patients and determine if there is any correlation with prognosis. This approach is being pursued with the pre-B subgroup of patients. In addition, C3 and Fc receptor expression on non-T, non-B cells may indicate more severe disease with a shorter remission (Esber et al. 1978, Richie et al. 1978). Although there are clues to the enigma, the heterogeneity of non-T, non-B ALL has not been sorted out completely. At present, it seems necessary to apply an ever increasing number of immunologic and other types of markers to the analysis of this major subgroup to derive a formula for identifying those markers that have prognostic significance.

It is clear that the knowledge derived from basic research concerning surface marker and functional characterization of normal lymphocyte subsets already has made a significant contribution to the defining of certain ALL subgroups (notably T cell leukemia), which require different therapeutic approaches to achieve optimal clinical responses. The current goals in understanding childhood leukemia include the following:

1. Specifically categorizing subgroups and their prognoses at the time of diagnosis;
2. Individualizing therapy to the needs of the subgroups;
3. Identifying relapse trends during and after therapy;
4. Extending therapeutic efficacy to benefit all patients.

In closing, a word of caution must be raised: we must avoid use of new markers as a basis for novel therapeutic approaches before significant clinical manifestations and response data can be correlated to establish that these markers indeed indicate distinct subgroups requiring type-specific therapy. Any attempts to do otherwise would jeopardize the benefits we have derived.

REFERENCES

Anderson, J. K., J. O. Moore, J. M. Falletta, W. F. Terry, and R. S. Metzgar. 1979. Acute lymphoblastic leukemia: Classification and characterization with antisera to human T-cell and Ia antigens. J. Natl. Cancer Inst. 62:293–298.

Balch, C. M., and E. W. Ades. 1979. Heterogeneity of cell surface xenoantigens on human T lymphocytes. J. Reticuloendothel. Soc. 25:635–651.

Balch, C. M., P. A. Dougherty, L. B. Vogler, E. W. Ades, and S. Ferrone. 1978. A new B-cell differentiation antigen (BDA) on normal and leukemic human B lymphocytes that is distinct from known Dr (Ia-like) antigens. J. Immunol. 121:2322–2328.

Borella, L., J. T. Casper, and S. J. Lauer. 1979. Shifts in expression of cell membrane phenotypes in childhood lymphoid malignancies at relapse. Blood 54:64–71.

Broder, S., D. Poplack, J. Whang-Peng, M. Durm, C. Goldman, L. Muul, and T. Waldman. 1978. Characterization of a suppressor cell leukemia. N. Engl. J. Med. 298:66–72.

Brouet, J. C., and M. Seligmann. 1978. The immunological classification of acute lymphoblastic leukemias. Cancer 42:817–827.

Brouet, J.-C., F. Valensi, M.-T. Daniel, G. Flandrin, J.-L. Preud'homme, and M. Seligmann. 1976. Immunological classification of acute lymphoblastic leukaemias: Evaluation of its clinical significance in a hundred patients. Br. J. Haematol. 33:319–328.

Cantor, H., and E. A. Boyse. 1977. Lymphocytes as models for the study of mammalian cellular differentiation. Immunol. Rev. 33:105–124.

Chess, L., R. Evans, R. E. Humphreys, J. L. Strominger, and S. F. Schlossman. 1976. Inhibition of antibody-dependent cellular cytotoxicity and immunoglobulin synthesis by an antiserum prepared against a human B-cell Ia-like molecule. J. Exp. Med. 144:113–122.

Chess, L., and S. F. Schlossman. 1977. Functional analysis of distinct human T-cell subsets bearing unique differentiation antigens, in Contemporary Topics in Immunobiology, O. Stutman, ed. Plenum Press, New York, pp. 363–378.

Crist, W., L. Vogler, A. Sorrit, J. Pullen, A. Bartolucci, J. Falletta, B. Humphrey, J. van Eys, and M. Cooper. 1979. Clinical and laboratory characterization of pre-B cell leukemia in children (Abstract). Blood 54:183a.

Esber, E. C., N. Movassaghi, and S. L. Leikin. 1978. Surface membrane determinants on childhood acute lymphocytic leukaemia cells: Immunoglobulin, Fc and C3 receptors. Clin. Exp. Immunol. 32:523–530.

Evans, R. L., H. Lazarus, A. C. Penta, and S. F. Schlossman. 1978. Two functionally distinct subpopulations of human T-cells that collaborate in the generation of cytotoxic cells responsible for cell-mediated lympholysis. J. Immunol. 120:1423–1428.

Flandrin, G., J.-C. Brouet, M. T. Daniel, and J. Preud'homme. 1975. Acute leukemia with Burkitt's tumor cells: A study of six cases with special reference to lymphocyte surface markers. Blood 45:183–188.

Galili, V., and H. Schlesinger. 1975. Subpopulations of human thymus cells differing in their capacity to form stable E-rosettes and in their immunologic reactivity. J. Immunol. 115:827–833.

Gatien, J. C., E. E. Schneeberger, and E. Merler. 1975. Analysis of human thymocyte subpopulations using discontinuous gradients of albumin: Precursor lymphocytes in human thymus. Eur. J. Immunol. 5:312–317.

Gelfand, M. D., C. J. Elfenbein, M. M. Frank, and W. Paul. 1974. Ontogeny of B lymphocytes. J. Exp. Med. 139:1125–1141.

Goldstone, A. H., B. A. McVerry, G. Janossy, and H. Walker. 1979. Clonal identification in acute lymphoblastic leukemia. Blood 53:892–898.

Greaves, M., G. Brown, N. Rapson, and T. A. Lister. 1975. Antisera to acute lymphoblastic leukemia cells. Clin. Immunol. Immunopathol. 4:67–84.

Greaves, M., and G. Janossy. 1978. Patterns of gene expression and the cellular origins of human leukaemias. Biochim. Biophys. Acta 516:193–230.

Hämmerling, U., A. F. Chin, and J. Abbott. 1976. Ontogeny of murine B lymphocytes: Sequence of B-cell differentiation from surface immunoglobulin-negative precursors to plasma cells. Proc. Natl. Acad. Sci. U.S.A. 73:2008–2012.

Horowitz, D., and M. A. Garrett. 1976. Distinctive functional properties of human blood lymphocytes: A comparison with T lymphocytes, B lymphocytes, and monocytes. J. Immunol. 118:1712–1721.

Janossy, G., F. J. Bollum, K. F. Bradstock, A. McMichael, N. Rapson, and M. F. Greaves. 1979. Terminal transferase-positive human bone marrow cells exhibit the antigenic phenotype of common acute lymphoblastic leukemia. J. Immunol. 123:1525–1529.

Kaplan, J., Y. Ravendranath, and W. D. Peterson. 1977. T and B lymphocyte antigen-positive null cell leukemias. Blood 49:371–378.

Kearney, J. F., M. D. Cooper, J. Klein, E. Abney, M. Parkhouse, and A. Lawton. 1977. Ontogeny of Ia and IgD on IgM-bearing B lymphocytes in mice. J. Exp. Med. 146:297–301.

Kung, P. C., G. Goldstein, E. L. Reinherz, and S. F. Schlossman. 1979. Monoclonal antibodies defining distinctive human T-cell surface antigens. Science 206:347–349.

Lin, P. S., and C. C. S. Hsu. 1976. Human leukaemic T cells with complement receptors. Clin. Exp. Immunol. 23:209–213.

MacDermott, R. P., L. Chess, and S. F. Schlossman. 1975. Immunologic functions of isolated human lymphocyte subpopulations. V. Isolation and functional analysis of a surface Ig negative, E-rosette negative subset. Clin. Immunol. Immunopathol. 4:415–424.

McCaffrey, R., T. A. Harrison, R. Parkman, and D. Baltimore. 1975. Terminal deoxynucleotidyl transferase in human leukemic cells and in normal human thymocytes. N. Engl. J. Med. 292:775–780.

Mills, B., L. Sen, and L. Borella. 1975. Reactivity of antihuman thymocyte serum with acute leukemic blasts. J. Immunol. 115:1038–1044.

Mohanakumar, T., and R. S. Metzgar. 1974. Human thymus-leukemia related antigen(s): Detection by a non-human primate antiserum. Cell. Immunol. 12:30–36.

Moretta, L., M. D. Mingari, A. Moretta, and P. Lydard. 1977a. Receptors for IgM are expressed on acute lymphoblastic leukemic cells having T-cell characteristics. Clin. Immunol. Immunopathol. 7:405–409.

Moretta, L., S. R. Webb, C. E. Grosse, M. Lydard, and M. Cooper. 1977b. Functional analysis of two human T-cell subpopulations: Help and suppression of B-cell responses by T-cells bearing receptors for IgM or IgG. J. Exp. Med. 146:184–200.

Nowell, P. C. 1976. The clonal evolution of tumor cell populations. Science 194:23–28.

Owen, J. T., D. E. Wright, H. Sonoko, M. Raff, and M. Cooper. 1977. Studies on the generation of B lymphocytes in fetal liver and bone marrow. J. Immunol. 118:2067–2072.

Perkins, W. D., M. J. Karnovsky, and E. R. Unanue. 1972. An ultrastructural study of lymphocytes with surface-bound immunoglobulin. J. Exp. Med. 135:267–276.

Raff, M. C., M. Megson, J. J. T. Owen, and M. Cooper. 1976. Early production of intracellular IgM by B-lymphocyte precursors in mouse. Nature 259:224–226.

Reinherz, E. L., P. C. Kung, G. Goldstein, and S. F. Schlossman. 1979a. A monoclonal antibody with selective reactivity with functionally mature thymocytes and all peripheral human T-cells. J. Immunol. 123:1312–1317.

Reinherz, E. L., L. M. Nadler, S. E. Sallen, and S. F. Schlossman. 1979b. Subset derivation of T-cell acute lymphoblastic leukemia in man. J. Clin. Invest. 64:392–397.

Reinherz, E. L., and S. F. Schlossman. 1979. Con-A inducible suppression of MLC: Evidence for mediation by the TH_2^+ T-cell subset in man. J. Immunol. 122:1335–1341.

Richie, E., S. J. Culbert, M. P. Sullivan, and J. van Eys. 1978. Complement-receptor positive, E-receptor negative lymphoblasts in childhood acute lymphocytic leukemia. Cancer Res. 38:3616–3620.

Richie, E., and M. Patchen. 1978. Correlation between temperature-stable E-rosette formation and lymphocyte commitment to activation. Clin. Immunol. Immunopathol. 11:88–97.

Richie, E. R., M. P. Sullivan, and J. van Eys. 1980. A unique surface marker profile in T-cell acute lymphocytic leukemia. Blood 55:702.

Roberts, M., M. Greaves, G. Janossy, R. Sutherland, and C. Pain. 1978. Acute lymphoblastic leukemia (ALL) associated antigen. I. Expression in different haematopoietic malignancies. Leuk. Res. 2:105–144.

Rosenberg, Y., and C. R. Parish. 1977. Ontogeny of the antibody-forming cell line in mice. IV.

Appearance of cells bearing Fc receptors, complement receptors, and surface immunoglobulin. J. Immunol. 118:612–617.

Ross, D. G. 1979. Identification of human lymphocyte subpopulations by surface marker analysis. Blood 53:799–808.

Scheid, M. P., G. Goldstein, V. Hammerling, and E. Boyse. 1975. Lymphocyte differentiation from precursor cells in vitro. Ann. N.Y. Acad. Sci. 249:531–538.

Schlossman, S. F., L. Chess, R. E. Humphreys, and J. L. Strominger. 1976. Distribution of Ia-like molecules on the surface of normal and leukemic human cells. Proc. Natl. Acad. Sci. U.S.A. 73:1288–1292.

Sen, I., and L. Borella. 1975. Clinical importance of lymphoblasts with T markers in childhood acute leukemia. N. Engl. J. Med. 292:828–832.

Shore, A., H.-M. Dosch, and E. W. Gelfand. 1979. Expression and modulation of C3 receptors during early T-cell ontogeny. Cell. Immunol. 45:157–166.

Siegal, F. P. 1978. Cytoidentity of the lymphoreticular neoplasms, in The Immunopathology of Lymphoreticular Neoplasms, J. J. Twomey and R. A. Good, eds. Plenum Medical Book Co., New York, pp. 281–323.

Stein, H., N. Peterson, G. Gaedicke, K. Lennert, and G. Landbeck. 1976. Lymphoblastic lymphoma of convoluted or acid phosphatase type-A tumor of T precursor cells. Int. J. Cancer 17:292–295.

Sullivan, M. P., and A. Frias. 1977. Convoluted cell lymphoma and T-cell leukemia: Survival patterns of relapse and rescue with LSA$_2$L$_2$ therapy (Abstract). Proc. Am. Soc. Clin. Oncol. 18:305.

Touraine, J.-L., J. W. Hadden, and R. A. Good. 1977. Sequential stages of human T lymphocyte differentiation. Proc. Natl. Acad. Sci. U.S.A. 74:3414–3418.

Tsukimoto, I., K. Y. Wong, and B. C. Lampkin. 1976. Surface markers and prognostic factors in acute lymphoblastic leukemia. N. Engl. J. Med. 294:245–248.

Tucker, L. W., J. Hozier, J. Minowada, and J. H. Kersey. 1979. Origin of chronic myelocytic leukemia in a precursor of pre-B lymphocytes. N. Engl. J. Med. 301:144–147.

Vogler, L. B., W. M. Crist, D. E. Bockman, E. R. Pearl, A. R. Lawton, and M. D. Cooper. 1978. Pre-B cell leukemia: A new phenotype of childhood lymphoblastic leukemia. N. Engl. J. Med. 298:872–878.

Winfield, J. B., P. I. Lobo, and M. E. Hamilton. 1977. Fc receptor heterogeneity: Immunofluorescent studies of B, T and "third population" lymphocytes in human blood with rabbit IgG b4/anti-b4 complexes. J. Immunol. 119:1778–1784.

Zuelzer, W. W., S. Inoue, R. I. Thompson, and M. J. Ottenbreit. 1976. Long-term cytogenetic studies in acute leukemia of children, the nature of the relapse. Am. J. Hematol. 1:143–190.

Status of the Curability of Childhood Cancers,
edited by J. van Eys and M. P. Sullivan.
Raven Press, New York © 1980.

Non-Hodgkin's Lymphomas in Children

James J. Butler, M.D.

*Department of Pathology, The University of Texas System Cancer Center M. D. Anderson
Hospital and Tumor Institute, Houston, Texas*

Recently published reports on lymphomas in children have reflected major disagreements over many aspects of the disease. Fundamental to these disagreements is the question of whether or not the classification and staging methods used for adults apply equally well to children. At one extreme is a series (Wollner et al. 1975) in which all the histologic types of disease seen in adults were also found in children. At the other extreme is the series reported by Lukes and Collins (1977), who state that, with rare exceptions, only four histologic types of lymphoma are commonly seen in children. Staging for the majority of the published series has followed the Ann Arbor system (Carbone et al. 1971), which was initially introduced for staging Hodgkin's disease in adults. Wollner et al. (1975), from Memorial Hospital, and Murphy (1978), from St. Jude's Hospital, felt that this staging system did not apply well to children and introduced major modifications.

The current controversy regarding which classification of non-Hodgkin's lymphomas is best also applies to lymphomas in children. It has been variously reported that the Rappaport classification does not predict behavior in children as well as it does in adults (Byrne 1977), that the Kiel classification shows previously undetected clinical correlations (Garwicz et al. 1978), and that the classification of Lukes and Collins is more efficient (Lukes and Collins 1977). The Rappaport classification has been used in most reports (Glatstein et al. 1974, Hausner et al. 1977, Hutter et al. 1975, Jaffe et al. 1977, Murphy et al. 1975, Pinkel et al. 1975, Wollner et al. 1975), the Kiel classification in two reports (Garwicz et al. 1978, Lennert 1977), and the Lukes and Collins classification in one (Lukes and Collins 1977). All the proposed classifications agree that Burkitt's lymphoma is a special type. Whether or not the closely related lymphoma designated undifferentiated lymphoma, non-Burkitt's type, in the Rappaport classification has the same prognosis as Burkitt's lymphoma is not clear, however. Large cell ("histiocytic") lymphoma is also recognized in all the classifications, but the term to be used to designate this type is in question. Much of the disagreement regarding the histologic classification of childhood lymphomas results from failure to identify the type of lymphoma described by Barcos and Lukes (1975) as convoluted lymphocytic lymphoma and later designated as lymphoblastic lymphoma by Nathwani et al. (1976). Cases of this type of lymphoma appear to have previously been designated as poorly differentiated lymphocytic lymphoma or undifferentiated lymphoma, non-Burkitt's type, in the classification of Rappaport and, therefore, not identified as a specific type of disease.

The present study was initiated in an attempt to determine the histologic types of lymphomas seen in childhood and to better define them as to sites of involvement, incidence of development of leukemia and central nervous system involvement, and prognosis, using the Lukes-Collins classification. The present report is preliminary, including all patients who presented with nodal or extranodal masses from January 1950 through December 1974. A final report, to include the findings at autopsy and to cover the period from January 1950 through December 1977, is in preparation.

MATERIALS AND METHODS

All patients less than 16 years of age seen at M. D. Anderson Hospital from January 1950 through December 1974 with non-Hodgkin's lymphoma form the basis for this report. All patients with nodal or extranodal masses as presenting signs or the cause of the presenting symptoms were included, regardless of whether or not they were leukemic or had bone marrow involvement. "Leukemic" is used here to mean that greater than 10% abnormal cells were present in the peripheral blood. Only those cases in which histologic material and follow-up information were available are included. Cases of lymphoma that could not be classified because of insufficient tissue or poor quality of available material were eliminated. The Lukes-Collins classification of lymphomas was used because the terms are more descriptive and immunologically accurate than those in the Rappaport classification. The corresponding terms in the Rappaport classification are given in parentheses and are shown in Table 1. A slightly modified version of the staging system proposed by Murphy (1978) was used (Table 2) because it was developed for childhood lymphomas and because the Ann Arbor

Table 1. *Comparison of Classifications of Childhood Lymphomas*

Rappaport	Lukes-Collins
Large cell ("histiocytic")	Large cleaved FCC Large noncleaved FCC Immunoblastic sarcoma True histiocytic
Burkitt's Undifferentiated, non-Burkitt's	Small noncleaved FCC
Lymphoblastic	Convoluted

Table 2. *Clinical Staging Classification for Non-Hodgkin's Lymphoma in Children**

Stage	Description
I	A single tumor (extranodal) or single anatomic area (nodal), with the exclusion of the mediastinum or abdomen.
II	A single tumor (extranodal) with regional lymph node involvement. Two or more nodal areas on the same side of the diaphragm. Two single (extranodal) tumors with or without regional lymph node involvement on the same side of the diaphragm. A resectable primary gastrointestinal tract tumor, usually in the ileocecal area, with or without involvement of associated mesenteric nodes only.
III	Two single tumors (extranodal) on opposite sides of the diaphragm. Two or more nodal areas above and below the diaphragm. All the primary intrathoracic tumors (mediastinal, pleural, thymic). All extensive, unresectable, primary intra-abdominal disease. All paraspinal or epidural tumors, regardless of other tumor site(s).
IV	Any of the above with initial involvement of the central nervous system, bone marrow, or liver.

* Modified from Murphy (1978).

staging system did not appear to accurately reflect the behavior of tumors confined to the mediastinum or abdomen. The proposed system was modified by including in stage IV those patients who presented with proven liver involvement.

Hematoxylin and eosin-stained sections were examined in every case. In selected cases, when material was available, sections were examined after staining with methyl green Pyronine (MGP), Giemsa, and naphthol AS-D chloroacetate esterase.

After the lesions were classified histologically, information was obtained from hospital charts. The duration of survival was calculated from the date of biopsy. All patients had been untreated except for two who had received local X-ray therapy to the site of biopsy prior to being referred to this hospital. Abdominal involvement was designated as involving intestine only when the tumor was removed. Other abdominal involvement was designated as abdomen, not otherwise specified (NOS); in some instances enlarged intra-abdominal lymph nodes were demonstrated by intravenous pyelograms, lower limb lymphangiograms, or gastrointestinal series. The first lower limb lymphangiogram on a patient in this series was performed in 1966. The method of Lee and Desu (1972) was used to evaluate differences in survival curves.

HISTOLOGY

The distribution of cases by histologic type is given in Table 3. Convoluted (lymphoblastic) lymphoma is composed of noncohesive cells (Figure 1) that vary greatly in size and have a very thin rim of cytoplasm that can only be seen with the oil immersion lens of the microscope or the MGP stain. The

Table 3. *Distribution of Childhood Lymphoma Cases (MDAH 1950–74)*

Type	No. of Cases (%)
Convoluted (Lymphoblastic)	54 (48)
Small noncleaved follicular center cell (Undifferentiated)	46 (41)
Burkitt's	11
Non-Burkitt's	25
NOS	10
Immunoblastic sarcoma (Large cell or "histiocytic")	12 (11)
Large cleaved follicular center cell, follicular (Nodular large cell or "histiocytic")	1 (1)
Total	113

nuclear chromatin is finely dispersed, as in blast cells, and nucleoli are not prominent in well-fixed material. The nuclei have convolutions that are best appreciated by focusing the microscope on the various levels of the nucleus. While the outlines of the nuclei are often irregular, producing peculiarly shaped cells, the nuclei may have regular outlines with convolutions present only in the inner portion. These cells show high mitotic activity. In lymph nodes, prolifer-

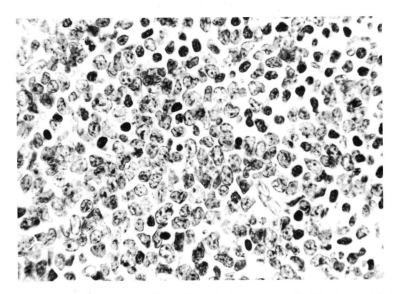

Figure 1. Convoluted (lymphoblastic) lymphoma in lymph node. Nuclei of convoluted cells vary in size and shape, while nuclei of small lymphocytes are small, dark staining, and relatively uniform in shape. Hematoxylin and eosin, reduced from ×400.

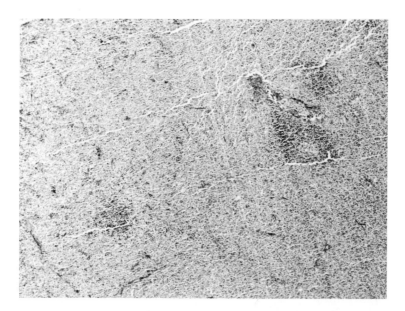

Figure 2. As a result of infiltration of lymph node by convoluted (lymphoblastic) lymphoma, islands of normal lymphocytes stand out. Hematoxylin and eosin, reduced from ×4.

ation of these cells seems to begin in the paracortical zone and then to extend to the cortex and medulla, isolating islands of normal lymphoid tissue (Figure 2). These cells are frequently associated with phagocytic histiocytes, producing the "starry sky" appearance that was once thought to be characteristic of Burkitt's tumor, but that may actually be seen in any lymphoma in which the cells have a high turnover rate. The nuclei of the phagocytic histiocytes serve as a reference for determining cell size. In well-fixed sections of convoluted lymphocytic lymphoma cells, the nuclei of the convoluted cells vary from slightly smaller than those of the phagocytic histiocytes to 1½ to 2 times as large. In poorly fixed material, the cells may be the size of small lymphocytes; this may result in an erroneous diagnosis of well-differentiated lymphocytic lymphoma.

Small noncleaved follicular center cell (SNCFCC) lymphoma, Burkitt's or non-Burkitt's (undifferentiated, non-Burkitt's) type, is composed of cells with a thin rim of amphophilic (plasma cell-like) cytoplasm that is strongly positive with the MGP stain and contains small vacuoles that can be demonstrated to contain neutral fat by special stains. The cells may be cohesive, if ideally fixed, and always exhibit high mitotic activity. The nuclei have coarsely reticulated chromatin and contain two to five small nucleoli. In the Burkitt's type, the nuclei of the tumor cells are all about the same size as the nuclei of the phagocytic histiocytes (Figure 3). In the non-Burkitt's type, the majority of the nuclei are the same size as or smaller than the nuclei of the phagocytic histiocytes, but a significant minority of the nuclei are distinctly larger and commonly

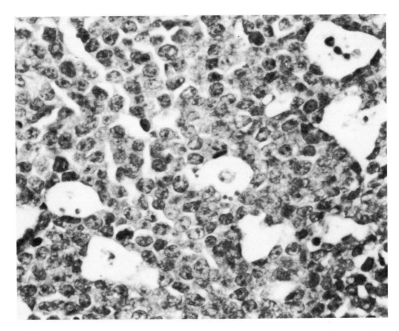

Figure 3. In SNCFCC lymphoma, Burkitt's type (Burkitt's lymphoma), nuclei of tumor cells are relatively uniform in size and about same size as nuclei of phagocytic histiocytes, one of which is in center. Hematoxylin and eosin, reduced from ×400.

have large nucleoli (Figure 4). In the present study, the poor quality of some sections of the older cases made it impossible to distinguish between these two types of disease; these cases were designated as SNCFCC lymphoma, NOS.

Immunoblastic sarcoma (IbS) of the B cell type (diffuse large cell or "histiocytic" lymphoma) is composed of transformed lymphocytes (immunoblasts) that have abundant amphophilic (plasmacytoid) cytoplasm that is frequently accentuated by eccentrically placed nuclei and is strongly pyroninophilic with the MGP stain. The nuclei are larger than those of the phagocytic histiocytes and have irregularly clumped chromatin and single prominent nucleoli (Figure 5). Nuclear pleomorphism, with occasional nuclei resembling those of Reed-Sternberg cells, is a common finding. Mature plasma cells are frequently found in varying numbers in association with the neoplastic cells.

One case of large cleaved follicular center cell (LCFCC), follicular (nodular large cell or "histiocytic"), lymphoma was also recognized. The follicular component was evident in only one part of the lymph node (Figure 6), with the remainder of the node showing a diffuse pattern. The cells making up this variant have irregular nuclear outlines, with the majority of nuclei larger than those of the phagocytic histiocytes. The cells have a thin, almost imperceptible, irregular rim of cytoplasm. The nuclei have clumped chromatin with small nucleoli (Figure 7).

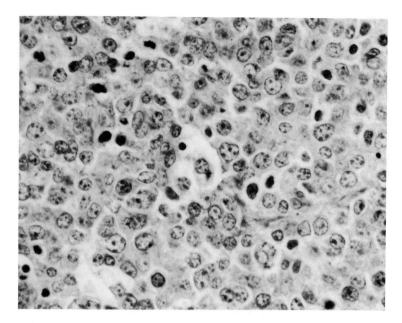

Figure 4. In SNCFCC lymphoma, non-Burkitt's type (undifferentiated, non-Burkitt's lymphoma), nuclei of lymphoma cells vary in size. Hematoxylin and eosin, reduced from ×400.

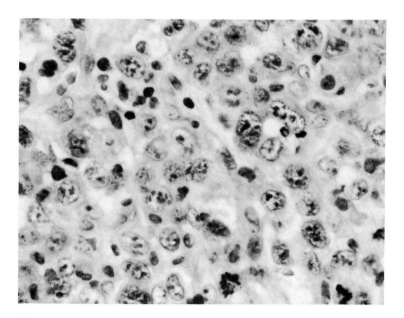

Figure 5. IbS, B cell type (large cell or "histiocytic" lymphoma). Many nuclei are large and have plasmacytoid cytoplasm. Several are lobulated. Hematoxylin and eosin, reduced from ×400.

Figure 6. LCFCC, follicular (nodular large cell or "histiocytic"), lymphoma. Poorly defined nodules of lymphoma cells are evident. Hematoxylin and eosin, reduced from ×4.

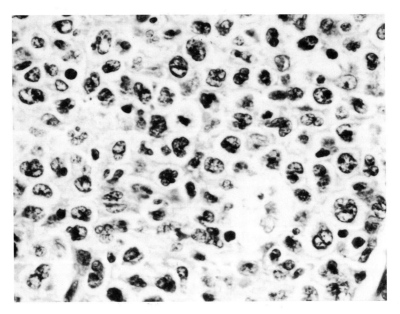

Figure 7. LCFCC, follicular (nodular large cell or "histiocytic"), lymphoma. Irregularities in nuclear size and shape are obvious. Hematoxylin and eosin, reduced from ×400.

CLINICAL FINDINGS

The patients were from 1 to 15 years of age when first seen, with the distributions for the three 5-year age groups given for the entire series and each histologic type in Table 4. The median age in both the convoluted and SNCFCC groups was 8 years. The median age for the IbS group was 12 years. The sex distribution and distribution by race are given in the same table. The large number of children of Spanish extraction in the present study is consistent with the percentage of children of Spanish extraction seen at the hospital with neoplasms of all types.

As indicated in Table 4, a marked male dominance was present in patients with two of the three histologic types, but not in the group with convoluted (lymphoblastic) lymphoma. Table 5 gives the sex distribution of the last group by anatomic site of involvement. While the sex distribution for the entire series of this histologic type shows almost equal numbers of males and females, more than twice as many males as females presented with mediastinal disease. Conversely, almost twice as many females as males presented without mediastinal disease.

According to the patients' histories, the presenting signs and symptoms of patients with SNCFCC lymphoma were abdominal pain in 25 patients, an abdominal mass in six, a mass in the neck in five, swelling of the jaw in three, and fever in two; axillary and cervical masses, constipation, nasal obstruction, and difficulty in swallowing were seen in one patient each.

In contrast, patients with convoluted lymphoma presented with a wide variety of signs and symptoms. Twelve patients presented with respiratory difficulties, and four with associated axillary masses; 21 patients presented with masses related to peripheral lymph nodes, localized to the cervical (12), inguinal (five),

Table 4. *Distribution of Lymphoma Patients by Age, Sex, and Race*

Variable	Convoluted (Lymphoblastic)	SNCFCC (Undifferentiated)	IbS (Large Cell)*	Total
Age (yrs)				
1–5	16	18	2	36
6–10	18	15	2	35
11–15	20	13	8	42†
Sex				
Male	28	38	9	76†
Female	26	8	3	37
Race				
White	39	35	11	85
Black	3	1	0	4
Latin	11	10	1	23†
Other	1	0	0	1
Total	54	46	12	

* "Histiocytic."
† One patient with LCFCC lymphoma, follicular.

Table 5. *Comparison of Sites of Involvement in Convoluted (Lymphoblastic) Lymphoma Patients by Sex*

	No. of Patients (%)	
Site	Male	Female
Mediastinum	17 (68)	8 (32)
Mediastinum normal	11 (38)	18 (62)
Generalized lymph nodes	7 (70)	3 (30)
Skin	2 (28)	5 (72)
Other	5 (33)	10 (67)
Total	28 (52)	26 (48)

or axillary (two) regions in 19. Four patients presented with tumors of the face, two with masses of the cheek, one with a soft tissue mass of the periorbital region, and one with a mass involving the lower jaw. Ten patients presented with nodules or masses involving skin (six patients) or soft tissue of the shoulder, chest, leg, or testis (one each). The chest mass was apparently edema secondary to a mediastinal mass, since it was not described on the admitting physical examination and the diagnosis was established by biopsy of a scalene lymph node. One patient presented with only fever. Pain was the presenting complaint in the final six patients. In three patients the pain was localized to the abdomen. One patient, who had epigastric pain and a mediastinal mass, never exhibited evidence of abdominal disease. A second patient, presenting with abdominal pain, was found to have necrosis of a portion of the small bowel without evidence of lymphoma in the bowel wall; an upper gastrointestinal series demonstrated extrinsic pressure on the duodenum, presumably by enlarged retroperitoneal lymph nodes. The cause of the abdominal pain in the third patient, who presented with masses in the cervical and inguinal regions and both breasts, was not apparent; the patient has never developed abdominal disease and is alive without evidence of lymphoma over 5 years after diagnosis. A fourth patient presented with leg pain associated with an osteolytic lesion of the long bones of the leg. The other two patients experienced chest pain (mediastinal mass) and pharyngeal pain (tonsils).

Patients with IbS also presented with a wide variety of signs and symptoms. Four patients presented with masses related to peripheral lymph nodes; two patients had masses in the axilla, one in the neck, and one in both the axilla and neck. Four patients presented with masses of soft tissue, one in the thigh, one in the calf and clavicular region, one in the lower jaw, and one in the lateral chest wall. One patient presented with an abdominal mass as a result of retroperitoneal lymph node enlargement. In two patients the presenting complaint was pain, one in the abdomen associated with intestinal involvement and the other in the chest associated with a mediastinal mass. The final patient had a skin lesion over the iliac crest associated with an axillary mass.

The patient with LCFCC, follicular, lymphoma presented with a left inguinal

Table 6. *Sites of Involvement on Physical and Laboratory Examination*

Site	Convoluted	SNCFCC	IbS
Mediastinum	25 (8)	1	2
Generalized lymph nodes	10 (5)	0	0
Cervical lymph nodes	20 (3)	5 (2)	6 (1)
Axillary lymph nodes	11	1	4 (1)
Retroperitoneal lymph nodes	3	2 (1)	1 (1)
Inguinal lymph nodes	6 (3)	0	0
Skin	7 (3)	0	2
Soft tissue	3 (2)	4	4 (3)
Intestine	0	20 (17)	1 (1)
Abdomen, NOS	1	15 (8)	0
Tonsils and nasopharynx	2	3 (1)	0
Pleural fluid	5	3	0
Bone	2	2	0
Jaw	2 (1)	4 (1)	0
Liver	0	1 (1)	0
Bone marrow	23	5	0
Leukemia	8	0	0

( ) Only finding.

mass. This was the only finding on physical examination also. The lower limb lymphangiogram, following biopsy of the left inguinal mass, showed abnormalities of the remaining inguinal lymph nodes on the same side.

The sites of involvement on physical and laboratory examination by histologic type are indicated in Table 6. It is apparent that convoluted lymphoma is a disease of lymph nodes, predominately above the diaphragm, and skin, while SNCFCC lymphoma is primarily infradiaphragmatic disease involving the intestines in addition to soft tissue and bone. Too few patients with IbS were in the study to determine a characteristic pattern of involvement.

The distributions of patients by stage for each histologic type are given in Figure 8. This figure also indicates the incidence of involvement of the mediastinum and abdomen for each stage. "Abdominal" is used here to indicate any type of abdominal involvement.

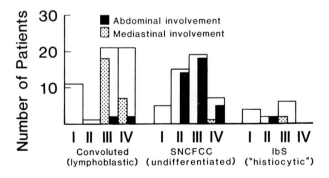

Figure 8. Distribution of patients by clinical stage.

Table 7. *Number of Patients with Leukemia and Bone Marrow Involvement by Histologic Type of Lymphoma*

Type	Leukemia	Bone Marrow Involvement*	Total
Convoluted (Lymphoblastic)	36 (67%)	43 (80%)	54
SNCFCC (Undifferentiated)	2 (4%)	7 (15%)	46
IbS (Large cell or "histiocytic")	1 (8%)	1 (8%)	12
LCFCC, follicular (Nodular large cell or "histiocytic" lymphoma)	0 (0%)	0 (0%)	1
Total	39 (35%)	51 (45%)	113

* One patient did not have a bone marrow examination.

The frequencies of development of leukemia for the entire series and for each histologic type are given in Table 7. It is apparent that leukemia occurs primarily in patients with convoluted lymphoma. Table 8 shows no significant differences in the incidence of leukemia by site of involvement or sex in patients with convoluted lymphoma. Although most patients showed leukemic conversion within 9 months of diagnosis, over 2 years elapsed before three patients became leukemic (Table 9). A comparison of patients seen in 1967 or before and those seen after that date (Table 9) shows that the incidences of leukemia on admission were essentially the same for the two time periods. The overall incidence of leukemia, however, was less for the latter period. Also, those who became leukemic during the 1968–74 period did so at a later date. The incidence of bone marrow involvement was less for the latter period, but not significantly so.

Nineteen of the 20 patients with convoluted lymphoma who developed bone marrow involvement after admission developed leukemia; the one exception developed bone marrow involvement 2 months after the diagnosis was established

Table 8. *Incidence of Leukemia Related to Site of Involvement and Sex of Patient with Convoluted (Lymphoblastic) Lymphoma*

Variable	Patients with Leukemia	Total
All patients	36 (67%)	54
Site		
Mediastinum	18 (72%)	25
Mediastinum normal	18 (62%)	29
Generalized lymph nodes	7 (70%)	10
Skin	3 (43%)	7
Sex		
Male	18 (64%)	28
Female	18 (69%)	26

Table 9. *Incidence of Leukemia and Bone Marrow and Cerebrospinal Fluid Involvement for Convoluted (Lymphoblastic) Lymphoma Patients*

Variable	1950–67	1968–74	Total Series
Total no. of patients	34*	20	54*
Leukemia	26 (76%)	10 (50%)	36 (67%)
On admission	6 (18%)	2 (10%)	8 (15%)
1–9 mo. later	17 (50%)	2 (10%)	19 (35%)
12–39 mo. later*	3 (9%)	6 (30%)	9 (17%)
CSF involvement	13 (38%)	7 (35%)	20 (37%)
CSF involvement, no leukemia	3 (9%)	2 (10%)	5 (9%)
Leukemia or CSF involvement	29 (85%)	12 (60%)	41 (76%)
BM involvement	29 (88%)	14 (70%)	43 (81%)
On admission	15 (45%)	8 (40%)	23 (43%)
Later	14 (42%)	6 (30%)	20 (38%)
BM involvement, no leukemia or CSF involvement	2 (6%)	3 (15%)	5 (9%)
Leukemia or CSF or BM involvement	31 (91%)	15 (75%)	46 (85%)

* One patient did not have a bone marrow examination.
CSF, cerebrospinal fluid; BM, bone marrow.

and died 2 months later. Fourteen patients who developed bone marrow involvement after admission developed leukemia within 2 months of bone marrow involvement. The five remaining patients developed leukemia within 4 to 24 months of bone marrow conversion.

One of the two patients with SNCFCC lymphoma who developed leukemia did so 8 months after diagnosis and 2 weeks prior to death. The other patient became leukemic 3 months after diagnosis and 2 months prior to death. One patient with IbS developed leukemia 2 months after diagnosis, 3 weeks prior to death. The patient with LCFCC, follicular, lymphoma has not developed leukemia or bone marrow involvement.

Involvement of the central nervous system (CNS), as evidenced by lymphoma cells in the cerebrospinal fluid (CSF), was most common in patients with convoluted lymphoma (37%) and was not seen in any of those with IbS; six (13%) of the 46 patients with SNCFCC lymphoma showed involvement of the CNS. As shown in Table 10, the CSF was positive most frequently in patients with convoluted lymphoma when the patient had positive bone marrow or leukemia. In contrast, the frequency of CNS involvement was not influenced by the presence or absence of mediastinal involvement, the stage of the disease, or the sex of the patient. Four of the six patients with SNCFCC lymphoma who developed CNS involvement also had bone marrow involvement by lymphoma, but only two of these patients were leukemic; five of the six had abdominal involvement.

SURVIVAL

Figure 9 compares the survival rates of patients by histologic type. The differences between the three types are not significant. In all three types a rapid

Table 10. *Relationship of Cerebrospinal Fluid Involvement to Other Factors in Patients with Convoluted (Lymphoblastic) Lymphoma*

Variable	Patients with CSF Involvement	Total No. of Patients
Mediastinal mass	10 (40%)	25
No mediastinal mass	10 (34%)	29
Leukemia	15 (42%)	36
No leukemia	5 (28%)	18
BM involvement	17 (40%)	43*
No BM involvement	2 (20%)	10
Stage I or II	5 (42%)	12
Stage III or IV	15 (36%)	42
Male	11 (39%)	28
Female	9 (35%)	26
Total	20 (37%)	54

* One patient did not have a bone marrow examination.
CSF, cerebrospinal fluid; BM, bone marrow.

drop occurs in the survival curve in the first 12 months, with less than 50% of the patients with all types alive after that time. While the curve for patients with IbS shows the most marked drop, with only three (25%) of the patients alive at 12 months, only one of the three patients has subsequently died. The survival curve for the SNCFCC group continues to fall rapidly until 18 months after diagnosis, then falls more slowly until 30 months, when it becomes flat. None of the patients surviving 30 months has subsequently died. In contrast, the survival of the convoluted group declines progressively less rapidly after it reaches a 50% level at 6 months, but continues to fall, even after 5 years.

In the SNCFCC group, the survival rates for patients with the Burkitt's,

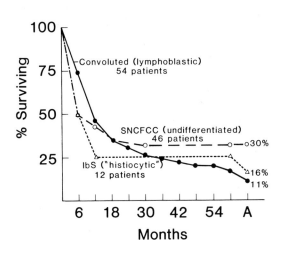

Figure 9. Survival rates for patients with convoluted (lymphoblastic), SNCFCC (undifferentiated), and IbS (large cell or "histiocytic") lymphoma. A = alive.

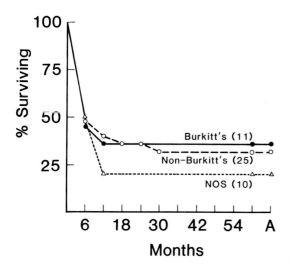

Figure 10. Survival rates for patients with various types of SNCFCC (undifferentiated) lymphoma.

non-Burkitt's, and NOS types were not significantly different (Figure 10). Because of this finding, the subtypes were not analyzed separately.

Since the last M. D. Anderson conference on tumors of the pediatric age group was held in 1967, a comparison was made between the survival of patients seen in the 1950–67 and 1968–74 time periods for both the convoluted (Figure 11) and SNCFCC (Figure 12) groups. For both groups the survival was significantly better for patients seen between 1968 and 1974 ($p = .05$ for the SNCFCC group and $p < .001$ for the convoluted group).

Staging predicts survival much better for patients with SNCFCC lymphoma (Figure 13) than for those with the convoluted type (Figure 14). For the SNCFCC group, the difference between stages I–II and III–IV is significant ($p < .001$).

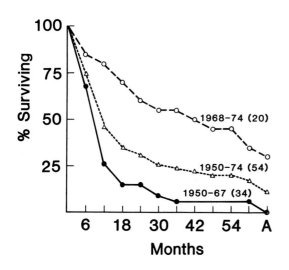

Figure 11. Survival rates for 1950–67, 1968–74, and 1950–74 for patients with convoluted (lymphoblastic) lymphoma.

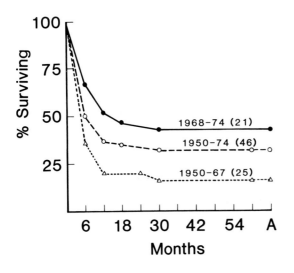

Figure 12. Survival rates for 1950–67, 1968–74, and 1950–74 for patients with SNCFCC (undifferentiated) lymphoma.

That between stages I–II and III of the convoluted group also is significant ($p = .007$), but that between stages I–II and IV is not. Patients with convoluted lymphoma and mediastinal disease have a significantly poorer survival rate ($p = .002$) than patients without mediastinal disease (Figure 15). The IbS group was too small to evaluate the effects of clinical stage on survival.

Figure 16 documents the importance of leukemia as a predictor of poor survival ($p = .04$) in patients with convoluted lymphoma. An involved bone marrow predicts almost as well; the difference between the two is not significant. The survival of patients who have leukemia when first seen is not significantly different from that of patients developing leukemia at any time during the course of the disease.

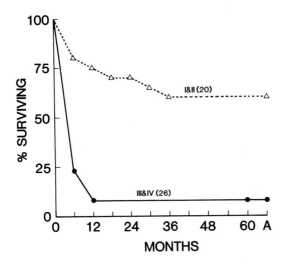

Figure 13. Survival rates for patients with SNCFCC (undifferentiated) lymphoma by clinical stage.

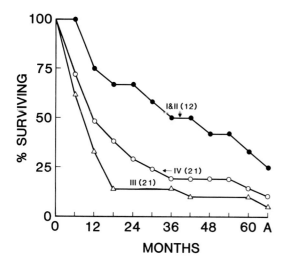

Figure 14. Survival rates for patients with convoluted (lymphoblastic) lymphoma by clinical stage.

A significant difference in survival related to age was not found in any of the three groups. A significant difference in survival related to the sex was not found in patients with convoluted lymphoma; the other two groups had too few females for an evaluation of this parameter. The presence of CNS involvement in patients with convoluted lymphoma did not correlate with a poorer survival.

DISCUSSION

A comparison of various series of children with non-Hodgkin's lymphoma is difficult for a number of reasons. Foremost among these is the failure to use an appropriate classification; any series that does not identify cases of convo-

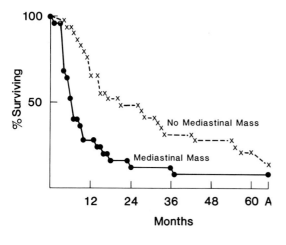

Figure 15. Survival rates for patients with convoluted (lymphoblastic) lymphoma with and without mediastinal mass.

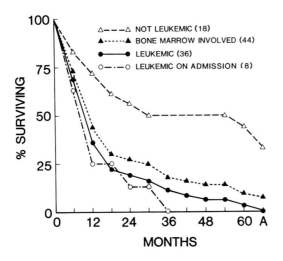

Figure 16. Survival rates for patients with convoluted (lymphoblastic) lymphoma with and without leukemia and bone marrow involvement.

luted (lymphoblastic) lymphoma fails to identify the most common lymphoma in childhood. Only the series reported by Lukes and Collins (1977) and the reports by Murphy et al. (1975) and Hausner et al. (1977) include this term in the classification used. The term is employed in the two reports using the Kiel classification (Garwicz et al. 1978, Lennert 1977), but the number of cases with this diagnosis in these studies suggests a more restrictive use of the term. The present report is also difficult to compare with others because it includes patients who were leukemic or who had bone marrow involvement at the time of diagnosis. Of 11 recent reports of childhood lymphoma, none included patients who were initially leukemic, four (Glatstein et al. 1974, Hausner et al. 1977, Jaffe et al. 1977, Wollner et al. 1975) accepted patients with bone marrow involvement of any type, two (Garwicz et al. 1978, Murphy et al. 1975) accepted only patients with focal bone marrow involvement, and three (Hutter et al. 1975, Lanerle et al. 1975, Pinkel et al. 1975) excluded all patients with bone marrow involvement. The status of the peripheral blood and bone marrow is not available in the study reported by Lukes and Collins (1977) and a study by Brecher et al. (1978). Finally, the upper ages accepted for inclusion in the reports on childhood lymphoma are not consistent; in three reports (Garwicz et al. 1978, Hutter et al. 1975, Murphy et al. 1975) it is 15 years, in one (Brecher et al. 1978) 16, in two (Glatstein et al. 1974, Pinkel et al. 1975) 17, in two (Hausner et al. 1977, Jaffe et al. 1977) 19, and in three (Lanerle et al. 1975, Lukes and Collins 1977, Wollner et al. 1975) it is not stated.

The question has been raised by others (Byrne 1977, Murphy et al. 1975) whether or not the Rappaport classification is applicable to childhood lymphomas. One reason for this doubt is the extreme rarity in children of nodular lymphoma, the most easily recognized type in the Rappaport classification and the one associated with a good prognosis. Also, as noted above, all but two of the published reviews of childhood lymphoma using the Rappaport classification have failed to recognize the convoluted (lymphoblastic) type of lymphoma, which is included in the modified Rappaport classification (Nathwani et al. 1978) and is the most common lymphoma in children reported in the present study and by Lukes and Collins (1977). The Rappaport classification is actually even better when applied to children than to adults since children do not manifest the variety of large cell or "histiocytic" lymphomas seen in adults; Strauchen et al. (1978) have shown that large cell ("histiocytic") lymphoma actually includes three different entities from the Lukes-Collins classification, IbS, large, noncleaved follicular center cell (LNCFCC) lymphoma, and LCFCC lymphoma, all with different prognostic implications. The Lukes-Collins classification was used in this study because it is more immunologically relevant.

The incidence of convoluted lymphoma in the present study (48%) is very similar to that reported by Lukes and Collins (1977) (49%). The incidence of SNCFCC lymphoma in the present study (41%) is also similar to that reported by Lukes and Collins (40%). The incidence of IbS was 10% in the present study and 7% in the earlier study. Lukes and Collins reported 1% of the patients had LCFCC lymphoma with sclerosis, as does the present report; the case in the present report had a follicular pattern, which was not found in the case in the earlier report. Lukes and Collins also reported two cases of true histiocytic lymphoma, none of which was seen in the present study.

The modified staging system used in this report was prognostically significant for children. In the SNCFCC group, only one stage III and no stage IV patients survived more than 10 months following diagnosis. The one living patient presented with a large unresectable abdominal mass that was biopsied. The patient is alive without evidence of disease at 118 months. In the convoluted group the results are not so striking, but the difference between stages I–II and III disease is significant ($p = .007$), whereas the difference between stages I–II and IV is not. The effect of stage on the IbS group cannot be determined because of the small size of the group. The three children in this group who survived more than 5 years were in stage I (two patients) or II (one patient) and were first seen after 1968. The other nine patients were in stages I–III and died in 12 months or less. The findings in the SNCFCC and convoluted lymphoma groups suggest that only two clinical stages need to be recognized in non-Hodgkin's lymphoma in children, one combining stages I and II and the other combining stages III and IV.

The overall age incidences in the present study are similar to those in three previous reports (Garwicz et al. 1978, Hutter et al. 1975, Lanerle et al. 1975) in that almost equal numbers of children were seen in each 5-year age group. They differ from those in five other studies (Brecher et al. 1978, Glatstein et al. 1974, Hausner et al. 1977, Jaffe et al. 1977, Murphy et al. 1975) in which only 20% or less of the children were under 6 years of age. The breakdown of patients according to age is not given in three studies (Lukes and Collins 1977, Pinkel et al. 1975, Wollner et al. 1975).

The sex distribution of the patients for the entire series is similar to that in five other series (Glatstein et al. 1974, Lanerle et al. 1975, Murphy et al. 1974, Pinkel et al. 1975, Wollner et al. 1975), where the male-to-female ratio was approximately 2 to 1. In four other series (Brecher et al. 1978, Garwicz et al. 1978, Hausner et al. 1977, Hutter et al. 1975) the ratio was greater than 3 to 1; in two of these series (Garwicz et al. 1978, Hutter et al. 1975) the age incidences were more similar to those in the present study. One study (Jaffe et al. 1977) contained only slightly more males than females. The sex distribution was not given in one study (Lukes and Collins 1977).

The convoluted group in the present series contained almost equal numbers of males and females because of the predominance of females among those in whom the mediastinum was not involved and a predominance of males among those in whom the mediastinum was involved, as indicated in Table 5. This predominance of females in patients who did not have mediastinal masses was also reported by Barcos and Lukes (1975) in their original article on convoluted lymphoma.

It is possible that the equal distribution by sex reflects an increased number of patients with non-T, non-B cell lymphomas in the group without mediastinal masses. Kersey et al. (1979) reported that the sex ratio was 1 to 1 in this group and that the median age of the patients was considerably less than for the T cell lymphoma group (6 vs. 12 years). In the present study the median age of the patients with convoluted lymphoma and mediastinal involvement was 9 years, while the median age of patients without mediastinal involvement was 7 years. The difference in sex distribution in the convoluted group may also be partially explained by the presence of two different subsets of T lymphocytes, as reported by Reinherz et al. (1979). In their report on acute lymphocytic leukemia, they identified a TH_2+ group, which had a male-to-female ratio of 0.66 to 1, with a mediastinal mass in only two of five patients and a mean survival of 36 months, and a TH_2- group, with a male-to-female ratio of 3.3 to 1, 11 of 13 patients with a mediastinal mass, and a mean survival of 11 months. In the present study the mean survival of patients with convoluted lymphoma who had a mediastinal mass was 13 months and the mean survival of those without a mediastinal mass was 34 months. These findings suggest an intermixture of non-T, non-B cell lymphoma with T cell lymphomas, with more of the former, together with the TH_2+ subset of T cell lymphomas reported by Reinherz et al. (1979), included in the nonmediastinal group. Unfortunately, cell surface marker studies are not available in this retrospective study.

The incidence of mediastinal involvement in this series, 25%, is slightly lower than the range of 29–36% reported in six other studies (Brecher et al. 1978, Glatstein et al. 1974, Hausner et al. 1977, Hutter et al. 1975, Jaffe et al. 1977, Pinkel et al. 1975), but slightly higher than the 16–20% found in two other studies (Murphy et al. 1975, Wollner et al. 1975). In the present study 46% of patients with convoluted lymphoma had mediastinal masses, compared with 52% in the study reported by Lukes and Collins (1977). The overall incidence of abdominal involvement in the present study, 39%, compares with the range of 19–55% in six other studies (Glatstein et al. 1974, Hausner et al. 1977,

Hutter et al. 1975, Jaffe et al. 1977, Murphy et al. 1975, Wollner et al. 1975). In the present series 80% of patients with SNCFCC lymphoma had abdominal involvement, compared to 72% in the study reported by Lukes and Collins (1977). Enlarged lymph nodes were the primary finding in 24% of the patients in the present study, which compares with a range of 16–26% in five other series (Brecher et al. 1978, Hutter et al. 1975, Jaffe et al. 1977, Murphy et al. 1975, Wollner et al. 1975).

It is not possible to compare the incidence of leukemic relapse in this study with that reported by others because it is not clear in the majority of studies if this term refers to the appearance of peripheral blood or to bone marrow involvement.

Central nervous system involvement occurred in 26 (23%) of the patients in the present series, 20 (37%) of the convoluted, six (13%) of the SNCFCC, and none of the IbS patients. In five other series (Garwicz et al. 1978, Glatstein et al. 1974, Hausner et al. 1977, Hutter et al. 1975, Murphy et al. 1975) the incidence varied from 10% to 32%. In one series (Hutter et al. 1975) all the patients with CNS involvement presented with both mediastinal masses and diffuse, poorly differentiated lymphocytic lymphoma. This combination was not found in any other series. In the present series 61% of the patients with CNS involvement did not have mediastinal masses. In the convoluted lymphoma group in the present series, 10 (40%) of the 25 patients who had mediastinal masses and 10 (35%) of the 29 patients who did not have mediastinal involvement had CNS disease. In the present series 84% of the patients with CNS involvement also had positive bone marrow at some time during the course of their disease, but only 65% had leukemia. Survival was the same, regardless of whether or not CNS involvement was present. There was no relationship between CNS involvement and the patient's sex or presenting clinical stage.

It is of interest that the median age of the IbS group is significantly older (12 years) than that of the other two groups (8 years each). This difference was also reported by Lukes and Collins (1977). As noted, the median age of patients in the convoluted group with mediastinal disease was 9 years and that of those without mediastinal disease was 7 years.

The relationship found between bone marrow involvement, leukemia, and mediastinal involvement in the convoluted group is an interesting one. In the group that presented with bone marrow involvement, 74% eventually developed leukemia and 39% had mediastinal masses. In contrast, 95% of patients who developed bone marrow involvement after admission developed leukemia and 60% had mediastinal involvement. The lower incidences of leukemia and me-diastinal masses in the first group also suggest some similarity to the non-T, non-B cell lymphoma–leukemia group described by Kersey et al. (1979). The higher incidences of leukemia and mediastinal involvement in the second group are similar to those in the T cell lymphoma group described by these authors. A significant difference in survival is not present between these groups, in spite of a somewhat higher incidence of leukemia in the second group.

Although the survival for the 1968–74 time period is significantly better for

Table 11. *Survival by Sex in Patients with Convoluted (Lymphoblastic) Lymphoma*

Years	Total No. of Patients	Patients Alive at 2 Years		Patients Alive at 5 Years	
		Male	Female	Male	Female
1950–67	34	1/17 (6%)	4/17 (24%)	0/17 (0%)	1/17 (6%)
1968–74	20	7/11 (64%)	5/9 (56%)	3/11 (27%)	4/9 (44%)
Total	54	8/28 (29%)	9/26 (35%)	3/28 (11%)	5/26 (19%)

all groups than that for 1950–67, the significance of mediastinal disease and leukemia as prognostic features is the same for both periods in the convoluted group. In the later period children with convoluted lymphoma continued to develop recurring disease and die, even after 24 months (Table 11). The survival of boys is significantly better for the later period, but still does not equal that of girls.

This review of childhood lymphomas seen at this hospital from 1950 to 1974 confirms that there are three main histologic types of lymphoma in children. Patients with convoluted (lymphoblastic) lymphoma presented primarily with involvement of the mediastinum, peripheral lymph nodes, and skin. These patients had a high incidence of leukemia and bone marrow and CNS involvement. Survival was poor in patients with leukemia or mediastinal masses. Relapse with death occurred in 11 patients who had survived more than 2 years and two patients who had survived more than 5 years. Convoluted (lymphoblastic) lymphoma appears to be the tissue counterpart of one type of acute lymphocytic leukemia.

Patients with SNCFCC (undifferentiated, non-Burkitt's, or Burkitt's) lymphoma presented primarily with involvement of the abdominal viscera. Leukemia, bone marrow involvement, and CNS involvement were each present in 15% or less of the patients in this study. Only one patient who survived more than 2 years has died.

IbS (large cell or "histiocytic" lymphoma) occurred in older children who presented primarily with involvement of lymph nodes and soft tissue. Leukemia and bone marrow involvement rarely developed in these patients. Involvement of the CNS was not seen. Patients relapsed even after surviving 5 years.

ACKNOWLEDGMENT

The author acknowledges the help of Barry W. Brown, Ph.D., who performed the statistical analysis.

REFERENCES

Barcos, M. D., and R. J. Lukes. 1975. Malignant lymphoma of convoluted lymphocytes: A new entity of possible T-cell type, *in* Conflicts in Childhood Cancer: An Evaluation of Current Management, vol. 4, L. F. Sinks and J. O. Godden, eds. Alan R. Liss, Inc., New York, pp. 147–178.

Brecher, M. L., L. F. Sinks, R. R. M. Thomas, and A. I. Freeman. 1978. Non-Hodgkin's lymphoma in children. Cancer 41:1997–2001.

Byrne, G. E. 1977. Rappaport classification of non-Hodgkin's lymphoma: Histologic features and clinical significance. Cancer Treat. Rep. 61:935–944.

Carbone, P. P., H. S. Kaplan, K. Musshoff, D. W. Smithers, and M. Tubiana. 1971. Report of the Committee on Hodgkin's Disease Staging Classification. Cancer Res. 31:1860–1861.

Garwicz, S., T. Landberg, L.-G. Lindberg, and M. Åkerman. 1978. Clinico-pathological correlations in the Kiel classification of non-Hodgkin's lymphomata in children. Scand. J. Haematol. 20:171–180.

Glatstein, E., H. Kim, S. S. Donaldson, R. F. Dorfman, T. J. Gribble, J. R. Wilbur, S. A. Rosenberg, and H. S. Kaplan. 1974. Non-Hodgkin's lymphomas. VI. Results of treatment in childhood. Cancer 34:204–211.

Hausner, R. J., A. Rosas-Uribe, D. A. Wickstrum, and P. C. Smith. 1977. Non-Hodgkin's lymphoma in the first two decades of life. Cancer 40:1533–1547.

Hutter, J. J., B. E. Fauara, M. Nelson, and C. P. Holton. 1975. Non-Hodgkin's lymphoma in children: Correlation of CNS disease with initial presentation. Cancer 36:2132–2137.

Jaffe, N., D. Buell, J. R. Cassady, D. Traggis, and H. Weinstein. 1977. Role of staging in childhood non-Hodgkin's lymphoma. Cancer Treat. Rep. 61:1001–1007.

Kersey, J. H., T. W. LeBiem, R. Hurwitz, M. E. Nesbit, K. J. Gajl-Peczalska, D. Hammond, D. R. Miller, P. F. Coccia, and S. Leikin. 1979. Childhood leukemia–lymphoma: Heterogeneity of phenotypes and prognosis. Am. J. Clin. Pathol. (suppl.) 72:746–752.

Lanerle, M., R. Gerard-Marchant, H. Sancho, and O. Schweisguth. 1975. Natural history of non-Hodgkin's malignant lymphomata in children. Br. J. Cancer 31(suppl. 2):324–331.

Lee, E., and M. Desu. 1972. A computer program for comparing K samples with right-censored data. Comput. Programs Biomed. 2:315–321.

Lennert, K. 1977. Klassifikation der non-Hodgkin-lymphome in kindesalter. Klin. Paediatr. 189:7–13.

Lukes, R. J., and R. D. Collins. 1977. Lukes-Collins classification and its significance. Cancer Treat. Rep. 61:971–979.

Murphy, S. B., G. Frizzera, and A. E. Evans. 1975. A study of childhood non-Hodgkin's lymphoma. Cancer 36:2121–2131.

Murphy, S. B. 1978. Current concepts in cancer: Childhood non-Hodgkin's lymphoma. N. Engl. J. Med. 299:1446–1448. 1978.

Nathwani, B. N., H. Kim, and H. Rappaport. 1976. Malignant lymphoma, lymphoblastic. Cancer 38:968–983.

Nathwani, B. N., H. Kim, H. Rappaport, J. Solomon, and M. Fox. 1978. Non-Hodgkin's lymphoma: A clinicopathologic study comparing two classifications. Cancer 41:303–325.

Pinkel, D., W. Johnson, and R. J. A. Aur. 1975. Non-Hodgkin's lymphoma in children. Br. Jr. Cancer 31(suppl. 2):298–323.

Reinherz, E. L., L. M. Nadler, S. E. Sallan, and S. F. Schlossman. 1979. Subset derivation of T-cell acute lymphoblastic leukemia in man. J. Clin. Invest. 64:392–397.

Strauchen, J. A., R. C. Young, V. T. DeVita, T. Anderson, J. C. Fantone, and C. W. Berard. 1978. Clinical relevance of the histopathological subclassification of diffuse "histiocytic" lymphoma. N. Engl. J. Med. 299:1382–1387.

Wollner, N., J. H. Burchenal, P. H. Lieberman, P. R. Exelby, G. J. D'Angio, and M. L. Murphy. 1975. Non-Hodgkin's lymphoma in children. Med. Pediatr. Oncol. 1:235–263.

Status of the Curability of Childhood Cancers,
edited by J. van Eys and M. P. Sullivan.
Raven Press, New York © 1980.

Lymphatic Leukemia: Spectrum of Outcome

Brigid G. Leventhal, M.D.

*The Johns Hopkins Oncology Center, The Johns Hopkins University School of Medicine,
Baltimore, Maryland*

The spectrum of outcome in the treatment of leukemia varies. In this review we will attempt to cite the factors that are important in evaluating outcome at each stage of the disease.

PREDISPOSING FACTORS

Exposure to ionizing radiation in childhood predisposes one to the development of acute lymphatic leukemia (ALL) (Miller 1977). This may be effected as a consequence of radiation damage to chromosome structure. Hereditary disorders involving chromosomal instability or defects in DNA repair also predispose one to neoplasia (Strong 1977). A number of these disorders, such as Down's syndrome, are associated with an increased incidence of acute lymphatic leukemia. In addition, a specific chromosome abnormality is associated with non-Hodgkin's lymphoma. A consistent translocation onto the long arm (q) of one chromosome in the number 14 pair was first noted in African Burkitt's lymphoma patients by Manolov and Manolova (1972). Since then, chromosome 14 abnormalities have been implicated in other lymphoid neoplasms, particularly those of B cell origin (Louie and Schwartz 1978). Chromosome abnormalities frequently involving the chromosome-14 pair have been revealed in lymphocytes from patients with ataxia-telangiectasia. The gradual rise of a single aberrant clone during the course of the disease and the development of chronic lymphatic leukemia (CLL) from this clone with tandem translocation 14q:14q have been reported by McCaw et al. (1975), who feel that abnormalities of chromosome 14 in lymphoma cells may represent a tissue-specific nonrandom characteristic of lymphocytic neoplasia (McCaw et al. 1977).

Klein (1979) has postulated that Burkitt's lymphoma develops in at least three steps. The first step would be the Epstein-Barr (EB) virus-induced immortalization of some B lymphocytes upon primary infection. The second step would be brought about by an environment-dependent factor, perhaps chronic holoendemic malaria, that would stimulate the latent EB virus-carrying cells frozen at a particular stage of B cell differentiation to chronic proliferation. By forcing the long-lived preneoplastic cells to repeated division, the environmental co-factor would provide the setting for cytogenetic diversification. The third and final step would take place if and when the "right" translocation occurred on chromosome 14 that would lead to the outgrowth of an autonomous monoclonal tumor. Klein feels that the frequent involvement of chromosome 14 in the genesis of human neoplasia of largely, if not exclusively, B cell origin suggests that one or more determinants on this chromosome are closely involved with the normal responsiveness of the B lymphocyte to growth-controlling mechanisms. Acute lymphoblastic leukemia with B cell characteristics and L3 morphology has also been reported to have a 14q+ chromosome (Roth et al. 1979) abnormality.

Less specific cytogenetic abnormalities in marrow cells have been found in approximately 50% of patients with acute leukemia (Bottomley 1976, Whang-Peng et al. 1969). Hyperdiploidy is more common in lymphatic than in myelogenous leukemia cells. In general, patients in whom abnormal chromosomes are detected in the marrow have the same prognosis as patients with diploid chromosomes in the marrow (Whang-Peng et al. 1976). Within the aneuploid-chromosome group, Secker-Walker et al. (1978) have suggested that patients with a hyperdiploid chromosome number may have a better prognosis than other patients.

CLINICAL FEATURES AT PRESENTATION

The single most important prognostic factor in terms of achieving an initial remission is probably the age of the patient. Survival is a decreasing function of age (except for patients under 1 year, who have poor survival). The best survival is observed in children 3–10 years old (George et al. 1973). In addition, the sex of the patient emerges as a significant clinical variable, with male patients achieving remission less often (Simone 1975). Race also appears to be a significant variable, with black children having consistently poorer survival than white children. Black children may suffer from more aggressive disease, as they generally have more advanced disease at diagnosis (Walters et al. 1972).

Probably the most significant single variable in prognosis is the tumor burden of the patient at the time of presentation. Patients with white blood cell counts over 100,000/mm³ present acute management problems that may result in early morbidity and sometimes mortality. These problems are related to cerebral hemorrhage and more particularly to metabolic difficulties that are a consequence of the inability of these patients to effectively excrete tumor breakdown products. This inability can lead to urate or xanthine nephropathy with diminished renal function and, less commonly, to hyperphosphatemia, hypocalcemia (Zusman et al. 1973), and hyperkalemia. Aside from the acute management problems, increased white blood cell counts ($> 20,000/mm^3$) at the time of diagnosis, even in patients who achieve remission, are associated with decreased survival (Chessells et al. 1977). Increased tumor load, as reflected in massive adenopathy and organomegaly, is also associated with a poor prognosis (Simone 1975). A special case in point is the thymic mass that is often present in patients with T cell tumors. It is of interest that bone pain and bone involvement at the time of diagnosis appear not to be correlated with prognosis (Hann et al. 1979).

West and co-workers (1972) have assigned prognostic significance to the platelet count at initial presentation. They feel patients with low platelet counts at presentation are more likely to have CNS involvement. The British Medical Research Council's (MRC) Working Party on Leukaemia in Childhood (1978) has noted an increased incidence of testicular involvement in patients with initial severe thrombocytopenia (platelet count under 20,000/mm³). It may be that small hemorrhages serve as seed points for leukemic cells in many areas of the body.

CELLULAR CHARACTERISTICS

Morphologic Studies

Recently the French-American-British (FAB) system of classifying blast morphology (Bennett et al. 1976) has been proposed as a uniform system of nomenclature in acute leukemias. The Children's Cancer Study Group (Miller et al. 1979) has classified 566 patients in its study CCG–141 with this system, using a score based on the amount of cytoplasm, number of nucleoli, and vacuolization. In this study, the L_1 morphologic type, with a uniform small cell population, represented 83.9% of the cases; L_2, with a more heterogeneous cell population, 15.0%; and L_3, a type similar to that of Burkitt's lymphoma, 1.1%. The L_3 morphologic type has been associated with a poor prognosis in all series. The L_2 type in this study was associated with other poor prognosis subsets of patients and a higher relapse rate in all patients. A number of other morphologic studies have shown an association between large cell size or increased number of nucleoli and poor prognosis, and this subject has been recently reviewed (Leventhal and Konior 1976).

Metabolic Studies

The rate of growth of leukemic cells, as reflected in the labeling index of the marrow, can be correlated with response to therapy. In general, patients with a high labeling index may go into remission quickly, but the remissions are short. Cells in DNA synthesis tend to be larger than those that are not. It is our feeling that many studies in which cell size has been considered a significant variable actually reflected rough measurements of the percent of cells in active DNA synthesis (Leventhal and Konior 1976).

Another method that can be used to determine the metabolic state of the cell employs the periodic acid-Schiff (PAS) stain for glycogen. Since glycogen is used as an energy source for the cell, it seems logical to assume that cells that are actively dividing with a high growth fraction and labeling index have low glycogen stores, resulting in a lack of PAS-positive material. This is the case for a tumor of known high growth fraction, Burkitt's lymphoma. It seems likely, then, that other patients with weak PAS staining in their lymphoblasts also have tumors with a high growth fraction and a poor prognosis. In fact, this association of high mitotic and labeling indices and low PAS positivity in leukemic cells with T cell markers and poor prognosis has been seen by Tsukimoto et al. (1976) and Heideman et al. (1978). Recently Murphy and co-workers (1979) have shown a good correlation between labeling index and cell subtype in patients with lymphoma and leukemia. Patients with B cell tumors had the highest labeling indices, with a median of 41%; those with T cell tumors had a median of 12%; finally, patients with newly diagnosed null cell ALL had the lowest labeling indices, with a 4.8% median.

Marker Studies on the Cells

Some markers that have been detected in lymphoid tumors are clearly found also in normal human lymphoid tissue. As these have been described, they aid in classifying the cell of origin of the tumor within the lymphoid system. This is useful in distinguishing one tumor from another and is further evidence that the vast majority of these tumors are of monoclonal origin (Stryckmans et al. 1978); in addition, these tumor cells may serve as purified cell populations that could permit the development of powerful reagents, such as specific antibodies, that would allow us to further dissect the nature of the immune system. The subject of markers has been recently reviewed (Leventhal et al. 1979).

T Cell Markers

The ability to bind sheep red blood cells to form E rosettes defines the normal, mature human T lymphocyte and thymocyte. In 15–25% of cases of ALL, significant percentages of patients' blast cells exhibit the E rosetting phenomenon (Humphrey and Lankford 1976). The sheep red cell receptor or its environment on the blast may differ from that on the normal T cell, since T cell ALL blasts form heat-stable E rosettes, whereas normal T cells do not (Borella and Sen 1973). In a recent study (Humphrey et al. 1979) it was suggested that the presence of blasts that form heat-stable rosettes results in a worse prognosis for the patient. Cases of ALL with E rosette-positive blasts are reliably detected by a number of antisera that recognize human T cells. However, some human T lymphocyte antigen (HTLA) antisera detect certain E rosette-negative cases (Borella et al. 1977). This fact and the similar clinical behavior of these fairly uncommon E rosette-negative, HTLA-positive leukemias suggest that the HTLA antisera recognize an antigen that appears before the sheep red blood cell receptor in T cell maturation. Such a malignant cell may have arisen from a normal thymic precursor or "pre-T cell."

Functional subcategorization of lymphoblasts is being studied. T lymphoblasts share with normal T lymphocytes the inability to stimulate allogeneic cells in mixed leukocyte culture (Leventhal et al. 1977). In addition, recent data suggest that T lymphoblasts bear receptors for the Fc portion of IgM, IgG, or both (Reaman et al. 1979b). Reinherz et al. (1979) have studied subsets of T cells in lymphoblastic malignant diseases. They feel that normal human peripheral blood T cells are composed of TH_2-positive (cytotoxic/suppressor) and TH_2-negative (helper) cells. Using heterospecific antisera, they classified 26 T cell ALL patients, and found that five were TH_2 positive. These five had a median age of 9.8 years; three were female and only two had mediastinal masses. Despite initial lymphoblast counts over 100,000/mm³, two are off treatment and disease free at 2 years. The TH_2-negative ALL patients were older and more often male, and had a worse prognosis. A recent report by Broder et al. (1978) describes a patient whose leukemia cells induced suppression of immunoglobulin production by pokeweed-stimulated lymphocytes in vitro. The prospect of further functional subcategorization of leukemias is exciting.

Clinically, T cell ALL is associated with several poor prognostic features, including high presenting white blood cell counts, mediastinal mass, male sex, and greater age. Most important, T cell ALL patients generally relapse early during conventional ALL chemotherapy (Tsukimoto et al. 1976, Frei and Sallan 1978).

B Cell Markers

In less than 5% of cases of ALL, the lymphoblasts bear surface immunoglobulin and complement receptors and have been considered to represent B cell ALL. These cells morphologically resemble Burkitt's lymphoma cells (Flandrin et al. 1975, Berger et al. 1979). B cell leukemia is associated with a poor prognosis, and these patients often fail to achieve even initial remissions.

Vogler et al. (1978) have identified cases of ALL in which the lymphoblasts were characterized by the presence of cytoplasmic immunoglobulin. These "pre-B" lymphoblasts are E rosette negative and SIg negative and appear to represent the neoplastic counterpart of a recently described B cell precursor in normal human bone marrow. Since these cases until recently were considered "null" ALL, it is likely that these patients will have a better prognosis than those with the B cell ALL described above.

Common ALL

In approximately 75% of cases of ALL, the blasts bear neither E rosette receptors, complement receptors, nor immunoglobulin. This phenotype is now referred to as common ALL (cALL). The ALL cells react with Ia antisera, and specific heteroantisera to cALL antigens have been prepared (Greaves et al. 1976, Billing et al. 1978). At present, cALL is treatable and often curable. These patients have the best prognosis, and over 50% have long-term remissions with current therapy.

Enzyme Levels in Leukemic Cells

Terminal deoxynucleotidyl transferase (TdT) has been identified in immature cells in the lymphoid line. It is present in large quantities in common ALL cells and in somewhat lesser quantities in T cells as they develop more differentiated characteristics (McCaffrey et al. 1975). Focal acid phosphatase and beta glucouronidase tend to be high in T cell ALL patients (Catovsky and Enno 1977). T phenotype lymphoblasts also demonstrate elevated levels of adenosine deaminase (Smyth et al. 1978) and markedly diminished activity of the plasma membrane-bound enzyme 5' nucleotidase (Reaman et al. 1979a) compared to normal lymphoid cells or to leukemic lymphoblasts, which lack T cell surface markers. In one study (Koller et al. 1979) an attempt was made to take advantage of these abnormalities and to selectively kill T lymphoblasts with a toxic accumulation of deoxyadenosine in the presence of the adenosine deaminase inhibitor 2' deoxycoformycin. This selective metabolic approach to therapy appears most promising.

Hormone Receptor Levels as Markers

Insulin-binding sites have been found in lower density in T lymphoblasts than in normal lymphocytes (Esber et al. 1976). In addition, Yarbro et al. (1977) have shown that glucocorticoid receptors are present in lower concentrations in the cytoplasm of T cell lymphoblasts than in that of "null" cell lymphoblasts. The pharmacologic importance of the latter observation is unclear, since most patients achieve remission at least once with a drug combination that includes vincristine and prednisone. When a larger series of patients was analyzed (Lippman et al. 1978), it was found that glucocorticoid receptor levels appeared to act as a prognostic variable independent of other facts such as cell subtype, white blood cell count, or age of patient. Overall remission duration tended to correlate with receptor level. Further clarification of the mechanism of glucocorticoid killing of the lymphoblast is needed for a better understanding of these results.

TREATMENT

Prognostic Significance

The single most significant variable in the patient's prognosis is response to treatment. Prognosis is best for those patients who are in remission after 4 weeks of vincristine and prednisone (Frei and Sallan 1978). Overall survival, even in patients who relapse, is related to the duration of the initial remission (Leventhal and Ziegler 1975), and in patients who manage to stay in remission for 2 years or more the weight of the early prognostic variables disappears (Sather et al. 1978).

In addition, it appears important that the patient be treated in a setting in which protocol therapy is used. Meadows et al. (1979) discovered that patients treated by trained personnel according to a cooperative group or nationally recognized protocol within or outside a national center are at greatly decreased risk of death from leukemia compared to those not treated on such a protocol.

Advances in Treatment

Great advances have been made in the treatment of leukemia in the past 30 years. These advances have come as investigators appreciated that maximum doses of single chemotherapeutic agents should be given (Pinkel et al. 1971) and that combinations of agents are superior to single agents. Later, the application of sanctuary therapy, particularly to the central nervous system, led to further advances in survival (Hustu et al. 1973).

Complications of Increasing Intensity of Therapy

Further addition of cytotoxic drugs to the combinations developed in the early 1970s has not led to further progress in the treatment of leukemia. With the conventional regimens, as reviewed by Frei and Sallan (1978), about 75% of patients with common ALL can expect to be disease free at 3 years, although T cell patients do not fare as well. The addition of more drugs to these regimens has resulted in problems, however, in that the patients in some studies have appeared to be at increased risk of infection without gaining any overall prolongation of remission (Hughes et al. 1975, Simone et al. 1972). In addition, increased intensity of therapy leads to a greater likelihood of long-term complications, particularly those disastrous events that occur in the central nervous system under the combined influence of radiotherapy and drugs and are called leukoencephalopathy (Hendin et al. 1974, Price and Jamieson 1975). Effects on growth, development, and endocrine function are also of concern (Meyer and Leventhal 1979).

Another potential complication of increasing the intensity of therapy is the interference of one drug with administration of the proper dosage of other drugs. The MRC Working Party on Leukemia in Childhood recently analyzed its data (1978) on testicular involvement with leukemia and discovered a high incidence, with 13% of first remissions being terminated by testicular relapse. The investigators felt that the incidence might be higher in patients who had received Cytoxan than in those who had not in a randomized study. They postulated that Cytoxan administration might have diminished the dose of more effective agents given, that drug interference might have occurred, that additional drugs might have induced neoplastic progression, and, finally, that Cytoxan might have induced destruction of other cells within the seminiferous tubules, which might have changed the microenvironment to allow proliferation of leukemic cells in that site. All these possibilities are interesting and deserve to be considered as we considered increasing the intensity of therapy.

FUTURE PROSPECTS

The Poor Prognosis Patient

We find ourselves in a dilemma, then, vis-à-vis the poor prognosis patient. To date, the addition of new cytotoxic agents has increased toxicity but not therapeutic effect. Immunotherapy with bacillus Calmette-Guérin (BCG) is thought by Mathé (1978) to improve the treatment of the good prognosis patient, but even in his hands patients with macrolymphoblastic disease do not respond. In several other trials using BCG with or without allogeneic cells in ALL, the BCG did not appear to add to the effects achieved with drugs alone (Poplack et al. 1978, Andrien et al. 1978, Heyn et al. 1978). Thus, at the moment it appears that immunotherapy is not the answer to the problem of the poor prognosis patient with ALL. The use of specific anti-T cell serum to clean malignant lymphoblasts from the marrow may represent a promising new immunologic approach to this tumor (Rodt et al. 1979).

The Good Prognosis Patient

We face a different dilemma with our good prognosis patients, i.e., those young patients with common ALL and low white blood cell counts. With these patients, we must be careful not to overtreat. We know that a certain percentage of patients will relapse within the 1st year after therapy is stopped, although continuing therapy beyond 5 years has not led to prolonged remissions (Cancer and Leukemia Group B, unpublished data). George et al. (1979) recently reanalyzed their data from St. Jude Children's Research Hospital and found that about 20% of patients in remission after 2½–3 years of therapy eventually relapse. It was striking that a greater percentage of those patients who relapsed were male than female and that the increased incidence of relapse was not accounted for by testicular relapse alone. The MRC (1978) has been concerned that the time to testicular relapse was equivalent in patients who underwent 86 and 150 weeks of therapy, which suggests that a residual, partially drug-sensitive population was being suppressed, but not eliminated. In these patients it appears that the most logical next step in treatment involves some intensification of therapy after 3 years of maintenance in an attempt to eradicate these residual cells in the 20% of patients who are fated to relapse.

CONCLUSIONS

In summary, then, we can describe a spectrum of responses in patients with acute lymphatic leukemia. We can identify a poor prognosis group of patients, who tend to be older and male, and who may have T cell disease. These patients are unlikely to be cured with current drug regimens, so new therapies must be developed. We can also identify a good prognosis group, who at the start of therapy are between 2 and 10 years old, have low white blood cell counts and common ALL, and are female. In this group about 75% can be expected to be in remission after 3 years of therapy.

The most important single prognostic variable for an individual patient, however, is his response to therapy. Once a patient has been in remission for over 2 years, the significance of all the early prognostic factors disappears (Sather et al. 1978) and the only variable that is important when therapy is discontinued is the sex of the patient (George et al. 1979), with girls managing to remain in remission longer than boys. In this group of patients, the main concern is to avoid overtreatment in terms of either time or drug dosage and it seems that an intensification of therapy after about 3 years of maintenance is the most logical next therapeutic approach to explore.

ACKNOWLEDGMENT

This investigation was partially supported by grant CA–06973–14 from the National Cancer Institute.

REFERENCES

Andrien, J. M., M. P. Beumer-Jockmans, J. Bury, C. Cauchie, J. L. David, M. J. Delbeke, R. Denolin, P. De Porre, D. Fiere, G. Flowerdew, S. L. George, H. Hainaut, J. Hughes, Y. Kenis, R. Masure, R. Maurus, J. Michel, J. Otten, M. E. Peetermans, M. B. Reginster-Bous, P. A. Stryckmans, R. Sylvester, M. Van Glabbeke, W. Van Hove, L. Verbist, A. Wennerholm, and H. Williaert. 1978. Immunotherapy vs. chemotherapy as maintenance treatment of acute lymphoblastic leukemia, *in* Immunotherapy of Cancer: Present Status of Trials in Man, W. Terry and D. Windhorst, eds. Raven Press, New York, pp. 451–470.

Bennett, J. M., D. Catovsky, M.-T. Daniel, G. Flandrin, D. A. G. Galton, H. R. Gralnick, and C. Sultan. 1976. Proposals for the classification of the acute leukemias. Br. J. Haematol. 33:451–458.

Berger, R., A. Bernheim, J. C. Brouet, M. T. Daniel, and G. Flandrin. 1979. t(8:14) translocation in Burkitt's type of lymphoblastic leukaemia (L3). Br. J. Haematol. 43:87–90.

Billing, R., J. Minowada, M. Cline, B. Clark, and K. Lee. 1978. Acute lymphocytic leukemia-associated cell membrane antigen. J. Natl. Cancer Inst. 61:423–429.

Borella, L., and L. Sen. 1973. T-cell surface markers on lymphoblasts from acute lymphocytic leukemia. J. Immunol. 111:1257–1260.

Borella, L., L. Sen, and J. T. Casper. 1977. Acute lymphoblastic leukemia (ALL) antigens detected with antisera to E rosette-forming and non-E rosette-forming ALL blasts. J. Immunol. 118:309–315.

Bottomley, R. H. 1976. Cytogenetic heterogeneity of the acute leukemias. Semin. Oncol. 3:253–257.

British Medical Research Council's Working Party on Leukaemia in Childhood. 1978. Testicular disease in acute lymphoblastic leukaemia in childhood. Br. Med. J. 1:334–338.

Broder, S., D. Poplack, J. Whang-Peng, M. Durm, C. Goldman, L. Muul, and T. A. Waldmann. 1978. Characterization of a suppressor-cell leukemia. N. Engl. J. Med. 298:66–72.

Catovsky, D., and A. Enno. 1977. Morphological and cytochemical identifications of lymphoid cells. Lymphology 10:77–84.

Chessells, J. M., R. M. Hardisty, N. T. Rapson, and M. F. Greaves. 1977. Acute lymphoblastic leukemia in children: Classification and prognosis. Lancet 2:1307–1309.

Esber, E. D., D. N. Buell, and S. L. Leikin. 1976. Insulin binding of acute lymphocytic leukemia cells. Blood 48:33–39.

Flandrin, G., J. C. Brouet, M. T. Daniel, and J. L. Preud'homme. 1975. Acute leukemia with Burkitt's tumor cells: A study of six cases with special reference to lymphocyte surface markers. Blood 45:183–188.

Frei, E., III, and S. Sallan. 1978. Acute lymphoblastic leukemia: Treatment. Cancer 42:828–838.

George, S. L., R. J. A. Aur, A. M. Mauer, and J. V. Simone. 1979. A reappraisal of the results of stopping therapy in childhood leukemia. N. Engl. J. Med. 300:269–273.

George, S. L., D. J. Fernbach, T. J. Vietti, M. P. Sullivan, D. M. Lane, M. E. Haggard, D. H. Berry, D. Lonsdale, and D. Komp. 1973. Factors influencing survival in pediatric acute leukemia: The SWCCSG experience 1958–1970. Cancer 32:1542–1553.

Greaves, M. F., G. Janossy, M. Robert, N. T. Rapson, R. B. Ellis, J. Chessels, T. A. Lister, and D. Catovsky. 1976. Membrane phenotyping: Diagnosis, monitoring and classification of acute lymphoid leukemias. Haematol. Bluttransfus. 20:61–75.

Hann, I. M., S. Gupta, M. K. Palmer, and P. H. Morris-Jones. 1979. The prognostic significance of radiological and symptomatic bone involvement in childhood acute lymphoblastic leukemia. Med. Pediatr. Oncol. 6:51–55.

Heideman, R. L., J. M. Falletta, N. Mikhopadhyay, and D. J. Fernbach. 1978. Lymphocytic leukemia in children: Prognostic significance of clinical and laboratory findings at time of diagnosis. J. Pediatr. 92:540–545.

Hendin, B., D. C. DeVivo, R. Torack, M. E. Lell, A. H. Ragab, and T. J. Vietti. 1974. Parenchymatous degeneration of the central nervous system in childhood leukemia. Cancer 33:468–482.

Heyn, R. M., P. Joo, M. Karon, M. Nesbit, N. Shore, N. Breslow, J. Weiner, A. Reed, H. Sather, and D. Hammond. 1978. BCG in the treatment of acute lymphocytic leukemia, *in* Immunotherapy of Cancer: Present Status of Trials in Man, W. D. Terry and D. Windhorst, eds. Raven Press, New York, pp. 503–512.

Hughes, W. T., S. Feldman, R. J. A. Aur, M. S. Verzosa, H. O. Hustu, and J. V. Simone. 1975. Intensity of immunosuppressive therapy and the incidence of *Pneumocystis carinii* pneumonitis. Cancer 35:2004–2009.

Humphrey, G. B., W. Crist, J. Falletta, E. Richie, A. Ragab, and J. Pullen. 1979. The implication of thermostable and thermolabile T cell leukemia in randomized trials (potential significance). Proc. Am. Assoc. Cancer Res. 20:289.

Humphrey, G. B., and J. Lankford. 1976. Acute leukemia: The use of surface markers in classification. Semin. Oncol. 3:243–251.

Hustu, H. O., R. J. A. Aur, M. S. Verzosa, J. V. Simone, and D. Pinkel. 1973. Prevention of central nervous system leukemia by irradiation. Cancer 32:585–597.

Klein, G. 1979. Lymphoma development in mice and humans: Diversity of initiations is followed by convergent cytogenetic evolution. Proc. Natl. Acad. Sci. U.S.A. 76:2442–2446.

Koller, C., M. Grever, and B. Mitchell. 1979. Treatment of acute lymphoblastic leukemia with the adenosine deaminase inhibitor 2′ deoxycoformycin. Proc. Am. Assoc. Cancer Res. 20:382.

Leventhal, B. G., C. I. Civin, and G. Reaman. 1979. Markers in human lymphoid tumors, *in* Oncofetal Markers in Human Tumors, S. Sell, ed. Humana Press, Clifton, N.J., in press.

Leventhal, B. G., and G. S. Konior. 1976. Prognostic factors in acute leukemia: A critical review. Semin. Oncol. 3:319–325.

Leventhal, B. G., E. Leung, G. Johnson, and D. G. Poplack. 1977. E rosette-forming lymphoblasts fail to stimulate allogeneic cells in mixed leukocyte culture (MLC). Cancer Immunol. Immunother. 2:21–25.

Leventhal, B. G., and J. L. Ziegler. 1975. The relation of duration of first remission to survival, *in* Advances in the Biosciences, vol. 14, T. M. Fliedner and S. Perry, eds. Pergamon Press, Oxford, pp. 83–89.

Lippman, M. E., G. K. Yarbro, and B. G. Leventhal. 1978. Clinical implications of glucocorticoid receptors in human leukemia. Cancer Res. 38:4251–4256.

Louie, S., and R. S. Schwartz. 1978. Immunodeficiency and the pathogenesis of lymphoma and leukemia. Semin. Hematol. 15:117–138.

Manolov, G., and Y. Manolova. 1972. Marker band in one chromosome 14 from Burkitt's lymphomas. Nature 237:33–34.

Mathé, G., L. Schwarzenberg, F. DeVassal, M. Delgado, J. PenaAngulo, D. Belpomme, P. Pouillart, D. Machover, J. L. Misset, J. L. Pico, C. Jasmin, M. Hayat, M. Schneider, A. Cattan, J. L. Amiel, M. Musset, and C. Rosenfel. 1978. Chemotherapy followed by active immunotherapy in the treatment of acute lymphoid leukemias for patients of all ages: Results of ICIG protocols 1, 9 and 10. Prognostic factors and therapeutic indications, *in* Immunotherapy of Cancer: Present Status of Trials in Man, W. D. Terry and D. Windhorst, eds. Raven Press, New York, pp. 451–470.

McCaffrey, R., T. A. Harrison, R. Parkman, and D. Baltimore. 1975. Terminal deoxynucleotidyl-transferase activity in human leukemic cells and in normal human thymocytes. N. Engl. J. Med. 292:775–780.

McCaw, B., A. L. Epstein, H. S. Kaplan, and F. Hecht. 1977. Chromosome 14 translocation in African and North American Burkitt's lymphoma. Int. J. Cancer 19:482–486.

McCaw, B., F. Hecht, D. G. Harden, and R. L. Teplitz. 1975. Somatic rearrangement of chromosome 14 in human lymphocytes. Proc. Natl. Acad. Sci. U.S.A. 72:2071–2075.

Meadows, A. T., R. Hopson, E. Lustbader, and A. E. Evans. 1979. Survival in childhood acute lymphocytic leukemia (ALL): The influence of protocol and place of treatment. Proc. Am. Assoc. Cancer Res. 20:425.

Meyer, W., and B. G. Leventhal. 1979. The late effects of therapy for cancer, *in* Complications of Cancer: Diagnosis and Management, M. D. Abeloff, ed. The Johns Hopkins University Press, Baltimore, pp. 397–416.

Miller, D. R., S. Leikin, V. Albo, and D. Hammond. 1979. Prognostic significance of lymphoblast morphology (FAB classification) in childhood leukemia (ALL). Proc. Am. Assoc. Cancer Res. 20:345.

Miller, R. W. 1977. Etiology of childhood cancer, *in* Clinical Pediatric Oncology, W. W. Sutow, T. J. Vietti, and D. J. Fernbach, eds. C. V. Mosby Co., St. Louis, pp. 16–32.

Murphy, S. B., S. L. Melvin, and A. M. Mauer. 1979. Correlation of tumor cell kinetic studies with surface marker results in childhood non-Hodgkin's lymphoma. Cancer Res. 39:1534–1538.

Pinkel, D., K. Hernandez, L. Borella, C. Holton, R. Aur, G. Samoy, and C. Pratt. 1971. Drug dosage and remission duration in childhood lymphocytic leukemia. Cancer 37:247–256.

Poplack, D. G., B. G. Leventhal, R. Simon, T. Pomeroy, R. G. Graw, and H. S. Henderson. 1978. Treatment of acute lymphatic leukemia with chemotherapy alone or chemotherapy plus immunotherapy, *in* Immunotherapy of Cancer: Present Status of Trials in Man, W. D. Terry and D. Windhorst, eds. Raven Press, New York, pp. 497–502.

Price, R. A., and P. A. Jamieson. 1975. The central nervous system in childhood leukemia. II. Subacute leukoencephalopathy. Cancer 35:306–318.

Reaman, G. H., N. Levin, A. Muchmore, B. J. Holiman, and D. G. Poplack. 1979a. Diminished lymphoblast 5' nucleotidase activity in acute lymphoblastic leukemia with T cell characteristics. N. Engl. J. Med. 300:1374–1377.

Reaman, G. H., W. J. Pichler, S. Broder, and D. G. Poplack. 1979b. Characterization of lymphoblast Fc receptor expression in acute lymphoblastic leukemia. Blood 54:285–291.

Reinherz, E., R. Parkman, J. Rappaport, F. S. Rosen, and S. F. Schlossman.1979. Aberrations of suppressor T cells in human graft-versus-host disease. N. Engl. J. Med. 300:1061–1068.

Rodt, H., B. Netzel, R. J. Haas, G. Janka, and S. Thierfelder. 1979. The concept of anti-leukemic, autologous bone marrow transplantation in acute lymphoblastic leukemia. Blut, in press.

Roth, D. G., M. C. Cimino, D. Variakojis, H. M. Golomb, and J. D. Rowley. 1979. B cell acute lymphoblastic leukemia (ALL) with a 14q+ abnormality. Blood 53:235–243.

Sather, H. N., P. Coccia, M. Nesbit, C. Level, and D. Hammond. 1978. Disappearance of the predictive value of prognostic factors for childhood acute lymphocytic leukemia (ALL). Proc. Am. Assoc. Cancer Res. 19:338.

Secker-Walker, L. M., S. D. Lawler, and R. M. Hardisty. 1978. Prognostic implications of chromosomal findings in acute lymphoblastic leukaemia at diagnosis. Br. Med. J. 2:1529–1530.

Simone, J. V. 1975. Prognostic factors in childhood acute lymphocytic leukemia, *in* Advances in the Biosciences, vol. 14, T. M. Fliedner and S. Perry, eds. Pergamon Press, Oxford, pp. 27–42.

Simone, J. V., E. Holland, and W. Johnson. 1972. Fatalities during remission of childhood leukemia. Blood 39:759–770.

Smyth, J. F., D. G. Poplack, B. J. Holiman, B. G. Leventhal, and G. Yarbro. 1978. J. Clin. Invest., 62:710–712.

Strong, L. C. 1977. Genetic considerations in pediatric oncology, *in* Clinical Pediatric Oncology, W. W. Sutow, T. J. Vietti, and D. H. Fernbach, eds. C. V. Mosby Co., St. Louis, pp. 16–32.

Stryckmans, P. A., L. Debusscher, C. Heyder-Bruckner, R. Heimann, I. M. Mandelbaum, and J. Wybran. 1978. Clonal origin of a T cell lymphoproliferative malignancy. Blood 52:69–76.

Tsukimoto, I., K. Y. Wong, and B. C. Lampkin. 1976. Surface markers and prognostic factors in acute lymphoblastic leukemia. N. Engl. J. Med. 294:828–832.

Vogler, L. B., W. M. Crist, D. E. Bockman, E. R. Pearl, A. R. Lawton, and M. D. Cooper. 1978. Pre-B cell leukemia: A new phenotype of childhood lymphoblastic leukemia. N. Engl. J. Med. 298:872–878.

Walters, T., M. Bushore, and J. Simone. 1972. Poor prognosis in Negro children with acute lymphocytic leukemia. Cancer 29:210–214.

West, R. J., J. Graham-Pole, and R. M. Hardisty. 1972. Factors in pathogenesis of central nervous system leukaemia. Br. Med. J. 3:311–314.

Whang-Peng, J., E. J Freireich, and J. J. Oppenheim. 1969. Cytogenetic studies on 45 patients with acute lymphocytic leukemia. J. Natl. Cancer Inst. 42:881–897.

Whang-Peng, J., T. Knutsen, J. Ziegler, and B. G. Leventhal. 1976. Cytogenetic studies in acute lymphocytic leukemia: Special emphasis on long-term survival. Med. Pediatr. Oncol., 2:333–351.

Yarbro, G. S. K., M. E. Lippman, G. E. Johnson, and B. G. Leventhal. 1977. Glucocorticoid receptors in subpopulations of childhood acute lymphocytic leukemia. Cancer Res. 37:2688–2695.

Zusman, J., D. M. Brown, and M. Nesbit. 1973. Hyperphosphatemia, hyperphosphaturia, and hypocalcemia in acute lymphoblastic leukemia. N. Engl. J. Med. 289:1335–1340.

Status of the Curability of Childhood Cancers,
edited by J. van Eys and M. P. Sullivan.
Raven Press, New York © 1980.

Renewed Momentum in Non-Hodgkin's Lymphomas

Margaret P. Sullivan, M.D., Antonio Frias, M.D.,* and Irma Ramirez, M.D.

*Department of Pediatrics, The University of Texas System Cancer Center M. D. Anderson Hospital and Tumor Institute, Houston, Texas, and *Dwight D. Eisenhower Army Medical Center, Fort Gordon, Georgia*

Recent discoveries in cellular immunology have provided insight into the fundamental nature of malignant lymphoid diseases. The ability to identify cells of the T and B lymphatic systems and an understanding of lymphocyte function in the two systems have resulted in a new pathologic classification system for non-Hodgkin's lymphomas that is gradually gaining acceptance. This revolutionary classification system (Lukes and Collins 1974, 1975) is based on a new concept relating lymphomatous diseases to the T and B lymphatic systems, alterations in lymphocyte transformation, and the morphology of the follicular center cells.

This presentation is restricted to a discussion of T and B cell characteristics and cellular attributes that relate to the outcome of therapy in non-Hodgkin's lymphomas of childhood.

The concept that malignant cells exert their deleterious effects by occupying space, crowding out normal cells, and exerting pressure on vital tissues and organs is insufficient for lymphoid malignancies; we now know that these malignant cells maintain the mobility of their normal counterparts and at least some of their functional capacity (de Sousa 1978, Broder et al. 1978). In addition, unequivocal maturation of malignant lymphoid cells has been noted. To better understand the nature of lymphoid malignancies, some knowledge of the behavior of normal lymphocytes is essential.

MOBILITY AND HOMING CHARACTERISTICS OF LYMPHOCYTES

Thymus-derived T lymphocytes are recognized by their ability to bind nonsensitized sheep red blood cells in a rosette distribution and by their lack of surface receptors for immunoglobulins. Under the influence of plant mitogens and of antigens to which there has been previous exposure, normal T cells transform in vitro from small, metabolically inactive lymphocytes to large, metabolically active forms (Lukes and Collins 1974).

Bone marrow–derived lymphocytes (B cells) are characterized by surface immunoglobulins, receptors for the third component of complement, and aggregated immunoglobulins. Under the influence of dendritic reticular cells, small lymphocytes undergo nuclear cleavage, enlarge, lose their cleaved appearance, and acquire prominent nucleoli (Lukes and Collins 1974). A normal lymphocyte, thus fully transformed, is four times the size of the normal small lymphocyte. Transformed cells may move out into interfollicular tissue and proliferate as immunoblasts, become plasma cells, or revert to a dormant state. A neoplastic clone may arise at any point in the differentiation process.

The number of lymphocytes in the blood is relatively small; they freely pass between the vascular and lymphatic systems (de Sousa 1978). In lambs, this circulation pattern between the two systems develops in fetal life. Lymphocyte traffic is orderly, with the traffic tempo and recirculation circuits differing between the immunologic types of lymphocytes. T cells are the more active: 70% are circulating, making four to six circuits daily (Lukes and Collins 1974). "In route" organs and tissues may be populated by the circulating cells. Lodging sites differ for T and B cells.

Laboratory investigations have demonstrated the following T cell lodging sites: the bone marrow where the cells are scattered, paracortical areas of lymph nodes, perivascular regions of the spleen, the tonsils, the gastrointestinal tract, and the skin (Lukes and Collins 1974, de Sousa 1978, Knowles and Holck 1978). Clinical observations would force the inclusion of the meninges and the testicles, high on the list of homing sites. The propensity of T cells for diapedesis through the walls of postcapillary venules in lymph nodes (de Sousa 1978) is well recognized. This phenomenon has been described in veins of the meninges as an early stage in the evolution of meningeal leukemia (Price and Johnson 1973).

Fewer B cells circulate and the tempo is slower, due to delays in major capillary networks. Most B cells reside in follicular centers of lymph nodes, the spleen, and the lamina propria; a few are scattered in the bone marrow (Lukes and Collins 1974). Major traffic is to these sites. The selectivity of homing is so great that immunoblasts from mesenteric nodes preferentially home to abdominal nodes, in contrast to somatic immunoblasts which home to peripheral somatic lymph nodes, the spleen and lungs (Hall et al. 1977).

Factors thought to influence the preferential migration of lymphocytes to homing sites are listed in Table 1; these include elements and cellular products of the microenvironment of the home, namely, the reticulin framework, the stroma, interdigitating cells, and "neighboring" cells, including permanent elements and other lymphocytes identical to or different from the homing cell (de Sousa 1978). T–T and T–B cell relationships are extremely complex (Broder and Waldmann 1978a, b, Gershorn 1979). Through these cell interactions, powerful immunoregulatory forces are exerted that are beyond the scope of this presentation.

The ability of T and B cells to home can be altered by substances that act

Table 1. *Factors Influencing Homing of Lymphocytes*

1. Microenvironment of the home
    a. Reticulin framework
    b. Stroma
    c. Interdigitating cells
    d. "Neighboring" cells
        i. Permanent elements
        ii. Other lymphocytes
2. Substances acting upon cell surface membranes
    a. Radioactive labels
    b. Neuraminadase
    c. Viral antigens
    d. Trypsin
    e. Concanavalin A
    f. Carbohydrates, lipopolysaccharides, phospholipase A
    g. *Bordetella pertussis* factor
    h. Antilymphocyte serum
3. Events altering the home
    a. Intravenously administered antigen
    b. Whole-body irradiation
    c. Stress or corticosteroids
    d. Locally injected antigen

upon cell surface membranes (de Sousa 1978). Alterations in the surface membranes reduce cell entry into lymph nodes, so that lymphocytes accumulate in capillaries of the liver, spleen, and lungs. A partial list of effector substances includes surface carbohydrates, lipopolysaccharides and phosphatases, neuraminadase, certain viral antigens, trypin, *Bordetella pertussis* factor, and antilymphocyte serum.

As also shown in Table 1, the homing process may also be altered by events of either a systemic or local nature that alter the home (de Sousa 1978). Systemic events, such as an intravenously administered antigen, whole-body irradiation, and stress or corticosteroid administration, result in a "hold-up" of lymphoid cells in the spleen; local events result in a "hold-up" of lymphocytes in the first-echelon nodes.

CLINICAL IMPLICATIONS

The two characteristics of lymphocytes just discussed, mobility and homing capacity, have important implications for the management of non-Hodgkin's lymphomas of children. As information on manipulations that affect the home and the homing process is fragmentary, these matters cannot be considered in depth at present. The interested reader is referred to the writings of Broder and Waldman (1979b) for a discussion of pharmacologic maneuvers that influence T–T and T–B interactions in the home.

The mobility of lymphocytes makes it necessary to consider lymphomatous malignancies as being dynamic with regard to the movement of cells from the tumor into the traffic circuits peculiar to the normal lymphoid counterpart.

Such cells would move freely back and forth from the lymphatic to the vascular system, lodging preferentially in favored sites that are known from either laboratory experimentation or clinical observation. A tumor formed by such cells would be disseminated almost from inception. The mechanism of disease extension would thus be quite different from the classic concept, exemplified by the solid tumors of adults, which spread in an orderly fashion from lymph node echelon to echelon and suddenly disseminate when a vessel wall is penetrated. Staging systems developed for adult solid tumors are thus not applicable to the non-Hodgkin's lymphomas of children. Efforts to apply the Ann Arbor Staging System have been so unsuccessful and useless that several alternative staging systems have been offered. In the case of Burkitt's tumor, the problem is compounded even further by the particularly short generation time of the tumor cell.

As the lymphomatous diseases of children are likely to be disseminated from inception and doubling times are short, prompt initiation of therapy is more helpful to the patient than attempts to precisely stage the disease. Due to the mobility of the malignant cells, chemotherapy should be the major treatment modality; treatment should be both prompt and intensive. Special therapeutic maneuvers should be employed to assure adequate therapy to homing sites in "sanctuary" areas protected partially by a blood:tissue barrier.

THERAPEUTIC APPLICATION

Using this information as a basis for therapeutic guidelines, it is instructive to consider the LSA_2–L_2 treatment regimen reported in 1974 to have achieved an overall long-term survival of 80% in children with non-Hodgkin's lymphomas (Wollner et al. 1974). The proportion surviving by histologic type in a subsequent report were: diffuse, poorly differentiated lymphocytic lymphoma, 87%; diffuse, undifferentiated lymphoma, 25%; and diffuse histiocytic lymphoma, 71% (Wollner et al. 1976). Whether through serendipity or intuition, the protocol provided for minimal staging and prompt, intensive multiagent chemotherapy with CNS prophylaxis (Figure 1). Provision was also made for radiotherapy to extra-abdominal disease sites and to residual abdominal disease sites identified by second-look surgery.

M. D. Anderson Hospital (MDAH) LSA_2–L_2 Field Trial

Initial results with LSA_2–L_2 therapy were so superior to those for all other treatment regimens for childhood non-Hodgkin's lymphomas that we abandoned our non-Hodgkin's lymphoma studies from October 1974 to October 1976 to conduct an LSA_2–L_2 field trial. In our study group of 32 children, nine had prior therapy differing from LSA_2–L_2. The other 23 were designated as having received no prior therapy, although some had received their first dose of Cytoxan immediately before admission to MDAH. Adherence to all other protocol provisions was strict.

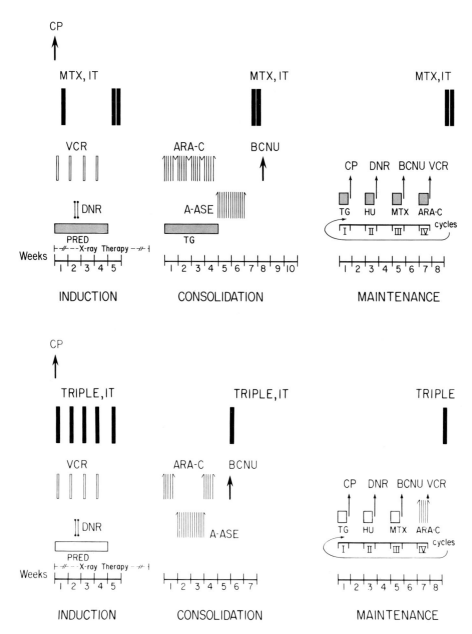

Figure 1. Top, Schematic representation of modified LSA$_2$–L$_2$ therapy for non-Hodgkin's lymphomas in children, M. D. Anderson Hospital field trial. Bottom, Schematic representation of M. D. Anderson Hospital second-generation LSA$_2$–L$_2$ therapy for non-Hodgkin's lymphomas in children (excluding those with diffuse undifferentiated lymphoma of the Burkitt's type). Abbreviations: CP, cyclophosphamide; MTX, methotrexate; IT, intrathecally; VCR, vincristine; DNR, daunomycin; PRED, prednisone; ARA-C, cytosine arabinoside; BCNU, bis-nitrosourea; A-ASE, L-asparaginase; TG, thioguanine; HU, hydroxyurea.

Therapeutic Results

The outcome of therapy was markedly different for previously untreated children and for those who had prior therapy, as shown in length of remission curves and survival curves (Figure 2). Fifty-seven percent of patients with no prior therapy survive; only one of nine patients with prior therapy survives.

Among patients with no prior therapy, lengths of remission exceed 2 years for 75% of those with undifferentiated lymphoma (non-Burkitt's), 65% of those with histiocytic lymphoma, and 62% of those with convoluted lymphoma. No child with Burkitt's lymphoma enjoyed a continuous complete remission (Figure 3 top). Treatment failures occurred early in patients with histiocytic and Burkitt's lymphomas. In convoluted lymphoma, relapses covered a greater time span, extending into the maintenance phase.

Survival curves show the successful retrieval of one patient with Burkitt's lymphoma, for a survival fraction of 20% (Figure 3 bottom). In general, survival time for relapsing patients exceeded remission time by 30–45 weeks.

Treatment Delays

As our results were not as good as the 70% survival with no evidence of disease (NED) reported by Wollner for histiocytic lymphoma and were significantly poorer than the 80% NED survival for convoluted lymphoma patients, our data were scrutinized to determine possible causes of treatment failure. Significant toxicity resulted in a failure to deliver prescribed therapy on schedule in most patients. Twenty doses of thioguanine and cytosine arabinoside were required by protocol, but the median number received by our patients was 12, (range 5–20). All discontinuations were due to myelosuppression. Twelve doses of L-asparaginase were prescribed, but the median number received was 9 (range 3–12). Hypersensitivity reactions were the cause of cessation of treatment with this agent. Primary disease sites were irradiated during induction or consolidation therapy. The subsequent myelosuppression often delayed chemotherapy, preventing initiation of the next phase of treatment. Such delays were particularly long in the children with convoluted lymphoma who received radiotherapy to the mediastinum. The reasons for the relative lack of tolerance for prescribed therapy in our patients are unknown.

In an effort to quantitate treatment delays, the median number of days to complete treatment phases was calculated and compared with the protocol time plan (Table 2). The median time for delivery of induction therapy exceeded the protocol time by 2 days, for consolidation by 9 days, and for the first maintenance cycle by 13 days. Thereafter, protocol and median times differed little. This apparent concordance is attributable to the elimination of cytosine arabinoside from maintenance therapy for three children who had severe toxicity with high fever and flulike symptoms, and to the deletion of hydroxyurea and daunomycin from maintenance therapy for another child who developed cardiop-

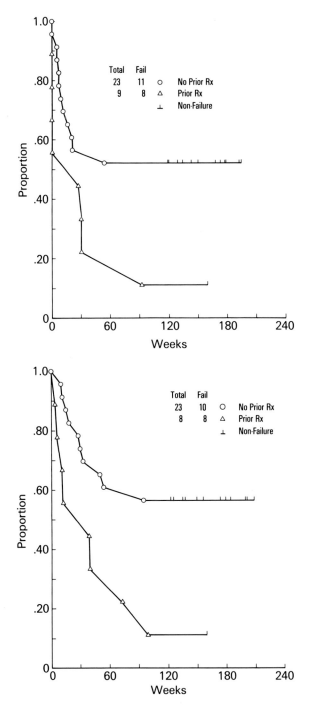

Figure 2. Length of remission curves (top) and survival curves (bottom) for children with no prior therapy and children with prior therapy, M. D. Anderson Hospital LSA$_2$–L$_2$ field trial.

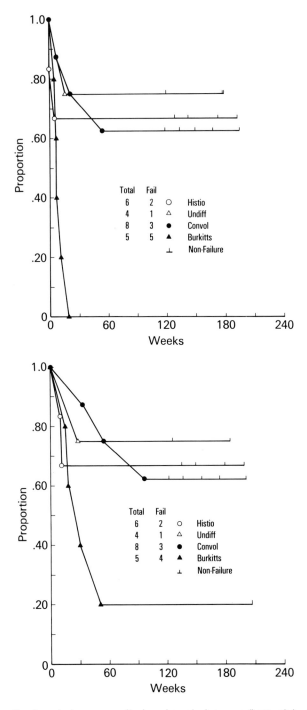

Figure 3. Length of remission curves (top) and survival curves (bottom) by histologic type for children with no prior therapy, M. D. Anderson Hospital LSA$_2$–L$_2$ field trial.

Table 2. *Median Number of Days for Various Phases of Treatment, LSA$_2$–L$_2$ Field Trial (MDAH)*

	INDN	CONS	M–1	M–2	M–3	M–4	M–5	M–6
Protocol time	35	51	65	65	65	65	65	65
Actual time	37	60	78	65	67	68	63	59
All agents received			78	67	71	70	81	71
Cytosar deleted				40	44	63	56	45
Hydroxyurea and daunomycin deleted					43	45	42	49

INDN—induction phase, CONS—consolidation phase, M—maintenance phase.

athy. When maintenance times for the 20 children receiving all chemotherapy agents are compared with the prescribed time, the difference for the first maintenance cycle was 13 days and for the fifth maintenance cycle, 16 days. Differences of 2–6 days were found for the other maintenance cycles. Patients completing 2 years of therapy received an average of 7½ maintenance cycles (range 6–8); had therapy proceeded according to protocol, they would have received 9 maintenance cycles.

Treatment Modifications

When considered with respect to the mobility and the homing propensities of malignant lymphoid cells, our poor therapeutic results could be attributed to (1) failure to provide continuous systemic therapy, which would protect homing sites from becoming populated with malignant cells, (2) lack of effective coordination of chemotherapy and radiotherapy so as to inactivate the primary tumor sites as a source of circulating malignant cells (in this regard it is of interest that our three children with convoluted lymphoma who relapsed all received mediastinal radiotherapy, 3,000 rad, and relapsed within the radiotherapy field), and (3) inadequate protection of the sanctuary meningeal homing site.

The following modifications of the regimen were made in an attempt to correct the deficiencies noted: (1) exclusion of patients with prior therapy; (2) exclusion of patients with abdominal Burkitt's lymphoma; (3) restriction of radiotherapy to patients with residual tumor at the completion of induction therapy; (4) administration of cytosine arabinoside by a more effective technique, viz., continuous infusion for 5 days; (5) reduction of the L-asparaginase dose from 60,000 u/m²/day to a more conservative 6,000 u/m²/day; and (6) reduction of maintenance doses for thioguanine, cyclophosphamide, hydroxyurea, and daunomycin by at least 25–30% to avoid prolongation of maintenance cycles, particularly the first.

Treatment modifications to insure protection from "in transit" and homing malignant cells have been incorporated into a second-generation non-Hodgkin's lymphoma protocol for all histologic tumor types of children except the abdominal presentation of Burkitt's tumor (Figure 1 bottom). Eight patients with no prior therapy have been entered in the pilot study; six have convoluted lymphoma and two have diffuse undifferentiated lymphoma (non-Burkitt's type). In addition, one patient with diffuse histiocytic lymphoma who had other induction therapy entered the second-generation protocol at the consolidation phase. All patients are doing well, but the on-study time is too short for conclusions to be drawn.

Four patients in relapse have also started second-generation therapy. Of this group, one with immunoblastic sarcoma (T cell) responded transiently, but died of a ruptured spleen when disease activity was again uncontrolled. One patient with histiocytic lymphoma and one with convoluted lymphoma appear to be responding well. The fourth patient, who also has convoluted lymphoma, is completing induction therapy with only a partial response. As with the parent LSA$_2$–L$_2$ regimen, previously treated patients appear to respond less satisfactorily. For this group, new therapeutic tactics are needed; hopefully, such tactics will become apparent as we learn to manipulate homing cells and their homes.

REFERENCES

Broder, S., D. Poplack, J. Whang-Peng, M. Durm, C. Godman, L. Muul, and T. A. Waldmann. 1978. Characterization of a suppressor-cell leukemia: Evidence for the requirement of an interaction of two T cells in the development of human suppressor effector cells. N. Engl. J. Med. 298:66–72.

Broder, S., and T. A. Waldmann. 1978a. The suppressor-cell network in cancer. Part I. N. Engl. J. Med. 299:1281–1284.

Broder, S., and T. A. Waldmann. 1978b. The suppressor-cell network in cancer. Part II. N. Engl. J. Med. 299:1335–1341.

de Sousa, M. 1978. Ecotaxis, ecotaxopathy, and lymphoid malignancy: Terms, facts, and predictions, *in* The Immunopathology of Lymphoreticular Neoplasms, vol. 4, Comprehensive Immunology, J. J. Twomey and Robert A. Good, eds. Plenum Press, New York, pp. 325–353.

Gershon, R. K. 1979. Immune regulation: Introduction. Fed. Proc. 38:2051–2052.

Hall, J. G., J. Hopkins, and E. Orlans. 1977. Migration pathways of lymphoid cells with reference to the gut immunoglobulins and lymphomata. Biochem. Soc. Trans. 5:1581.

Knowles, D. M., and S. Holck. 1978. Tissue localization of T-lymphocytes by the histochemical demonstration of acid alpha-naphthyl acetate esterase. Lab. Invest. 39:70–76.

Lukes, R. J., and R. D. Collins. 1974. Immunologic characterization of human malignant lymphomas. Cancer 34:1488–1503.

Lukes, R. J., and R. D. Collins. 1975. New approaches to the classification of the lymphomata. Br. J. Cancer 31:1–28.

Price, R. A., and W. W. Johnson. 1973. The central nervous system in childhood leukemia. I. The arachnoid. Cancer 31:520–533.

Wollner, N., J. H. Burchenal, P. Exelby, P. H. Lieberman, G. D'Angio, and M. L. Murphy. 1974. Non-Hodgkin's lymphoma in children, *in* Conflicts in Childhood Cancer, L. F. Sinks and J. O. Gooden, eds. Alan R. Liss, New York, pp. 179–223.

Wollner, N., J. H. Burchenal, P. H. Lieberman, P. Exelby, G. D. D'Angio, and M. L. Murphy. 1976. Non-Hodgkin's lymphoma in children: A comparative study of two modalities of therapy. Cancer 37:123–134.

Status of the Curability of Childhood Cancers,
edited by J. van Eys and M. P. Sullivan.
Raven Press, New York © 1980.

Pediatric Hodgkin's Disease: Focus on the Future

Sarah S. Donaldson, M.D.

*Department of Radiology, Division of Radiation Therapy, Stanford University School of
Medicine, Stanford, California*

During the last decade, major therapeutic advances have resulted in dramatic improvements in cure rates for a broad spectrum of pediatric cancers, including the malignant lymphomas and Hodgkin's disease. It was less than 150 years ago that Thomas Hodgkin initially described the disease that later came to bear his name. Hodgkin's historic paper, "On Some Morbid Appearances of the Absorbent Glands and Spleen," was read before the Medical-Chirurgical Society in London on January 10 and 24, 1832. During the subsequent decades there was improved recognition of this disease, but a general belief persisted that this dreaded disorder was uniformly fatal. However, dramatic discoveries during the past 2 decades have solved many of the puzzles related to Hodgkin's disease, leading to higher control rates and cures for the majority of those afflicted. It is now clear that pediatric Hodgkin's disease can be likened to the disease in the adult in terms of natural history and response to treatment.

This chapter will summarize several recent advances in the treatment of pediatric Hodgkin's disease and explain how they are responsible for our current excellent results and how they have directed our thinking in the development of new treatment programs.

PROGRESS IN THERAPY

Large series of children with Hodgkin's disease have been reported recently with overall survival rates of about 90% (Donaldson et al. 1976, Jenkin et al. 1979, Botnick et al. 1977). Table 1 summarizes the data from some representative series. The Stanford series, the largest for pediatric Hodgkin's disease, extends over a 10-year period, during which time staging procedures and treatment policies varied (Donaldson et al. 1976). In this group, 52% of the patients underwent surgical staging with both laparotomy and splenectomy. The treatment policies used have been described previously and consisted largely of radiotherapy for stage I–III disease, MOPP chemotherapy (nitrogen mustard, vincristine, procarbazine, and prednisone) for stage IV, and combined therapy for subsets of each stage as that therapy was determined by ongoing clinical trials. In the Princess Margaret Hospital experience with 42 children, 64% of

Table 1. Results with Three Series of Pediatric Hodgkin's Disease Patients*

Series	Years	No. of Patients	Stages	Survival/DFS	No. of Patients Surgically Staged	Treatment
Stanford (Donaldson et al. 1976b)	1962–72	79	I–IV	89%/66%	41 (52%)	Radiotherapy, IF, STL, TLI—depending on stage MOPP—advanced stages
Princess Margaret Hospital (Jenkin et al. 1979)	1969–72	42	I–IV	90%/56%	27 (64%)	Radiotherapy, STL—all patients
Joint Center (Botnick et al. 1977)	1969–75	52	I–III	98%/90%	52 (100%)	Radiotherapy STL—IA, IIA TLI—IIIA TLI + MOPP—IIB, IIIB

* DFS—disease-free survival; IF—involved field; STL—subtotal lymphoid; TLI—total lymphoid irradiation.

whom were surgically staged, extended-field irradiation was used, with control rates produced similar to those in the Stanford series (Jenkin et al. 1979). More recently, the Joint Center in Boston has described its experience with 52 children with stage I–III disease, all of whom underwent surgical staging and achieved a 90% disease-free survival rate (Botnick et al. 1977). Thus, data are emerging from several centers that suggest that nine out of 10 children with Hodgkin's disease who are managed with appropriate staging and treatment will achieve long-term survival.

CONTRIBUTIONS TO THE PRESENT STATUS

It is evident that significant advances have been made in a number of areas that have contributed to the current improved state of these children.

Histopathology

By using the Rye modification of the Lukes and Butler histologic classification (Lukes and Butler 1966), one can detect a clear relationship between tumor histology and the age of the patient. The lymphocyte-predominant subtype is seen more often in patients in the early decades of life, while the lymphocyte-depletion variety is unusual in this age group. The majority of pediatric cases fall into the nodular sclerosis or mixed cellularity subgroups, with nodular sclerosis being the most frequent type seen in the adolescent. In a population of 105 children 15 years of age or less from Stanford, lymphocyte predominance accounted for approximately 15% of the cases. While 58% of the children had the nodular sclerosis subtype, this was less frequently seen in children under 10 than in adolescents. Mixed cellularity, however, appeared more often in those under 10 than it did in those over 10 (Parker et al. 1976).

Diagnostic Studies

Improvements in diagnostic evaluation, particularly radiographic studies, have greatly increased our ability to detect Hodgkin's disease at the time of presentation, to follow the results of therapy, and to detect early relapse. The studies recommended in the routine work-up and clinical staging of children have been described (Donaldson et al. 1976b). Plain chest radiographs with whole-lung tomography are essential in ascertaining the extent of intrathoracic disease, an important consideration when radiotherapy is to be used in the treatment program. A lymphogram is an indispensible guide to initial staging and radiotherapy treatment planning, an aid to the surgeon during surgical staging, and a means of following the status of the opacified lymph nodes by serial surveillance of abdominal radiographs. The lymphogram should be performed on all children with Hodgkin's disease, irrespective of age. Particular expertise is required for the correct lymphographic interpretation, as the changes associated with reactive hyperplasia are more commonly seen in young patients than in adolescents or adults. With experienced radiologists, the correlation between lymphographic staging and histologic findings in children who later underwent surgical staging has been shown to be excellent, with 95% accuracy (Dunnick et al. 1977). Experience with computerized tomography (CT) in preoperative staging is now being obtained. While a CT scan is easier to perform than a lymphogram, it has not been shown to be as sensitive a detector of minimal disease. Therefore, until its value is demonstrated in the pediatric population with Hodgkin's disease, the CT scan should not replace the lymphogram and other established staging procedures. Isotopic scans, abdominal ultrasonograms, and miscellaneous radiographic studies have not been demonstrated to be useful in the routine staging of large series of asymptomatic patients, but may be employed when patients have signs or symptoms referable to a particular organ system.

Surgical Staging

Surgical staging with splenectomy came into wide use in 1968, and has been a principal factor in improved cure rates. In the Stanford series of 79 children, a marked difference in relapse-free survival was seen at 5 years, with 82% of surgically staged patients relapse free, as compared to only 55% of those clinically staged (Donaldson et al. 1976b). In addition, in this series no relapses were seen after 2 years in patients staged surgically. The clinical stage is altered in approximately 30% of pediatric patients on the basis of surgical staging (Jenkin and Berry 1979, Donaldson et al. 1976b, Cohen et al. 1977). In the Stanford series of 41 surgically staged patients, in 14 cases (34%) a change in stage was made based upon pathologic findings, and six patients (15%) had treatment modifications made on the basis of the detection of unsuspected splenic involvement that did not change the numerical stage (Donaldson et al. 1976b).

In girls and young women, if there is a possibility of using pelvic irradiation, an oophoropexy should be performed at the time of staging laparotomy (Ray et al. 1970). If one designs a therapy program based upon the extent of disease, surgical staging is mandatory. For example, if a staging laparotomy is not performed and radiotherapy is used as the primary therapeutic modality, the upper abdomen should be irradiated to cover the 30% probability of occult splenic or upper abdominal lymph node disease. In the pediatric population, a *major* value of the staging laparotomy is to define the extent of disease so that abdominal-pelvic radiation can be carefully planned and administered selectively, thus avoiding the need for total lymphoid irradiation in all children.

Therapy

Treatment philosophies for children with Hodgkin's disease generally have reflected those for adults with the disease. Major advances were made with the introduction of megavoltage therapy units, specifically the linear accelerator, permitting treatment of large fields, carefully shaped to encompass multiple lymph node chains in continuity, and the use of sufficiently high doses. Sophisticated set-up techniques now permit treatment of all major lymphoid regions in the body to tumoricidal dose levels. As a result, total lymphoid irradiation or slight modifications thereof have become the established treatment of choice for essentially all adults with stage I–IIA or B and IIIA or III_sA disease, and are incorporated in combined modality therapy for IIIB and III_sB disease (Kaplan 1972). The use of extended-field, high-dose radiation produces excellent survival rates, as shown in Table 1. Some investigators, recognizing the high potential of salvage treatment, question whether less aggressive initial radiotherapy with treatment to smaller fields might be appropriate, delaying maximal therapy until the first relapse. This question of therapeutic philosophy has not been answered, but is currently being investigated in clinical trials.

Series in which patients have been treated with chemotherapy alone are few. While a number of chemotherapy programs have been successful, none has been demonstrated to be superior to the MOPP program as described by DeVita and co-workers (1970). In Uganda, where radiotherapy facilities are nonexistent, 48 children have been treated with MOPP chemotherapy alone. Forty-two children (88%) achieved a complete response, and 31 of the 42 (74%) remain in complete remission. Actuarial survival for the group is 67%, 75% for those with stages I–IIIA and 60% for those with stages IIIB and IV (Olweny et al. 1978). However, the adult experience in Uganda with MOPP alone is less successful. Of 17 patients (14 with stage IV disease), 13 (76%) obtained a complete remission, with a mean remission duration of 16 months, and 61% are alive at 2 years (Olweny et al. 1971). Thus, in view of the effectiveness of both radiotherapy and chemotherapy in the control of Hodgkin's disease, a number of investigators now look toward various combinations of these two therapeutic modalities. Jenkin and co-workers have described 27 children who were not surgically staged and who were treated with subtotal lymphoid radiotherapy to a mantle, spleen, and para-aortic field to doses of 2,000–3,500 rad and six cycles of MOPP chemotherapy. They have reported actuarial 3- and 5-year survival and relapse-free survival rates of 91% (Jenkin et al. 1979). The major advance in this series compared to their initial experience was the improvement in 5-year relapse-free survival from 57% to 91% (Jenkin et al. 1975, 1979).

THE PRICE OF SUCCESS

Since the present results of treatment are so gratifying in children, we are in the fortunate position of being able to look to reducing the severity of therapy programs with the intent of minimizing complications. To evaluate the relative effectiveness of our treatment, we must look criticially at the price paid for long-term survival. Such successes must be weighed against acute and long-term complications. The acute complications of therapy generally are reversible. While they are of major importance at the time of therapy, they assume less importance as recovery from acute normal tissue injury occurs. The potential late effects of the treatment become significant in children, who are undergoing active growth and development at the time of treatment and in whom long-term survival is expected.

Complications of Staging

The work-up and evaluation for Hodgkin's disease are now quite standard and nonmorbid. In experienced hands there is a high degree of accuracy and low complication rate with the radiographic evaluations, including lymphograms, in the young child (Castellino et al. 1975). While surgical staging and splenectomy remain routine for the adult population, their place has been questioned in the management of children, particularly children under the age of 5 (Sullivan et al. 1975), because of the concern for overwhelming infection in the asplenic child. However, there is no evidence that the age of 5 is a critical time, beyond which one is at a lesser degree of risk. The incidence of surgical complications following laparotomy, such as bowel obstruction, has been low in experienced hands (Rosenstock et al. 1974) and not significantly associated with mortality. The risk of severe infection in children with Hodgkin's disease is about 10% (Chilcote et al. 1976, Donaldson et al. 1978).

Infections

Of particular concern in treating children with Hodgkin's disease is the incidence of viral and bacterial infections. Serious bacterial infections in children with Hodgkin's disease are caused most frequently by encapsulated organisms, with *Streptococcus pneumoniae* being the most common offending organism. The incidence of serious bacterial infections appears related more to the aggressiveness of treatment than to the presence or absence of the spleen (Donaldson et al. 1978). Among 181 children treated at Stanford, 27 episodes of serious bacterial infection (bacteremia, meningitis, pneumonia, or acute pyelonephritis) occurred in 22 children, of which 15 episodes in 14 children involved bacteremia, meningitis, or both. The incidence of infection in splenectomized children treated with radiotherapy alone was 1.4%, compared to 2.8% among nonsplenectomized children treated with radiotherapy. However, when chemotherapy was added to the treatment regime there was an 18% incidence of infection among splenectomized children and 23% among those nonsplenectomized. There was no difference in the probability of infection as a function of splenectomy, although all children with *Streptococcus pneumoniae* or *Hemophilus influenzae* meningitis had their spleens removed. There were three septic episodes, in this series among patients who were off all treatment with no evidence of disease and in whom the asplenic state was the only parameter felt responsible for the infection, an incidence of 1.67% of all patients (Donaldson et al. 1978). It is important to note that functional asplenia with overwhelming sepsis and death occurred in a young woman at Stanford in whom no splenectomy was performed but who had undergone splenic irradiation (Dailey et al. 1980).

Many investigators now recommend the use of prophylactic penicillin to decrease the incidence of infection. While this appears to be beneficial, quantitative data are not yet available. Factors relevant to antibiotic therapy include patient compliance, length of time antibiotics should be administered, optimum dosage, and risk of secondary infection. Polyvalent pneumococcal vaccine currently is being investigated. Patients undergoing or recently completing active immunosuppressive treatment who have been given the pneumococcal vaccine after splenectomy have been shown to have an impaired antibody response and occasionally reduced antibody levels due to immune tolerance (Siber et al. 1978). The optimal timing and potential efficacy of administering the vaccine prior to splenectomy and the value of booster immunization need to be defined.

The incidence of herpes zoster–varicella among children with Hodgkin's disease has been reported as high as 35% in the Stanford series of 181 children, of whom 46 (25%) had localized infections and 17 (9%) had generalized infections (Reboul et al. 1978). This incidence correlates with stage of disease and aggressiveness of treatment, with a 24% incidence after extended-field radiotherapy, 11% after involved-field radiotherapy, and 56% after extended-field radiotherapy plus chemotherapy. Of these episodes, 80% occurred within the 1st year after completion of treatment. Splenectomy did not increase the incidence of infection. Thus, the incidence of bacterial and viral infections is greatly increased by combined modality treatment, as are other infections seen in the immunosuppressed host, including opportunistic, fungal, and *Pneumocystis carinii.*

Long-Term Complications

The major long-term complications of treatment include abnormalities in growth and development and organ function, fertility and genetic abnormalities, and second malignant tumors. These will be discussed individually as they relate to children.

Growth and Development

The long-term effects of treatment upon growth and development are of great significance to this group of patients, who have a high probability of long-term survival. Many late effects secondary to radiotherapy can be minimized by careful attention to such treatment techniques as the use of megavoltage beams, meticulous treatment planning, individualized blocks and beam-shaping devices, and multiple simulations and the shrinking-field approach (Donaldson et al. 1976a). The radiation effects on growing bone are related directly to the radiation dose and the patient's age at the time of treatment. The major impact upon the axial skeleton among long-term survivors of Hodgkin's disease seems to occur during the time of active bone growth, i.e., before 6 years of age and during the adolescent growth spurt, between 11 and 13 years (Probert and Parker 1975, Probert et al. 1973). The alteration produced is a disproportionate decrease in sitting as compared to standing height, and is greatest among children receiving axial skeleton doses greater than 3,500 rad. In addition, soft tissue changes and fibrosis occur and are particularly apparent in the thorax following mantle field irradiation, with shortened clavicles and a small neck produced but unaffected upper extremities.

Organ Function

Physiologic impairment of organ growth, with attendant cardiac, pulmonary, neurologic, and vascular complications, may occur in children as well as in adults and may be enhanced by combined modality therapy. However, with attention to treatment techniques and the proper use of pulmonary, cardiac, laryngeal, and spinal cord blocks, the incidence of complications secondary to mantle therapy has been greatly reduced. In the Stanford series, the incidence of symptomatic pulmonary radiation reaction has decreased from 26% to 4%, and pericarditis from 17% to 2.5%, with newer techniques of treatment (Carmel and Kaplan 1976). Despite this lower complication rate, the incidence of thoracic relapse has not increased, and in fact has decreased from 13% to 7.6%. It is important to note that both pneumonitis and carditis may be activated by the rapid tapering off of corticosteroids (Castellino et al. 1974). Prednisone should be omitted from the MOPP regimen if the lungs or heart are to receive a moderate radiation dose. It has previously been demonstrated that prednisone itself does not appear to add to the chemotherapy-induced remission rate or length of remission in Hodgkin's disease patients (Jacobs et al. 1976).

Radiation-induced chemical or clinical hypothyroidism has been well documented in patients receiving radiation to the thyroid (Glatstein et al. 1971, Shalet et al. 1977), and is most pronounced in those who have undergone a previous lymphogram, presumably because of the associated iodine load. The incidence of thyroid dysfunction in children following neck irradiation has been reported to be as high as 91% (Shalet et al. 1977). The impact of the sustained stimulation of the thyroid gland by thyroid stimulating hormone (TSH) is unknown. Therefore, patients with low serum thyroxine (T 4), elevated TSH levels, or both, should receive thyroid replacement to achieve a clinical and chemical euthyroid state. However, the natural history of chronic radiation-induced thyroid dysfunction is not known, nor are the risk of thyroid neoplasia and its relationship to hormonal replacement quantitated.

Fertility and Genetic Abnormalities

Gonadal dysfunction following therapy has a major impact on children. The combination of oophoropexy and appropriate gonadal shielding during pelvic radiation has allowed approximately 75% of menstruating women to maintain menses with apparently normal ovarian function (Donaldson et al. 1976b). With these techniques, 21 women who underwent oophoropexy followed by high-dose pelvic radiotherapy have become pregnant, and 15 have given birth to 20 healthy children (Donaldson 1979). The remaining six had abortions. There have been no observed abnormalities in the offspring or in the products of conception. Approximately 50% of women maintain or resume normal menses following combination chemotherapy. These women are also capable of having normal pregnancies and deliveries, and producing normal offspring. In male patients treated with an inverted-Y treatment field, transient aspermia occurs, but spermatogenesis is often recovered and many male patients have fathered normal offspring within a few years of completion of radiotherapy.

There is, however, increasing evidence documenting a depletion of testicular germ cells with subsequent sterility following combination chemotherapy in boys and men. Of 19 Uganda boys treated with MOPP, nine of 13 pubertal boys (age 11–16) developed gynecomastia and germinal aplasia, with elevated follicle stimulating hormone and lutenizing hormone and reduced serum testosterone levels (Sherins et al. 1978). It is not known if prepubescent boys experience the same degree of testicular injury following combination chemotherapy. In the Uganda experience, the six prepubertal boys did not develop the hormonal changes or gynecomastia that the pubertal boys did; however, Arneil (1972) has discussed reports of prepubertal therapy with Cytoxan resulting in postpubertal azoospermia. Thus, MOPP chemotherapy is associated with germ cell depletion and Leydig cell dysfunction in adolescent boys and men, which to date do not appear to be reversible.

While a possibility of genetic risk secondary to current therapy certainly does exist, it is unlikely to be observed for several generations. Holmes and Holmes (1978) compared pregnancy outcomes for treated Hodgkin's disease patients with those for matched sibling controls and were unable to detect differences in numbers of spontaneous abortions or abnormal offspring between irradiated patients and controls; however, they did observe an increased risk of both in 13 patients treated with chemotherapy and radiotherapy.

Second Malignant Tumors

A new concern for survivors of Hodgkin's disease is the rising incidence of second malignant tumors, particularly acute myelogenous leukemia (AML) and non-Hodgkin's lymphoma (NHL), which are usually unresponsive to conventional therapy. Among 579 consecutive adult patients with Hodgkin's disease treated at Stanford, the actuarial risk of developing AML is 2% and NHL 4% at 7 years' follow-up. These hematologic neoplasms have not been observed in patients receiving radiotherapy alone. Among those who have received combined modality therapy with irradiation and combination chemotherapy, the incidence of AML is 3.9% and NHL approximately 8%; both incidences appear to be rising at 7 years (Coleman et al. 1977, Krikorian et al. 1979). Among

79 consecutive children at Stanford, we have observed two who developed second malignant solid tumors, one an undifferentiated sarcoma of the abdomen and the other a soft tissue sarcoma of the neck. A third child has developed AML. All three children had been given radiotherapy and MOPP chemotherapy.

FUTURE

With current treatment results showing long-term survival and disease-free survival rates of approximately 90%, it will be difficult to demonstrate any further improvement in outcome. The major concern now is the *quality* of survival, with appropriate efforts being taken to minimize the acute and long-term complications of treatment without compromising these excellent results of therapy. Our future focus for the pediatric population must be on cautiously modifying our therapies with this goal in mind.

The major questions in treating children with Hodgkin's disease are the following:

1. *Can we omit some of the diagnostic tests or substitute less invasive tests?* The lymphogram is indispensable in evaluating the lymph node status of children. The accuracy of CT scanning in large groups of children is not known. It appears that CT scanning of the abdomen may be complementary to lymphography by providing information on the status of lymph nodes in the celiac axis area, a location poorly visualized by lymphography. However, the CT scan does not provide the ease of follow-up or the details of lymph node morphology and architecture that can be provided by a lymphogram. This information is essential in staging, particularly in differentiating between abnormalities of reactive hyperplasia, which are so common in the pediatric population, and filling defects from Hodgkin's disease. Thus, at present one should not omit the lymphogram in favor of abdominal CT scanning.

It is possible to omit a prelaparotomy bone marrow biopsy in a child who has clinical stage IA or IIA disease and an unequivocally normal lymphogram if surgical staging with open bone marrow biopsy is planned. At Stanford, we have never identified bone marrow involvement at the time of presentation in any patient who was asymptomatic and had stage I or II supradiaphragmatic disease following complete clinical staging (Rosenberg 1971).

2. *Can we eliminate surgical staging?* Surgical staging can be defended only if treatment policies are selected on the basis of the extent of disease. Since in approximately 30% of children the stage is changed on the basis of surgical findings, to omit surgical staging makes necessary the use of more extensive treatment. With respect to radiotherapy, extended-field treatment is treatment to a mantle and the upper abdomen at a minimum, with at least a splenic field and para-aortic irradiation. If chemotherapy is not used, the liver, and probably the pelvis as well, should be treated. At present, the staging laparotomy in children provides data otherwise unobtainable, but at some risk of morbidity and mortality, primarily from septicemia, and continued investigation is required.

The mortality from postsplenectomy septicemia is in the 1–2% range. Perhaps this will be reduced by the routine use of prophylactic antibiotics and better knowledge about the timing and use of polyvalent pneumococcal vaccine.

3. *Should we give MOPP alone to all children?* The complete response rates with MOPP are about 80%, and cure rates are approximately 50% (DeVita et al. 1970, Olweny et al. 1971, Young et al. 1978). These figures are not as favorable as those reported following therapy by extended-field radiotherapy alone or combined modality programs for stages I–III disease. Therefore, at present MOPP cannot be recommended as the sole treatment in areas where adequate radiotherapy facilities exist.

4. *Can we permit relapse to occur? If so, how can we improve our salvage or cure rates for patients who have relapsed?* When planning therapy for children, the question invariably is asked, can we limit our initial treatment and save aggressive staging and therapy for those who will relapse? To save aggressive therapy for those who relapse requires the availability of salvage treatment that is nearly 100% effective. At present, chemotherapy for salvage treatment can cure only about one half of those patients (Young et al. 1978, Portlock et al. 1978). Thus, it is essential to maximize the effectiveness of a first course of treatment and to prevent relapse.

5. *How can we improve our cure rates for stage IV marrow disease?* While multiple chemotherapeutic agents produce responses in Hodgkin's disease, our success with patients with marrow involvement is still disappointing. At present, multiagent chemotherapeutic programs such as MOPP produce cure rates of only about 20–25% for patients with stage IV disease involving the bone marrow (Portlock et al. 1978). Other combination programs, such as Bonadonna's ABVD regimen (Bonadonna et al. 1975) or B-CAVe (Porzig et al. 1978), have had some success in patients who have suffered a relapse. Perhaps combining these agents in an alternating program at the initiation of therapy will improve the outlook for this subset of patients.

6. *Can we decrease the dose or the volume of radiotherapy?* The sequelae of radiotherapy in children have been discussed and are directly related to dose and volume and inversely related to age. While a dose-response curve with radiotherapy alone is known, an established dose-response curve for irradiation in combination with chemotherapy is not yet known. However, such data are being obtained. At Stanford, an innovative protocol was initiated 10 years ago combining low-dose radiation (1,500, 2,000 or 2,500 rad) and MOPP chemotherapy for surgically staged children. To date, 35 children have been treated using this program, described in Table 2. Figure 1 illustrates a survival rate of 94% and a relapse-free survival rate of 90% for these 35 children, with a maximum follow-up of 9½ years. These data are comparable to those described by Jenkin and co-workers (1979), who advocated extended-field radiotherapy (subtotal lymphoid) at doses of 2,000–3,500 rad and six cycles of MOPP for all children who were not surgically staged. In the Stanford series of surgically staged children, 17 of the 35 (49%) were demonstrated to have localized disease, stage

Table 2. *Pediatric Hodgkin's Disease Protocol*

	Treatment		
Pathologic Stage	Radiation	and	Chemotherapy
IA, IIA	Involved field	and	MOPP × 6
I_EA, II_EA	Subtotal lymphoid	and	MOPP × 6
IB, II_EB	Total lymphoid	and	MOPP × 6
I_EB, II_EB	Total lymphoid	and	MOPP × 6
IIIA, III_EA, III_SA	Total lymphoid	and	MOPP × 6
IIIB, III_EB, III_SB	Alternating MOPP and radiotherapy*		
Multiple E, IV	Alternating MOPP and radiotherapy*		
IV_M	MOPP × 6, radiotherapy, and maintenance MOPP		

Radiation Dose
　　Bone age—less than 6 years　　1,500 rad
　　　　　　　　　6–10 years　　2,000 rad
　　　　　　　　　11–14 years　　2,500 rad

MOPP Dose
　Nitrogen mustard, 6 mg/m² i.v. days 1, 8
　Vincristine, 1.4 mg/m² i.v. days 1, 8 (limit 2 mg)
　Procarbazine, 100 mg/m² days 2–14
　Prednisone, 40 mg/m² p.o. days 1–14 with rapid tapering, cycles 1 and 4;
　　omit in children who receive mantle irradiation

　　* MOPP × 2 cycles, followed by radiotherapy to one region, followed by MOPP × 2 cycles, followed by radiotherapy to a second region, with a total of 6 cycles of MOPP, as described by Hoppe et al. (1979).

IA or IIA, and were treated with low-dose involved-field or mantle therapy alone. Thus, half of the patients received a more limited volume and lower dose of radiation than in Jenkin's experience, further minimizing the potential morbidity from treatment. The two deaths in the Stanford series (Figure 1) occurred in patients with surgical stage IV marrow-positive disease who died within 6 months of diagnosis, never responding to MOPP therapy. The one patient who relapsed had stage $III_{SE}B$ disease with extranodal involvement of the pericardium and lung and failed at 22 months in an irradiated lymph node. Thus, of these 35 patients, the only failures were in those with very unfavorable stage IIIB and IV marrow-positive disease. Such an approach of low-dose radiation plus MOPP would seem appropriate for most children with Hodgkin's disease.

　　Some subsets of patients may, after careful staging, be candidates for even less aggressive therapy, such as radiotherapy alone. Such patients might include those with high right neck disease with a lymphocyte-predominant histology. However, these cases must be approached on an individual basis, taking into account the patient's age, disease stage, histology, and potential morbidity of treatment. Careful definition is now required of the subsets in whom the dose and volume of radiotherapy may be reduced, keeping as the constant goal cure

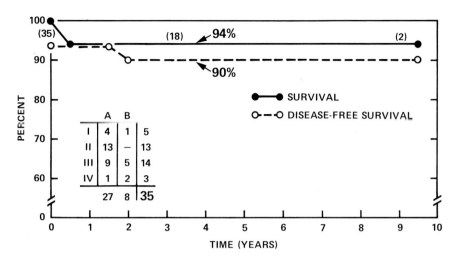

Figure 1. Actuarial survival and disease-free survival curves for 35 surgically staged children with Hodgkin's disease as of September 1979, treated on current protocol (Table 2). ( ) indicates number of children at risk.

and an improved quality of survival, while minimizing complications from treatment.

Still unknown are all the long-term effects of chemotherapy and combined modality therapy. We must continue to investigate less toxic combinations of drugs. The probability of sterility for the male and the increased risk of second malignant tumors following high-dose total nodal radiotherapy and MOPP must be kept in mind when planning therapy programs. Until chemotherapy programs are developed that improve upon the complete response rate and duration of the response produced by MOPP, and thus improve the outlook for stage IV marrow-positive patients, radiotherapy will remain a major modality in the treatment of Hodgkin's disease. However, at this time a reduced dose-volume of radiotherapy with planned chemotherapy is appropriate for the majority of children afflicted with this challenging disorder.

ACKNOWLEDGMENTS

I wish to thank Drs. J. Wilbur and F. Ralph Berberick for their aid in caring for some of the patients, Drs. R. Hoppe, S. A. Rosenberg, and H. S. Kaplan for their help in reviewing the manuscript, and Ms. Meg Rose for her secretarial assistance.

This investigation was supported in part by Research Grant CA-05838 from the National Cancer Institute, National Institutes of Health, Department of Health, Education and Welfare, Bethesda, Maryland.

REFERENCES

Arneil, G. C. 1972. Cyclophosphamide and the prepubertal testis. Lancet 2:1259–1260.

Bonadonna, G., R. Zucali, S. Monfardini, M. DeLena, and C. Uslenghi. 1975. Combination chemotherapy of Hodgkin's disease with Adriamycin, bleomycin, vinblastine and imidazole carboxamide versus MOPP. Cancer 36:252–259.

Botnick, L. E., R. Goodman, N. Jaffe, R. Filler, and J. R. Cassady. 1977. Stages I–III Hodgkin's disease in children: Results of staging and treatment. Cancer 39:599–603.

Carmel, R. J., and H. S. Kaplan. 1976. Mantle irradiation in Hodgkin's disease: An analysis of technique, tumor eradication, and complications. Cancer 37:2813–2825.

Castellino, R. A., F. F. Bellani, M. Gasparini, G. Terno, and R. Musumeci. 1975. Lymphography in childhood: Six years experience with 242 cases. Lymphology 8:74–83.

Castellino, R. A., E. Glatstein, M. M. Turbow, S. A. Rosenberg, and H. S. Kaplan. 1974. Latent radiation injury of lungs or heart activated by steroid withdrawal. Ann. Intern. Med. 80:593–599.

Chilcote, R. R., R. L. Baehner, and D. Hammond. 1976. Septicemia and meningitis in children splenectomized for Hodgkin's disease. N. Engl. J. Med. 295:798–800.

Cohen, I. T., G. R. Higgins, D. R. Powars, and D. M. Hays. 1977. Staging laparotomy for Hodgkin's disease in children. Arch. Surg. 112:948–951.

Coleman, C. N., C. J. Williams, A. Flint, E. J. Glatstein, S. A. Rosenberg, and H. S. Kaplan, 1977. Hematologic neoplasia in patients treated for Hodgkin's disease. N. Engl. J. Med. 297:1249–1252.

Dailey, M., Coleman, C. N., and Kaplan, H. S. 1980. Functional asplenia in patients undergoing splenic irradiation: A case report and a review of autopsy cases. N. Engl. J. Med., 302:215–217.

DeVita, V. T., A. A. Serpick, and P. P. Carbone. 1970. Combination chemotherapy in the treatment of advanced Hodgkin's disease. Ann. Intern. Med. 73:881–895.

Donaldson, S. S. 1980. The preservation of ovarian function in patients undergoing pelvic radiation, *in* Controversies in Gynecologic Oncology, S. Ballon, ed. G. K. Hall and Co., Boston, in press.

Donaldson, S. S., E. Glatstein, and H. S. Kaplan. 1976a. Radiotherapy of childhood lymphoma, *in* Trends in Childhood Cancer, M. H. Donaldson and H. G. Seydel, eds. John Wiley & Sons, New York, pp. 37–60.

Donaldson, S. S., E. Glatstein, S. A. Rosenberg, and H. S. Kaplan. 1976b. Pediatric Hodgkin's disease. II. Results of therapy. Cancer 37:2436–2447.

Donaldson, S. S., E. Glatstein, and K. L. Vosti. 1978. Bacterial infections in pediatric Hodgkin's disease. Cancer 41:1949–1958.

Dunnick, N. R., B. R. Parker, and R. A. Castellino. 1977. Pediatric lymphography: Performance, interpretation, and accuracy in 193 consecutive children. Am. J. Roentgenol. 129:639–645.

Glatstein, E., S. McHardy-Young, N. Brast, J. R. Eltringham, and J. P. Kriss. 1971. Alterations in serum thyrotropin (TSH) in thyroid function following radiotherapy in patients with malignant lymphoma. J. Clin. Endrocrinol. Metab. 32:833–841.

Holmes, G. E., and F. F. Holmes. 1978. Pregnancy outcome of patients treated for Hodgkin's disease. Cancer 41:1317–1322.

Hoppe, R. T., C. S. Portlock, E. Glatstein, S. A. Rosenberg, and H. S. Kaplan. 1979. Alternating chemotherapy and irradiation in the treatment of advanced Hodgkin's disease. Cancer 43:472–481.

Jacobs, C., C. S. Portlock, and S. A. Rosenberg. 1976. Prednisone in MOPP chemotherapy for Hodgkin's disease. Br. Med. J. 2:1469–1471.

Jenkin, D., M. Freedman, P. McClure, V. Peters, F. Saunders, and M. Sonley. 1979. Hodgkin's disease in children: Treatment with low dose radiation and MOPP without staging laparotomy. A preliminary report. Cancer 44:80–86.

Jenkin, R. D. T., and M. P. Berry. 1979. Hodgkin's disease in children. Semin. Oncol. (in press).

Jenkin, R. D. T., T. C. Brown, M. V. Peters, and M. J. Sonley. 1975. Hodgkin's disease in children. A retrospective analysis: 1958–73. Cancer 35:979–990.

Kaplan, H. S. 1972. Hodgkin's Disease. Harvard University Press, Cambridge, Mass., 452 pp.

Krikorian, J. G., J. S. Burke, S. A. Rosenberg, and H. S. Kaplan. 1979. Occurrence of non-Hodgkin's lymphoma after therapy for Hodgkin's disease. N. Engl. J. Med. 300:452–458.

Lukes, R. J., and J. J. Butler. 1966. The pathology and nomenclature of Hodgkin's disease. Cancer Res. 26:1063–1081.

Olweny, C. L. M., E. Katongole-Mbidde, C. Kiire, S. K. Lwanga, I. Magrath, and J. L. Ziegler. 1978. Childhood Hodgkin's disease in Uganda: A ten-year experience. Cancer 42:787–792.

Olweny, C. L. M., J. L. Ziegler, C. W. Bernard, and A. C. Templeton. 1971. Adult Hodgkin's disease in Uganda. Cancer 27:1295–1301.

Parker, B. R., R. A. Castellino, and H. S. Kaplan. 1976. Pediatric Hodgkin's disease. I. Radiographic evaluation. Cancer 37:2430–2435.

Portlock, C. S., S. A. Rosenberg, E. Glatstein, and H. S. Kaplan. 1978. Impact of salvage treatment on initial relapses in patients with Hodgkin's disease, stage I–III. Blood 51:825–833.

Porzig, K. J., C. S. Portlock, A. Robertson, and S. A. Rosenberg. 1978. Treatment of advanced Hodgkin's disease with B-CAVe following MOPP failure. Cancer 41:1670–1675.

Probert, J. C., and B. R. Parker. 1975. The effects of radiation therapy on bone growth. Radiology 114:155–162.

Probert, J. C., B. R. Parker, and H. S. Kaplan. 1973. Growth retardation in children after megavoltage irradiation of the spine. Cancer 32:634–639.

Ray, G. R., H. W. Trueblood, L. P. Enright, H. S. Kaplan, and T. S. Nelsen. 1970. Oophoropexy: A means of preserving ovarian function following pelvic megavoltage radiotherapy for Hodgkin's disease. Radiology 96:175–180.

Reboul, F., S. S. Donaldson, and H. S. Kaplan. 1978. Herpes zoster and varicella infections in children with Hodgkin's disease. Cancer 41:95–99.

Rosenberg, S. A. 1971. Hodgkin's disease of the bone marrow. Cancer Res. 31:1733–1736.

Rosenstock, J. G., G. J. D'Angio, and W. B. Kiesewetter. 1974. The incidence of complications following staging laparotomy for Hodgkin's disease in children. Am. J. Roentgenol. 120:531–535.

Shalet, S. M., J. D. Rosenstock, C. G. Beardwell, D. Pearson, and P. H. Morris-Jones. 1977. Thyroid dysfunction following external irradiation to the neck for Hodgkin's disease in childhood. Clin. Radiol. 28:511–515.

Sherins, R. J., C. L. M. Olweny, and J. L. Ziegler. 1978. Gynecomastia and gonadal dysfunction in adolescent boys treated with combination chemotherapy for Hodgkin's disease. N. Engl. J. Med. 299:12–16.

Siber, G. R., S. A. Weitzman, A. C. Aisenberg, H. J. Weinstein, and G. Schiffman. 1978. Impaired antibody response to pneumococcal vaccine after treatment for Hodgkin's disease. N. Engl. J. Med. 299:442–448.

Sullivan, M. P., L. M. Fuller, and C. Fernandez. 1975. Prognostic factors and late effects: Innovative guidelines for selective, age-conditioned therapy for Hodgkin's disease in children, *in* Conflicts in Childhood Cancer: An Evaluation of Current Management, L. F. Sinks and J. O. Gooden, eds. Alan R. Liss, Inc., New York, pp. 103–115.

Young, R. C., G. P. Canellos, B. A. Chabner, S. M. Hubbard, and V. T. DeVita. 1978. Patterns of relapse in advanced Hodgkin's disease treated with combination chemotherapy. Cancer 42:1001–1007.

Status of the Curability of Childhood Cancers,
edited by J. van Eys and M. P. Sullivan.
Raven Press, New York © 1980.

The Challenge in Granulocytic Leukemia Research

F. Leonard Johnson, M.D.

*University of Washington and Children's Orthopedic Hospital and Medical Center,
Seattle, Washington*

It is certainly a very important fact that we have in it [acute leukemia]
to deal with conditions which, when abandoned to themselves, or subjected to any one of the hitherto known methods of treatment, continually grow worse and ultimately lead to death.

Rudolf Virchow (1860)

FROM VIRCHOW TO TIVEY

The basic challenge in acute granulocytic leukemia is that over 130 years
after Virchow's first description of the disease, his gloomy conclusion still holds
true for the majority of patients suffering with acute granulocytic leukemia
(AGL). Osler's recommended treatment in 1897 was "fresh air, good diet, and
absentation from mental worry and care. . . . There are certain remedies which
have an influence upon the disease. Of these, arsenic, given in large doses, is
the best" (Osler 1897).

In fact, for over 80 years the main advances in our understanding of AGL
consisted of better definitions of the disease. The specific "myelogenous" form
of the disease was detected by Neumann in 1878, and Ehrlich's introduction
of staining techniques enabled cytologic differences between various types of
leukemic cells to be defined.

In 1953 Burchenal and co-workers reported that 6-mercaptopurine was the
first chemotherapeutic agent to show any influence in treating AGL, but by
1954 Tivey, in analyzing the "duration of survival time from diagnosis to death
. . . in several hundred cases in both adults and children with acute granulocytic
leukemia," found this duration was 1–2 months for children.

THE ERA OF CHEMOTHERAPY

The discovery of 6-mercaptopurine led to accelerated development of other
agents, including cytosine arabinoside, the anthracyclines (Adriamycin and daunomycin), and 5-azacytidine, which over the past 2 decades have proved to

251

be the most effective single agents, producing complete remissions in 25–40% of patients with AGL (Ellison et al. 1968, Weil et al. 1973, Vogler et al. 1976). In contrast, drugs such as vincristine, prednisone, and methotrexate, vital in the treatment of acute lymphoblastic leukemia (ALL), did not appear to produce a significant number of remissions in AGL (Karon et al. 1966, Wolff et al. 1967, Vogler et al. 1967).

Marked improvements in supportive care with more effective antibiotic and blood component therapy enabled more marrow-suppressive and effective combination-drug regimens to be introduced (Whitecar et al. 1972, Gale and Cline 1977, Rai et al. 1975, Chard et al. 1978), which have confirmed the observation by Freedman and his colleagues in 1971 that combination chemotherapy is more effective than single-drug therapy in childhood AGL.

Use of these various combination regimens, such as cytosine arabinoside, daunomycin, and thioguanine (Gale and Cline 1977) or cytosine arabinoside and daunomycin (Rai et al. 1975), has made possible the first significant therapeutic advance in AGL—the ability to produce complete remissions in over 60% of afflicted children.

Unfortunately, this is the only therapeutic advance that has been afforded by chemotherapy, for we are still without an established, effective method of maintaining remissions in most children with AGL. At best, only one in six patients attains a continuous complete remission of sufficient duration (over 2–3 years) to consider cessation of chemotherapy (Chard et al. 1978), and controversy continues as to whether maintenance chemotherapy actually prolongs remissions.

Recent studies in adults with AGL have shown no advantage in giving maintenance chemotherapy after an initial intensive induction course. In one study (Lewis et al. 1979) the median survivals with and without maintenance chemotherapy were identical, and there was no increase in remission duration in patients under 50 years of age who were given chemotherapy. A second study comparing the remission durations of patients given immunotherapy alone or immunotherapy with maintenance chemotherapy following the same intensive chemotherapeutic induction regimen produced initial remission durations of 8 months for both groups (Powles et al. 1979). As shall be discussed, the increased remission durations produced by marrow transplantation without remission maintenance by systemic chemotherapy after an initial preparative regimen of cyclophosphamide and total body irradiation also raise the question of the role of maintenance chemotherapy in AGL (Thomas et al. 1979).

ALTERNATIVE METHODS OF MAINTAINING REMISSIONS

In response to the current lack of effective chemotherapeutic agents for the maintenance of AGL remissions, other methods of treatment aimed at prolonging remissions have been tried over the past decade. These include splenectomy, manipulation of the mitotic cycle of the leukemia cell, adjuvant treatment to the central nervous system, and immunotherapy.

The median remission duration in 14 children who underwent splenectomies after they had obtained complete remissions was 14.5 months (Fleming et al. 1974), not greatly different from the 11–12-month median first-remission duration in most chemotherapy-maintained studies (Chard et al. 1978).

An attempt to manipulate the mitotic cycle of the leukemic cell with constant infusions of cytosine arabinoside resulted in a remission rate of 75%, but a median remission duration of only 6 months (Lampkin et al. 1976). Such an approach, however, is appealing, and with increasing knowledge of the biology of the cancer cell may find increasing application, replacing the more empirical approaches that have so far characterized the chemotherapy of AGL.

At the present time, the role of adjuvant treatment to the central nervous system (CNS) with radiation therapy, intrathecal chemotherapy, or both, remains unclear. This is partly because the exact incidence of CNS involvement in AGL remains to be defined.

In a recently published study by the Children's Cancer Study Group (CCSG) (Chard et al. 1978), seven of 94 children (7.4%) obtaining complete remissions developed isolated CNS relapses after a median of 16 months. The median first marrow remission duration in this study was 11.5 months. In childhood ALL it was not until the median first marrow remission duration had approached 12 months that isolated CNS leukemia became a major problem. Thus, we may only now be reaching the median remission duration, when localized CNS disease will become more apparent.

Smaller series have shown up to 50% of patients developing CNS involvement either in isolation or associated with marrow relapse as the median remission duration exceeded 1 year (Fleming et al. 1974, Peterson and Bloomfield 1977). The effect of early adjuvant therapy to the CNS is currently being investigated in several studies, but while early marrow relapse remains the major cause of therapeutic failure, its impact on the prognosis of children with AGL may be difficult to discern.

Perhaps the greatest disappointment of all the methods introduced to prolong AGL remission durations during the 1970s has been immunotherapy. The early promise of initial studies that suggested bacillus Calmette-Guérin (BCG) or allogeneic AGL cells helped prolong remissions (Vogler and Chan 1974, Gutterman et al. 1974) has not been fulfilled with longer follow-up (Powles 1976). A CCSG study in childhood AGL in which the results in 47 children maintained with chemotherapy alone were compared with those in 39 children given immunotherapy with BCG and allogeneic AGL cells in addition to chemotherapy showed median remission durations of 11 and 7 months, respectively (Baehner et al. 1979).

BONE MARROW TRANSPLANTATION

On a more optimistic note, another therapeutic approach offering the possibility of prolonged, maintenance-free remissions has emerged from experience with bone marrow transplantation over the past decade. Marrow toxicity remains one of the major factors limiting the use of larger doses of chemotherapy and irradiation therapy, which have a greater chance of leukemic cell kill. Use of marrow transplantation following high-dose chemotherapy and irradiation therapy enables this limiting factor to be overcome.

Early experience with transplantation in AGL was in late-stage, relapsed patients refractory to available conventional chemotherapy, whose expectation of disease-free survival without further therapy was nil. Eleven percent of these patients obtained remissions of at least 4 years (Thomas et al. 1977, Schulman et al. 1978).

This result led to the performance of marrow transplantations, provided suitable donors were available, much earlier in the course of AGL. Current studies are demonstrating that 60% of patients treated with high-dose cyclophosphamide, total body irradiation, and marrow transplantation during their first marrow remission can anticipate long-term, continuous complete remissions, and 40% of all children treated by transplantation are well without evidence of chronic graft-versus-host disease (GVHD) (Thomas et al. 1979). Seven of eight remain in remission, with the median remission duration not yet reached at 21 months. Five have no significant medical problems and two have chronic GVHD. These numbers are small and longer follow-up is necessary to define the true impact of marrow transplantation on the prognosis of patients with AGL.

Many problems are associated with marrow transplantation, not the least being that it is available to only a limited number of patients with AGL, theoretically one in four, and from practical experience with patients typed at the Puget Sound Blood Center, Seattle, one in three. Fatal acute GVHD, interstitial pneumonia, and relapse, though apparently less common with remission transplants in AGL (Thomas et al. 1979), are the commonest causes of early failure. More disturbing is the problem of chronic GVHD, which produces debilitating medical problems in patients otherwise apparently free of leukemia (Thomas et al. 1979, Schulman et al. 1978). Despite these problems, marrow transplantation offers results as good as, if not better than, the best results in patients treated with conventional chemotherapy, with the obvious additional advantage of not requiring maintenance chemotherapy.

These current data on transplantation also raise several questions. If these results are confirmed in other studies, then we must ask ourselves why these patients have done better. Is it because they have been treated with more aggressive chemotherapy and irradiation when their leukemic cell load is small? If so, would more aggressive conventional chemotherapy protocols produce better results? Confusing this issue is the fact that GVHD may play a role in the prevention of leukemic recurrence.

The antileukemic effect of GVHD in rodent leukemia models has been known since 1957, when Barnes and Loutit demonstrated in CBA leukemic mice that cure was not produced by syngeneic transplants, and although allogeneic grafts produced fatal GVHD, afflicted animals were leukemia free. Bortin and his colleagues (1973) similarly demonstrated in the AKR leukemic mouse model that absence of GVHD correlated with absence of a graft-versus-leukemia effect. A similar effect in humans has recently been reported (Odom et al. 1978, Weiden et al. 1979). Weiden and his colleagues demonstrated that the relapse rate in leukemia patients in whom bone marrow transplants were performed and who recovered from moderate to severe GVHD was 2½ times less than that in similarly treated patients who developed little or no GVHD.

The incidence of severe GVHD appears lower when transplants are performed during remission (Thomas et al. 1979). This is perhaps because the preparative chemotherapy and radiotherapy are sufficient to eradicate the small leukemic cell population present at the time of transplantation, and GVHD is not required for an antileukemic effect. It still may be, however, that clinically inapparent GVHD plays a role in eradicating leukemia in these patients. This possibility is supported by current data on twins undergoing transplants for acute leukemia when GVHD is not a clinical problem; the relapse rate is 50–70% for patients in whom transplants are performed in remission or relapse. If GVHD plays an antileukemic role in allogeneic transplants, then transplantations confront us with a double-edged sword—too severe GVHD may produce a fatal complication in a leukemia-free patient, but no GVHD produces a high risk of leukemic relapse. For the conventional treatment of AGL, this implies an even more difficult problem than developing more aggressive cytotoxic regimens to cure AGL.

A quarter of a century after the development of specific agents that can modify the course of AGL, we continue to face many therapeutic challenges. Further research should be directed toward developing the following:

1. More effective, less toxic induction regimens, and particularly more effective maintenance chemotherapy;

2. A better understanding of leukemic cell kinetics to produce more specific chemotherapeutic regimens;

3. A deeper understanding of how to manipulate the body's immune system and how to use the exciting potential of monoclonal antibodies in leukemia therapy (Bernstein et al. 1980);

4. Ways of applying the lessons currently being learned from marrow transplantations to the treatment of AGL, including techniques for performing mismatched transplants successfully (Clift et al. 1979).

A role for autologous marrow infusion in AGL remains to be established, and is unlikely to become practical unless marrow stored in remission can be rendered leukemia free prior to reinfusion, perhaps with specific antileukemic sera, or after reinfusion by maintenance chemotherapy.

REDEFINING THE DISEASE

Complementing our current approaches to advancing the treatment of AGL are attempts to better define the disease so as to recognize specific characteristics that may lead to improved therapy. Such an approach in childhood ALL has made possible the definition of several subgroups based on age, white blood cell count at diagnosis, and immunological and enzyme markers, and has led to attempts to define more specific and effective therapy for each subgroup. Such well-defined subgroups have yet to emerge in AGL. One large study suggesting that children between the ages of 5 and 10 years have a better prognosis (Chard et al. 1978) is countered by a smaller study in which children under 5 years of age were reported to have the best outlook (Madanat and Sullivan 1979). Such discrepancies raise the question of whether we are really studying the same disease in different oncology centers, and recent international collaborative studies aimed at better defining the various subgroups in acute nonlymphoblastic leukemia can only ensure more accurate comparisons of different therapies (Gralnick et al. 1977). In the interim, certain prognostic indicators are being defined, including serum lysozyme activity (Alsabti 1979), chromosome banding (Golomb et al. 1978), and in vitro leukemic cell growth characteristics (Moore et al. 1974). In one study eight patients with chromosome banding abnormalities had a median survival of only 2 months, compared with 13 months in 16 patients without abnormalities (Golomb et al. 1978).

One source of vital information about AGL is a population in which from 10% to as many as 25% will likely develop AGL. This population consists of persons treated for Hodgkin's disease, a long-term, increasingly worrisome complication of which is acute nonlymphoblastic leukemia (Cadman et al. 1977). Collaborative prospective studies of this unique population may provide insight not only into the development of chemotherapy- and radiotherapy-associated cancer, but also into the very pathogenesis of AGL in the general population.

As we enter the 1980s, AGL remains a major problem and presents a major challenge. In the past, some have met the challenge by ignoring it. Cahen stated in 1856 that "leukemia has no special causes, special symptoms, particular anatomic lesions or specific treatment, and I thus conclude that it does not exist as a distinct malady" (quoted in Gunz and Baike 1974). Over the past 130 years since its first description, we have come to understand that leukemia unfortunately does exist as a distinct malady and, for children afflicted with AGL, remains a major scourge. Nevertheless, more progress in understanding and treatment of this disease has been made over the last 25 years than in the previous 105, and there is every reason to be confident that the challenge of AGL will eventually be met.

REFERENCES

Alsabti, E. 1979. The prognostic value of serum lysozyme activity in acute myelogenous leukemia. Med. Pediatr. Oncol. 6:189–194.

Baehner, R. L., I. D. Bernstein, G. Higgins, S. McCreadie, R. L. Chard, and D. Hammond. 1979. Addition of immunotherapy to chemotherapy to prolong maintenance duration and survival in childhood acute non-lymphoblastic leukemia (ANLL) (Abstract C-608). Proc. Am. Soc. Clin. Oncol. 20:437.

Barnes, D. W. H., and J. F. Loutit. 1957. Treatment of murine leukemia with X-rays and homologous bone marrow. Br. J. Haematol. 3:241–252.

Bernstein, I. D., M. R. Tam, and R. C. Nowinski. 1980. Mouse leukemia: Therapy with monoclonal antibodies against a thymus differentiation antigen. Science, in press.

Bortin, M. M., A. A. Rimm, E. C. Saltzstein, and G. E. Rodey. 1973. Graft versus leukemia. III. Apparent independent antihost and antileukemic activity of transplanted immunocompetent cells. Transplantation 16:182–188.

Burchenal, J. H., M. L. Murphy, R. R. Ellison, M. P. Sykes, T. C. Tan, L. A. Leone, D. A. Karnofsky, L. F. Craver, H. W. Dargeon, and C. P. Rhoads. 1953. Clinical evaluation of a new antimetabolite, 6-mercaptopurine, in the treatment of leukemia and allied diseases. Blood 8:965–969.

Cadman, E. C., R. L. Capizzi, and J. R. Bertino. 1977. Acute nonlymphocytic leukemia: A delayed complication of Hodgkin's disease therapy. Analysis of 109 cases. Cancer 40:1280–1296.

Chard, R. L., Jr., J. Z. Finkelstein, M. J. Sonley, M. Nesbit, S. McCreadie, J. Weiner, H. Sather, and G. D. Hammond. 1978. Increased survival in childhood acute nonlymphocytic leukemia after treatment with prednisone, cytosine arabinoside, 6-thioguanine, cyclophosphamide, and Oncovin (PATCO) combination chemotherapy. Med. Pediatr. Oncol. 4:263–273.

Clift, R. A., J. S. Hansen, E. D. Thomas, C. D. Buckner, J. E. Sanders, E. M. Mickelson, R. Storb, F. L. Johnson, J. W. Singer, and B. W. Goodell. 1979. Marrow transplantation for donors other than HL-A identical siblings. Transplantation 28:235–242.

Ellison, R. R., J. F. Holland, M. Weil, C. Jacquillat, M. Boiron, J. Bernard, A. Sawitsky, F. Rosner, B. Gussoff, R. Silver, A. Karanas, J. Cuttner, L. Spurr, D. M. Hayes, J. Blom, L. A. Leone, H. Farid, R. Kyle, J. L. Hutchinson, R. Jackson Forcier, and J. H. Moon. 1968. Arabinosyl cytosine: A useful agent in the treatment of acute leukemia in adults. Blood 32:507–523.

Fleming, I., J. Simone, R. Jackson, W. Johnson, T. Walters, and C. Mason. 1974. Splenectomy and chemotherapy in acute myelocytic leukemia of childhood. Cancer 33:427–434.

Freedman, M. H., J. Z. Finklestein, G. D. Hammond, and M. Karon. 1971. The effects of chemotherapy on acute myelogenous leukemia in children. J. Pediatr. 78:526–528.

Gale, R. P., and M. J. Cline. 1977. High remission induction rate in acute myeloid leukemia. Lancet 1:497–499.

Golomb, H. M., J. W. Vardiman, J. D. Rowley, J. R. Testa, and U. Mintz. 1978. Correlation of clinical findings with quinacrine banding in acute nonlymphocytic leukemia. N. Engl. J. Med. 299:613–619.

Gralnick, H. R., D. A. G. Galton, D. Catovsky, C. Sultan, and J. M. Bennett. 1977. Classification of acute leukemia. Ann. Intern. Med. 87:740–753.

Gunz, F., and A. Baike. 1974. Leukemia. 3rd ed. Grune and Stratton, New York, 841 pp.

Gutterman, J. U., E. M. Hersh, V. Rodriquez, K. B. McCredie, G. Mavligit, R. Reed, M. A. Burgess, T. Smith, E. Gehan, G. P. Bodey, and E. J Freireich. 1974. Chemoimmunotherapy of adult acute leukemia: Prolongation of remission in myeloblastic leukemia with B.C.G. Lancet 2:1405–1409.

Karon, M., E. J Freireich, E. Frei III, R. Taylor, I. J. Wolman, I. Djerassi, S. S. Lee, A. Sawitsky, J. Hananian, O. Selawry, D. James, P. George, R. B. Patterson, O. Burgert, F. I. Havrani, R. A. Oberfield, C. T. Macy, B. Hoogstraten, and J. Blom. 1966. The role of vincristine in the treatment of childhood acute leukemia. Clin. Pharmacol. Ther. 7:332–339.

Lampkin, B. C., N. B. McWilliams, A. M. Mauer, H. C. Flessa, D. A. Hake, and V. Fisher. 1976. Manipulation of the mitotic cycle in the treatment of acute myelogenous leukemia. Br. J. Haematol. 32:29–32.

Lewis, J. P., J. W. Linman, and J. R. Bateman. 1979. Impact of maintenance chemotherapy on survival in acute nonlymphocytic leukemia (Abstract). Proc. Am. Soc. Clin. Oncol. 20:326.

Madanat, F. F., and M. P. Sullivan. 1979. Improved survival in young children with acute granulocytic leukemia treated with combination chemotherapy using cyclophosphamide, Oncovin, cytosine arabinoside and prednisone. Cancer 44:819–823.

Moore, M. A. S., G. Spitzer, N. Williams, D. Metcalf, and J. Buckley. 1974. Agar studies in 127 cases of untreated acute leukemia: The prognostic value of reclassification of leukemia according to its in vitro growth characteristics. Blood 44:1–18.

Neumann, E. 1878. Ueber myelogene Leukamie. Berl. Klin. Wochenschr. 15:69–71.

Odom, L. F., C. S. August, J. H. Githens, J. R. Humbert, H. Morse, D. Peakman, B. Sharma, S. Rusnack, and F. B. Johnson. 1978. Remission of relapsed leukemia during graft-versus-host reaction: A "graft-versus-leukemia reaction" in man? Lancet 2:537–540.

Osler, W. 1897. The Principles and Practice of Medicine. 2nd ed. Appleton, New York, 1,143 pp.

Peterson, B. A., and C. D. Bloomfield. 1977. Asymptomatic central nervous system (CNS) leukemia in adults with acute non-lymphocytic leukemia (ANLL) in extended remission. Proc. Am. Soc. Clin. Oncol. 18:341.

Powles, R. 1976. Pitfalls in analysis of survival in clinical trials. Biomedicine 24:327–328.

Powles, R. L., P. J. Selby, G. Palu, G. Morgenstern, T. J. McElwain, H. M. Clink, and P. Alexander. 1979. The nature of remission in acute myeloblastic leukemia. Lancet 2:674–676.

Rai, K. R., J. F. Holland, and O. Glidewell. 1975. Improvement in remission induction therapy of acute myelocytic leukemia. Proc. Am. Soc. Clin. Oncol. 16:265.

Schulman, H. M., G. E. Sale, K. G. Lerner, E. A. Barker, P. L. Weiden, K. Sullivan, B. Gallucci, E. D. Thomas, and R. Storb. 1978. Chronic cutaneous graft-versus-host disease in man. Am. J. Pathol. 91:545–570.

Thomas, E. D., C. D. Buckner, M. Banaji, R. Clift, A. Fefer, N. Flournoy, B. W. Goodell, R. O. Hickman, K. G. Lerner, P. E. Neiman, G. E. Sale, J. E. Sanders, J. Singer, M. Stevens, R. Storb, and P. L. Weiden. 1977. One hundred patients with acute leukemia treated by chemotherapy, total body irradiation, and allogeneic marrow transplantation. Blood 49:511–533.

Thomas, E. D., C. D. Buckner, R. A. Clift, A. Fefer, F. L. Johnson, P. E. Neiman, K. G. Lerner, and H. Glucksberg. 1979. Marrow transplantation for acute nonlymphoblastic leukemia in first remission. N. Engl. J. Med. 301:597–600.

Tivey, H. 1954. The natural history of untreated acute leukemia. Ann. N.Y. Acad. Sci. 60:322–358.

Virchow, R. 1860. Blood and lymph, *in* Cellular Pathology as Based on Physiological and Pathological Histology, F. Chance, trans. John Churchill, London, pp. 156–176.

Vogler, W. R., and Y. Chan. 1974. Prolonging remission in myeloblastic leukaemia by Tice-strain bacillus Calmette-Guérin. Lancet 2:128–131.

Vogler, W. R., C. M. Huguley, Jr., and R. W. Rundles. 1967. Comparison of methotrexate with 6-mercaptopurine–prednisone in treatment of acute leukemia in adults. Cancer 20:1221–1226.

Vogler, W. R., D. S. Miller, and J. W. Keller. 1976. 5-Azacytidine (NSC 102816), a new drug for the treatment of myeloblastic leukemia. Blood 48:331–337.

Weiden, P. L., N. Flournoy, E. D. Thomas, R. Prentice, A. Fefer, C. D. Buckner, and R. Storb. 1979. Antileukemic effect of graft-versus-host disease in human recipients of allogeneic-marrow grafts. N. Engl. J. Med. 300:1068–1073.

Weil, M., O. J. Glidewell, C. Jacquillat, R. Levy, A. A. Serpick, P. H. Wiernick, J. Cuttner, B. Hoogstraten, L. Wasserman, R. R. Ellison, S. Gailani, K. Brunner, R. T. Silver, V. B. Rege, M. R. Cooper, L. Lowenstein, N. I. Nissen, F. Haurani, J. Blom, M. Boiron, J. Bernard, and J. F. Holland. 1973. Daunorubicin in the therapy of acute granulocytic leukemia. Cancer Res. 33:921–928.

Whitecar, J. P., G. P. Bodey, E. J Freireich, K. B. McCredie, and J. S. Hart. 1972. Cyclophosphamide (NSC-26271), vincristine (NSC-67574), cytosine arabinoside (NSC-63878) and prednisone (NSC-10023) (COAP) combination chemotherapy for acute leukemia in adults. Cancer Chemother. Rep. 56:543–550.

Wolff, J. A., C. A. Brubaker, M. L. Murphy, M. I. Pierce, and M. Severo. 1967. Prednisone therapy of acute childhood leukemia: Prognosis and duration of response in 330 treated patients. J. Pediatr. 70:626–631.

THE FUTURE BEYOND CURE

Status of the Curability of Childhood Cancers,
edited by J. van Eys and M. P. Sullivan.
Raven Press, New York © 1980.

The Future Beyond Cure

Margaret P. Sullivan, M.D.

*Department of Pediatrics, The University of Texas System Cancer Center M. D. Anderson
Hospital and Tumor Institute, Houston, Texas*

For patients, what is beyond cure? *Life* is beyond cure, *living* once more!

We need to remind ourselves of the difference between the adolescent's or the child's and our adult concepts of "living." Adults are "living" when professional goals are being achieved, real property reflects this success, and fiscal planning provides financial assurance; when there is security and love within family relationships; and when a comfortable, understanding, even amusing, circle of friends exists. But this is not "living" to the teen-ager, nor would hope of achieving all this offer the teen-ager or younger child an incentive to continue cancer therapy. "Living," to children and teen-agers with cancer, is no more stringy, thin hair or wigs, no more steroid-induced acne and prednisone-associated weight gain, no more nausea and vomiting, no more clinic or hospital visits. "Living" is not being "weird" or different. It is being one of the group again, it is doing everything everyone else is doing, it is being accepted, it is dating, and it is being "promised"—that's *living!*

I dwell on this because physicians look upon the fact of living as being reward enough for the patient with severe late effects of cancer therapy. But these children are not really alive—they are existing outside the mainstream and they feel that life is passing them by.

We must bear the responsibility of at least relieving these patients of the psychological effects of their therapy, even though we cannot alleviate the physical and hormonal changes resulting from treatment. Better still, we should prevent the cancers in the first place rather than trying to ameliorate the effects of cancer treatment. This is a large order, given the present state of our knowledge. Genetic counseling can be successful in only a few cases. We seem powerless to control our environment so as to eliminate the carcinogens therein. Have we even tried to do anything to prevent the epidemic of lung cancer that will surely occur in teen-agers and college students as smoking becomes more and more common in our elementary schools? No, we have done nothing—we may not have even noticed. As a matter of fact, many of us have not even stopped smoking ourselves. Cancer prevention has not really been our concern, but perhaps this is the time for it to *become* our concern!

In this section, Dr. Meadows will describe what the body must give to be cured of cancer, and Dr. Zwartjes, what the psyche must give. Objective data in both areas are sorely needed. Dr. Draper will describe how characteristics of groups and populations of people relate to the occurrence of childhood cancer. Dr. Knudson will describe those individual governors of our individuality, our genes, and how they may be altered sequentially in the oncogenic process. By this time we shall be grateful to Dr. Miller if he will only explain how the whole malignant process can be prevented. And finally an overview by Dr. Hartmann, who is tempered with wide experience and mellowed by expectations unfulfilled and successes unexpected, will bring reason and promise to our work, which now appears only half finished.

Status of the Curability of Childhood Cancers,
edited by J. van Eys and M. P. Sullivan.
Raven Press, New York © 1980.

The Medical Cost of Cure: Sequelae in Survivors of Childhood Cancer

Anna T. Meadows, Nancy L. Krejmas, and Jean B. Belasco for
the Late Effects Study Group*

*Department of Pediatrics, University of Pennsylvania School of Medicine and Children's
Cancer Research Center, The Children's Hospital of Philadelphia,
Philadelphia, Pennsylvania*

Mortality from childhood cancer has declined dramatically in the past 20 years (Myers et al. 1975). While this decline has not characterized all pediatric neoplasms, significant proportions of children with acute lymphocytic leukemia, Wilms' tumor, Hodgkin's and non-Hodgkin's lymphoma, and soft tissue and bone sarcomas can be expected to be cured of their childhood cancers (Hammond et al. 1978).

Approximately one third of children with neoplastic disease have acute lymphocytic leukemia (Young and Miller 1975). Prior to 1965, only 20% of these children were expected to live more than 2 years. The long-term disease-free survival rate for this group of children now approximates 50% or more (Pinkel 1979). Among children with solid tumors, the long-term disease-free survival following Wilms' tumor has escalated to more than 80% (D'Angio et al. 1976a). These remarkable improvements are balanced by diseases, such as metastatic neuroblastoma, in which therapeutic interventions have been considerably less effective (Finklestein et al. 1979). We now estimate that, overall, 60% of childhood cancer patients will be cured. We are cautious in estimating the likelihood of eventual cure for children with some neoplasms, such as brain tumors and osteogenic sarcomas, since late relapses may occur (Sutow 1976). Nevertheless, if one in 600 children between birth and 15 years of age acquires some form of neoplastic disease (Young and Miller 1975) and 60% can be expected to be cured, then in approximately 10 years one in 1000 individuals reaching the age of 20 will be a survivor of childhood cancer and its therapy. Hence, we have become concerned not only with the development of effective therapy for cancer, but also with the effects of our therapy on the long-term quality of the patients' lives.

Concern for the long-term survivors of pediatric cancer arises from the known and suspected sequelae of disease and of therapeutic intervention. Examples

---

*The LESG members are listed in the appendix to this chapter.

of such potential sequelae include learning dysfunctions after cranial irradiation, myocardial dysfunction following anthracycline therapy, and sterility from alkylating agents. There is also concern that organ damage may predispose survivors to malignant transformation. The incidence of second tumors in survivors of childhood cancer has been reported to be as high as 12% by 20 years after irradiation (Li 1977). Such a high rate, while generally attributed to therapy, may also reflect a predisposition to specific neoplasms or to neoplasia in general (Meadows et al. 1977).

METHODS

This report presents the results of a retrospective survey by the Late Effects Study Group (Appendix), a 13-institution consortium, which recorded systematically the sequelae encountered in 5-year survivors of childhood cancer. The group attempted to systematically analyze the reported and observed late sequelae in children who had been free of disease following a diagnosis of cancer made in 1972 in order to (1) develop methods for detecting potential medical problems so that we might prevent, reverse, or ameliorate sequelae of disease or therapy, (2) assess the relationship of the more commonly occurring sequelae to disease, therapy, and patient characteristics, (3) determine a minimal estimate of the frequency and severity of treatment-related effects to provide a rational basis for calculating the medical needs of these survivors, (4) determine the incidence of second malignant neoplasms (SMN) in a designated cohort of long-term survivors of childhood cancer, and (5) provide improved clinical care and counseling to long-term survivors.

The reasons for selecting disease-free survivors diagnosed in 1972 were as follows: (1) the therapy given in 1972 for most pediatric neoplasms is very similar to present therapy, (2) all patients would be at least 5 years from diagnosis in 1978, the year of the review, and (3) many sequelae would be expected to develop within this elapsed time from therapy. It was anticipated that this cohort would provide preliminary data that could be used in the development of follow-up techniques for many institutions and multi-institution groups.

A total of 369 children comprised the study population, and their records were reviewed for demographic and disease characteristics, as well as treatment and late effects. The diagnoses of the survivors studied are listed in Table 1. The distribution of tumor types reflects incidence, survival, and referral patterns in the collaborating institutions. Clinically significant late effects were those that were considered moderate to severe. Problems that very likely existed prior to the diagnosis of cancer or that could be irrelevant to treatment were excluded.

In addition, all cases of SMN in individuals whose first cancer occurred in childhood were recorded. We attempted to determine whether therapy with surgery, radiation, and chemotherapy or a history of genetic diseases predisposing to cancer could be invoked in the etiology of these SMN.

Table 1. *Five-Year Survivors of Child-hood Cancer by Disease Type—1972 Cohort*

Acute leukemia	110
Lymphomas	59
Wilms' tumor	54
Soft tissue sarcomas	46
Neuroblastoma	31
Brain tumors	30
Bone sarcomas	16
Histiocytosis	6
Retinoblastoma	6
Others	11
Total	369

RESULTS

Leukemia

One hundred ten patients comprised the cohort of acute leukemia survivors. The majority had had acute lymphocytic leukemia and 21 (19%) were noted to have significant sequelae (Table 2). The most frequently occurring sequelae were those related to the nervous system, with eight patients reported affected. Learning disability was reported in five, encephalopathy in two, and a seizure disorder in one. All of these children had received radiotherapy and chemotherapy for prevention of CNS leukemia. Although 57% of the children were less than 5 years of age at diagnosis, seven of the eight patients with nervous system sequelae were in that age group. Hence, at least 11% of the children diagnosed before the age of 5 had ongoing deficits of intellectual functioning presumed

Table 2. *Significant Late Effects in 21 of 110 5-Year Survivors of Leukemia*

Learning disability	5
Amenorrhea	3
Testicular failure	3
Encephalopathy	2
Chronic lung disease	2
Seizure disorder	1
Chronic liver disease	1
Bowel resection	1
Chronic dental and gingival disease	1
Splenectomy	1
Facial (jaw) contractures	1
Growth retardation, severe	1
Osteoporosis	1
Hearing loss	1

Table 3. *Significant Late Effects in 15 of 54 5-Year Survivors of Wilms' Tumor*

Splenectomy	4
Bowel resection–obstruction	3
Impaired renal function	3
Scoliosis, severe	3
Amenorrhea	1
Restrictive lung disease	1
Liver disease	1

secondary to therapy. Only one of these children had had CNS leukemia at initial diagnosis, at age 4½ years.

Gonadal failure was clinically obvious in six postpubertal 5-year survivors. Some of the cohort had received radiation to the gonads and all had received chemotherapy. Gonadal dysfunction was unrelated to sex, as equal numbers of boys and girls were affected and all were prepubertal when treatment was given.

Chronic lung disease was seen in two survivors, both of whom had suffered from *Pneumocystis carinii* pneumonia during their therapy course. Other sequelae found to be significant covered a wide range of organ systems and could not be correlated with specific therapy. Minor abnormalities of various organ systems at 5-year follow-up included elevated thyroid stimulating hormone in two children who were clinically euthyroid, mild scoliosis in two, alopecia in two, and minor coordination problems, emotional immaturity, excessive dental caries, mild conductive hearing loss after repeated episodes of otitis, and cysts on the thigh secondary to intramuscular pentamidine in one each.

Wilms' Tumor

There were 54 survivors of Wilms' tumor, 15 of whom had significant late effects (Table 3). The most common effects were splenectomy and gastrointestinal disturbance. Splenectomy was required for children whose tumors involved or

Table 4. *Significant Late Effects in 25 of 46 5-Year Survivors of Soft Tissue Sarcomas*

Pelvic exenteration	7
Facial cosmetic	6
Severe sensory deficits	5
Bony deformities	4
Gastrointestinal tract disorders	4
Soft tissue abnormalities	3
Urinary tract disorders	3
Severe growth failure	1
Sterility	1
Severe learning disability	1

abutted on the spleen so that complete tumor resection required removal of this organ. Residual gastrointestinal disease resulted primarily from bowel resections performed when postsurgical adhesions caused obstruction and required lysis. Renal impairment, defined as creatinine clearance of less than 50 ml/min/1.73 m², affected three survivors. Two of the three had had bilateral Wilms' tumor. Significant musculoskeletal abnormalities, such as scoliosis, were present in three children, while an additional 13 had mild scoliosis or atrophy of the soft tissues of the flank. All children with significant late effects had been treated with surgery, radiation, and drugs.

Soft Tissue Sarcomas

More than 50% of children with soft tissue sarcomas (25 of 46) showed substantial residual deficits secondary to therapy for their disease (Table 4). These sequelae reflected the sites of primary disease and radiation therapy, compounded by local or regional surgery. Pelvic exenterations were performed on seven of the 46 children, who later developed persistent urologic, gastrointestinal, reproductive, sexual, and in some cases psychological problems. Isolated reproductive, urinary, and gastrointestinal disorders were noted in one, three, and four patients, respectively. Facial deformities comprised 13% of the late effects in this group. Many of these will require surgical correction, and their economic and psychological costs to the patients cannot yet be calculated. Severe sensory deficits were seen in 11% of the patients. Most involved conductive hearing and visual loss, which can be expected to be permanent. Musculoskeletal deficits were seen in seven patients and occurred in both bony structures and soft tissue. Not all of these children have reached their maximum growth, so the full magnitude of these disabilities may become apparent only in the future. Late effects in this cohort appear unrelated to age and sex, except for the severity of the musculoskeletal defects seen in younger children.

Lymphoma

Fifty-nine patients had had lymphoma, including 13 who had had non-Hodgkin's lymphoma and 46 who had had Hodgkin's disease (Table 5). This disproportion seems to be related to the better survival rate for patients with Hodgkin's

Table 5. *Significant Late Effects in 47 of 59 5-Year Survivors of Lymphomas*

Splenectomy	37
Musculoskeletal abnormality	7
Amenorrhea	5
Bowel obstruction	4
Pulmonary fibrosis	3
Hypothyroidism	2
Marrow suppression	1

disease. Asplenia was the most frequent late effect (63%), as most patients had undergone splenectomy for staging. Residual musculoskeletal defects were noted in seven patients, and largely involved tissues receiving radiation therapy. All patients known to be sterile (8.5%) had received radiation and chemotherapy and were pubertal or postpubertal at diagnosis. Bowel obstructions requiring surgical intervention occurred in four patients who had undergone staging laparotomies and three patients showed persistent restrictive pulmonary disease 5 years after radiation to the mediastinum. Paradoxically, only two patients were clinically hypothyroid, despite the large number who had received neck radiation. Six other children were noted to have elevated thyroid stimulating hormone levels despite their euthyroid clinical state. Among the other minor deficits encountered in the 5-year survivors of Hodgkin's disease were dental caries in ten, breast atrophy or asymmetry in two, and X-ray evidence only of pulmonary fibrosis in two.

Bone Tumors

Thirteen of the 16 patients with bone tumors had significant sequelae and, as expected, these sequelae were of the musculoskeletal system. Ten of the 13 had had ablative surgery, ten had had radiation therapy, and 13 had also received chemotherapy. Only two patients were less than 5 years of age at the time of diagnosis. Amputations and growth abnormalities following irradiation accounted for the large number of musculoskeletal sequelae, which were severe in 11 cases and minor in five. Facial, cosmetic, and neurosensory late effects were seen in this group and again were associated with the sites of surgery and radiation therapy. Chemotherapy could be associated with the two cases of cystitis and the solitary cases of sterility and esophagitis.

Brain Tumors

More than half of the children with brain tumors (16/30) had late effects, and these primarily involved the central nervous system. It is difficult, therefore, to determine whether the disease or the therapy was responsible for the current status of these patients. The 21 residual deficits seen in these 16 survivors consisted of intellectual dysfunction (eight cases), growth disorder (three), motor dysfunction (three), panhypopituitarism (two), personality disorders (two), and seizure disorder, visual impairment, and hearing loss (one each). As a consequence of radiation therapy, one patient had kyphoscoliosis and two had permanent alopecia.

Neuroblastoma

Relatively few of the 31 survivors of neuroblastoma had severe sequelae of therapy. In six of the seven affected patients the sequelae were of the musculoskeletal system and were related to combined surgical and radiation effects on the spine. All these children were less than 5 years of age at diagnosis, with the average age being 18 months. Five other patients had minor musculoskeletal defects. One child continued to have opsoclonus and demonstrated a learning disorder, but this may have been related to the syndrome associated with neuroblastoma, rather than to the therapy.

Other Tumors

In the remaining patients the most severe late effects appeared in the six retinoblastoma patients, all of whom had undergone a single enucleation and five of whom had received radiation to the remaining eye. As a consequence, all had mild to severe visual problems. These patients were under 5 years of age at diagnosis. This was also true of the two patients with histiocytosis who showed severe late effects, one of whom showed a severe learning disorder and the other significant dental disease following radiation to the cranium.

In the remaining 11 patients, growth retardation was seen in two and severe facial cosmetic defect, asplenia, sterility, and hypothyroidism in one each. Surgery and radiation therapy caused these defects.

Oncogenic Late Effects

The Late Effects Study Group investigators have now registered 200 individuals with second malignant neoplasms. The tumors were grouped according to presumptive etiology (genetic susceptibility and association with radiation) (Table 6). Fewer than 50% (94) could be accounted for by radiation alone. Leukemias and second neoplasms that arose in irradiated sites in children without known genetic disease were included in this category. Of special interest are the 39 children who had no known genetic disease and in whom radiation could not be invoked as a possible etiologic agent. Eleven of the 39 had received chemotherapy only, and their neoplasms, the intervals between tumors, and the drugs administered are summarized in Table 7. As shown in the table, many alkylating agents were used. It is also noteworthy that two of these patients with Wilms' tumor developed brain tumors, as did another child with Wilms' tumor who had not received drugs. This association may be nonrandom, as is

Table 6. *Presumptive Etiology of Second Malignant Neoplasms in Children*

Genetic Disease	Radiation Associated (132)	Not Radiation Associated (68)
Known (67)	38	29
(Retinoblastoma 35)	(21)	(14)
Not known (133)	94	39

Table 7. *Second Malignant Neoplasms in Children Treated by Chemotherapy Alone*

Neoplasm 1	Neoplasm 2	Interval (Yrs)	Drugs
Wilms' tumor	Brain tumor	2	Actinomycin D (AMD)
Wilms' tumor	Brain tumor	3	AMD
Wilms' tumor	Basal cell carcinoma	7	AMD
Acute myelogenous leukemia (AML)	Ewing's sarcoma	4	Vincristine (VCR), prednisone, 6-mercaptopurine, methotrexate (MTX), cytosine arabinoside, cyclophosphamide (CPM)
Osteosarcoma	Pancreatic sarcoma	7	AMD, mitomycin C
Hodgkin's disease	AML	10	Mustard, CPM, chlorambucil, vinblastine (VBL), VCR, procarbazine, Adriamycin (ADR), L-asparaginase
Hodgkin's disease	Osteosarcoma	8(3)*	CPM, VBL, chlorambucil
Hodgkin's disease	Acute myelomonocytic leukemia	3	Cyclophosphamide, Oncovin, prednisone, and procarbazine (COPP), ADR
Hodgkin's disease	AML	5	COPP, ADR, CCNU
Histiocytosis X	Hepatoma	18	MTX
Medulloblastoma	Melanoma	4	CCNU, VCR

* Eight years from diagnosis, 3 years from chemotherapy.

that between Hodgkin's disease and acute nonlymphocytic leukemia, and may reflect specific susceptibilities. We have seen a similar association in patients with retinoblastoma who developed osteogenic sarcomas as a preferential second neoplasm, regardless of whether or not they had received radiation. Sixteen of the retinoblastoma patients developed SMN; 11 neoplasms arose in irradiated bones and five did not (Meadows et al. 1979). Neither radiation, chemotherapy, nor genetic disease could explain the SMN in 28 children. It is possible that some of these individuals have an as yet unidentified cancer predisposition. The combination of brain tumor and leukemia or lymphoma in five individuals and in five families in which siblings were affected may reflect such a susceptibility.

The distribution of first neoplasms in these 200 children reflects the survival rates and proportions with known genetic predisposition to other tumors, rather than the incidence (e.g., more retinoblastoma and Wilms' tumor than leukemia) (Table 8). The second neoplasms are listed according to whether or not radiation was associated with their development in Table 9. There were 207 neoplasms because five children had more than two each. With a single exception, these children appeared to be at exceptional risk of malignant disease (Table 10).

The current status of children who developed second neoplasms is noted in Table 11. Half have survived their SMN, reflecting the relatively good outlook for those with thyroid and skin neoplasms, while those who developed leukemia or bone or soft tissue sarcoma fared considerably less well.

Table 8. *First Neoplasms in 200 Children Who Later Developed Second Neoplasms*

Retinoblastoma	35
Wilms' tumor	32
Brain tumor	24
Hodgkin's disease	22
Neuroblastoma	20
Soft tissue sarcoma	20
Bone tumor	9
Leukemia	8
Non-Hodgkin's lymphoma	7
Gonadal tumor	6
Skin	5
Histiocytosis X	4
Colon carcinoma	4
Nasopharyngeal carcinoma	2
Adrenocortical carcinoma	2

Table 9. *Etiology of Second Malignant Neoplasms in 200 Children*

Second Neoplasm	Radiation Associated	Not Radiation Associated
Bone sarcoma	34	9
Soft tissue sarcoma	31	11
Leukemia/lymphoma	21	12
Thyroid carcinoma	15	3
Skin carcinoma	11	11
Brain tumor	5	16
Breast carcinoma	4	2
Others	12	10
Total	133	74

Table 10. *Neoplasms in Patients with More Than Two Neoplasms Each*

Neoplasms	Association
Rhabdomyosarcoma, neurofibrosarcoma, osteogenic sarcoma	Neurofibromatosis
Medulloblastoma, basal cell carcinoma, ovarian fibrosarcoma	Nevoid basal cell carcinoma syndrome
Colon carcinoma, thymoma, glioma, squamous cell carcinoma	Sibling with lymphoma, familial immunoglobulin deficiency
Colon carcinoma, spongioblastoma, junctional melanoma	Siblings (3) with brain tumors
Glioblastoma, lymphoma, adenocarcinoma of rectum	Siblings (2) with lymphoma
Neuroblastoma, glioma, thyroid carcinoma	—

Table 11. *Survival in Children with Second Malignant Neoplasms*

Second Neoplasm	Alive	Dead	
		SMN	Other Cause
Bone	12/42	30	0
Soft tissue	16/38	17	5
Leukemia/lymphoma	7/31	22	2
Thyroid	15/17	0	2
Skin	16/23	6	1
Brain	6/22	12	4
Other	9/23	9	5
Total	81/196	96	19

Table 12. *Incidence of Second Malignant Neoplasms in Children*

Interval (Yrs)	No. SMN	Average Annual Rate*
0–5	26	75
5.1–10	26	302
10.1–15	27	479
15.1–20	9	307
20.1–25	5	935
25.1–30	2	1,204

* Per 100,000 person-years at risk.

Estimates of survival according to primary tumor made it possible to estimate the number of survivors at risk each year from diagnosis for which patients with SMN were registered. From diagnosis to 5 years, the incidence of SMN averages 75 per 100,000 per year, or a sixfold increase over the rate of 12 per 100,000 in the pediatric population as a whole (Table 12). The incidence continues to rise, so that 20 years from diagnosis the rate is approximately 300 per 100,000 per year, or ten times greater than that reported for 20–24-year-olds in the Third National Cancer Society Survey (1975).

DISCUSSION

Pediatricians have witnessed a dramatic decline in the mortality of their patients from all causes during the last 25 years. Pediatric oncologists have been able to reduce mortality from cancer, and can therefore begin to appreciate the medical costs of having effected this improvement. The Late Effects Study Group was organized to study systematically the long-term disabilities these cured patients face, to follow them over time, and to observe the natural history of untoward sequelae. By relating these sequelae to therapeutic intervention, we may be able to help investigators select new therapies that are likely to be less toxic in the future. Concern for the quality of life of children cured of cancer is consistent with the philosophy inherent in pediatrics, which recognizes the importance of preventive medicine.

This survey of 369 patients diagnosed in 1972 suggests the disabilities likely to be encountered in the future by children treated with modern methods of combined therapy. We previously observed that these figures may underestimate what would be seen with more specific examinations (Meadows et al. 1975). This survey reflects clinical observations primarily, laboratory investigations being left to the discretion of individual investigators. Investigations that were apt to reflect organ dysfunctions, such as creatinine clearance and pulmonary function tests, were not uniformly performed on all patients at risk. Some organ functions cannot yet be assessed because the individuals at risk have not reached the age at which defects might become apparent. Most notable among these are gonadal functions relating to hormone secretion and fertility, which cannot be predicted in prepubertal children (Shalet and Beardwell 1979). Five years from the diagnosis of cancer, most pediatric patients are still prepubertal. Effects on learning ability and other neuropsychologic functions, unless grossly obvious, become apparent only after the ages at which these abilities might be expected to be present normally. In a group of children studied at the Children's Hospital of Philadelphia, we have observed unsuspected learning disabilities in the early school grades, 2 to 4 years after irradiation. The incidence of intellectual handicaps might, therefore, be minimal.

The progressive nature of sequelae to radiation therapy and surgery in children whose growth potential has not yet been realized must also be considered (Heaston et al. 1979). This progressive nature is particularly evident in very young children, such as those with neuroblastoma or retinoblastoma, who have been treated with radiation that affects bone and soft tissue. The loss of organs or extremities and the sequelae of surgery and radiation that impair sensory functions are permanent, and their effects on productivity and self-esteem are inestimable. The absence of a spleen in 12% of our survivors poses the threat of overwhelming infection in these children (Chilcote et al. 1976). Likewise, the psychological impact of cosmetic disabilities cannot be gauged, but may be considerable.

Abnormalities that occur because of acute secondary sequelae of disease or therapy can also persist. These include chronic pulmonary dysfunction following *Pneumocystis carinii* pneumonia or other severe pneumonias.

Controversy persists over whether or not persons with one neoplasm are more likely to develop a second as a consequence of a general or specific susceptibility (Moertel 1977). Therapeutic agents such as radiation and drugs may be associated with an increased incidence of second cancers (Li 1977, Reimer et al. 1977). At least one chemotherapeutic agent, however, actinomycin D, has been associated with a decreased oncogenic risk from radiation (D'Angio et al. 1976b). Children might be an excellent group in which to observe the effects of "therapeutic" carcinogens with long latent periods. If cured, children survive for many years. In addition, they have relatively little exposure to the extraneous oncogens to which adults are exposed, such as those in the workplace.

Children with SMN may also provide clues to new "genetic diseases" that reflect a neoplastic predisposition. We and others have observed the effects of a "cancer gene" that accompanies retinoblastoma and produces osteogenic sarcoma, regardless of therapy (Abramson et al. 1979). This may be only one of several such genes that will become apparent as the cure rates for other childhood neoplasms approach that for retinoblastoma. The possibility also exists that we may recognize some children with a genetic disease who are more susceptible to the effects of mutagenizing therapies. Such a susceptibility is obvious in patients with the nevoid basal cell carcinoma syndrome who develop basal cell carcinoma soon after irradiation (Strong 1977). As the number of long-term survivors increases, children with SMN may lead us to an understanding of both therapeutic and host factors that place some individuals at high risk of cancer.

Individuals who plan therapy for children with cancer should not be discouraged by these results. They should continue to develop new treatment methods that are likely to cure children with resistant disease. But they should also develop, with the same aggressive zeal, ways of reducing therapy in children whose clinical outlook is excellent and who have more to lose because of the long-term effects of treatment that is more aggressive than their disease warrants. Only by evaluating the efficacy and sequelae of various treatments can progress be made toward the realization of normal, healthy adults.

ACKNOWLEDGMENTS

The studies described herein were made possible through the efforts of the Late Effects Study Group investigators and Valerie Miké of the Biostatistics Laboratory, Memorial Sloan-Kettering Cancer Institute.

This investigation was supported in part by Contract CP65803 and Grant CA14489 from the National Institutes of Health.

REFERENCES

Abramson, D. H., H. J. Ronner, and R. M. Ellsworth. 1979. Second tumors in nonirradiated bilateral retinoblastoma. Am. J. Ophthalmol. 87:624–627.

Chilcote, R. R., R. L. Baehner, and D. Hammond. 1976. Septicemia and meningitis in children splenectomized for Hodgkin's disease. N. Engl. J. Med. 295:798–800.

D'Angio, G. J., A. E. Evans, N. Breslow, B. Beckwith, H. Bishop, P. Feigl, W. Goodwin, L. L. Leape, L. F. Sinks, W. Sutow, M. Tefft, and J. Wolff. 1976a. The treatment of Wilms' tumor: Results of the National Wilms' Tumor Study. Cancer 38:633–646.

D'Angio, G. J., A. T. Meadows, V. Miké, C. Harris, A. Evans, N. Jaffe, W. Newton, O. Schweisguth, W. Sutow, and P. Morris-Jones. 1976b. Decreased risk of radiation-associated second malignant neoplasms in actinomycin-D-treated patients. Cancer 37:1177–1185.

Finklestein, J. Z., M. R. Klemperer, A. E. Evans, I. Bernstein, S. Leikin, S. McCreadie, J. Grosfeld, R. Hittle, J. Weiner, H. Sather, and D. Hammond. 1979. Multiagent chemotherapy for children with metastatic neuroblastoma: A report from the Children's Cancer Study Group. Med. Pediatr. Oncol. 6:179–188.

Hammond, G. D., W. A. Bleyer, J. R. Hartmann, D. M. Hays, and R. D. T. Jenkin. 1978. The team approach to the management of pediatric cancer. Cancer 41:29–35.

Heaston, D. K., H. I. Lipshitz, and R. C. Chan. 1979. Skeletal effects of megavoltage irradiation in survivors of Wilms' tumor. Am. J. Roentgenol. 133:389–395.

Li, F. P. 1977. Second malignant tumors after cancer in childhood. Cancer 40:1899–1902.

Meadows, A. T., G. J. D'Angio, A. E. Evans, C. C. Harris, R. W. Miller, and V. Miké. 1975. Oncogenesis and other late effects of cancer treatment in children: Report of a single hospital study. Radiology 114:175–180.

Meadows, A. T., G. J. D'Angio, V. Miké, A. Banfi, C. Harris, R. D. T. Jenkin, and A. Schwartz. 1977. Patterns of second malignant neoplasms in children. Cancer 40:1903–1911.

Meadows, A. T., L. C. Strong, F. P. Li, G. J. D'Angio, O. Schweisguth, A. I. Freeman, R. D. T. Jenkin, P. Morris-Jones, and M. E. Nesbit. 1979. Bone sarcoma as a second malignant neoplasm in children: Influence of radiation and genetic predisposition. Cancer, in press.

Moertel, C. G. 1977. Multiple primary malignant neoplasms. Cancer 40:1786–1792.

Myers, M. H., H. W. Heise, F. P. Li, and R. W. Miller. 1975. Trends in cancer survival among U.S. white children, 1955–1971. J. Pediatr. 87:815–818.

Pinkel, D. 1979. The Ninth Annual David Karnofsky Lecture: Treatment of acute lymphocytic leukemia. Cancer 43:1128–1136.

Reimer, R. R., R. Hoover, J. F. Fraumeni, Jr., and R. C. Young. 1977. Acute leukemia after alkylating-agent therapy of ovarian cancer. N. Engl. J. Med. 297:177–215.

Shalet, S. M., and C. G. Beardwell. 1979. Endocrine consequences of treatment of malignant disease in childhood: A review. J. R. Soc. Med. 72:39–41.

Strong, L. C. 1977. Theories of pathogenesis—Mutation and cancer, *in* Genetics of Human Cancer, J. Mulvihill, R. W. Miller, and J. F. Fraumeni, Jr., eds. Raven Press, New York, pp. 401–415.

Sutow, W. W. 1976. Late metastases in osteosarcoma. Lancet 1:856.

Third National Cancer Survey: Incidence Data. 1975. DHEW Publication No. (NIH) 75–787. Monograph 41. National Cancer Institute, Bethesda, Md., 454 pp.

Young, J. L., and R. W. Miller. 1975. Incidence of malignant tumors in U.S. children. J. Pediatr. 86:254–258.

Appendix: *Late Effects Study Group*

Participating Institutions	*Investigators*
Sidney Farber Cancer Institute Boston, Mass.	Dr. Frederick Li Dr. Steve Sallan
Columbus Children's Hospital Columbus, Ohio	Dr. William Newton
Children's Hospital of Philadelphia Philadelphia, Penn.	Dr. Audrey Evans
Children's Memorial Hospital Chicago, Ill.	Dr. Edward Baum
Institut Gustave-Roussy Villejuif, France	Dr. Jean Lemerle
Istituto Nazionale Tumori Milano, Italy	Dr. Alberto Banfi Dr. Franca Fossati-Bellani Dr. Marco Gasparini
M. D. Anderson Hospital Houston, Texas	Dr. Jan van Eys Dr. Louise Strong
Princess Margaret Hospital Toronto, Canada	Dr. R. D. T. Jenkin
Roswell Park Memorial Institute Buffalo, N.Y.	Dr. Daniel Green
Royal Manchester Children's Hospital Manchester, England	Dr. Patricia Morris-Jones
Emma Kinderziekenhuis Amsterdam, The Netherlands	Dr. P. A. Voute
University of Minnesota Minneapolis, Minn.	Dr. Mark Nesbit
Los Angeles Children's Hospital Los Angeles, Calif.	Dr. Stuart Siegel Dr. Gussie Higgins

Chairman: Dr. Giulio J. D'Angio; coordinator: Dr. Anna T. Meadows

Status of the Curability of Childhood Cancers,
edited by J. van Eys and M. P. Sullivan.
Raven Press, New York © 1980.

The Psychological Costs of Curing the Child with Cancer

William J. Zwartjes, M.D.

Department of Oncology and Hematology, The Children's Hospital, Denver, Colorado

In recent years, dedication to the study of medical needs has led to a dramatic improvement in the physical care of children with cancer and higher survival rates. This success, however, has created new concerns for these children, since it has not been accomplished without a price. Perhaps the area about which we know the least is that which holds the answer to the question of whether the cure is worth the price. Since the ultimate goal is not simply to preserve a life, but to do so while facilitating a quality existence, the psychological costs to the patient of such an accomplishment are of utmost importance.

Unfortunately, the study of these phenomena is much more difficult than the evaluation of concrete physical side effects of disease or therapy. Psychology is defined as the science that deals with the mind and mental processes. Thus, its study encompasses a multitude of higher brain functions, many of which are poorly understood and all of which are intricately interdependent. The wide variety of variables involved in the etiology of any single human action prevents the elucidation of a simple cause-and-effect relationship. It is the complex interaction of many factors that leads to a certain behavioral pattern. While the malignant illness and its therapy cannot be considered the sole causes of any single action or manner of behaving, they are substantial modifiers of behavior.

The manner in which such modifications are evaluated varies even as the changes themselves. While some direct effects of the disease, such as involvement of the brain, can alter all brain functions, others may interfere only with certain parameters, such as memory, intellectual ability, or personality. In the case of the last, effects may be subtle and related to a complex interplay of social and emotional variables. The significance of such effects for the patient's long-term functioning in society is difficult to measure. Even functions such as intellectual performance, while subject to relative measurement, may be altered by pressures exerted by the social and emotional phenomena associated with the illness.

While analysis of the psychological costs of the cure of childhood cancer is difficult, it behooves those of us in the oncology field to attempt such an evaluation. Only through an understanding of the problems of these individuals can we eliminate or amend the obstacles to their achievement of a normal lifestyle following their cure.

DIRECT EFFECTS ON THE CHILD'S MENTAL ABILITIES

Though very complex, changes in mental abilities are perhaps the easiest to understand of the modifications to the patient's mental processes. However, even when the trauma directly involves the brain, as in patients with central nervous system (CNS) tumors, attendant social and emotional factors alter the child's psychological state as well. While long-term survivors of brain tumors have been reported for years, little attention has been paid to the quality of their lives. Bamford et al. (1976) suggest that this most severe of insults to the brain by childhood cancer results in substantial impairment. Of 33 long-term survivors in their study, three had been committed to mental institutions, six others were profoundly disabled, and only six had no residual problems. Seventeen were considered below average academically and only three were above average. While other studies (e.g., Bloom et al. 1969) suggest the effects are not so severe, evaluations at The Children's Hospital in Denver (DCH) substantiate the findings of Bamford and co-workers. In a study of educational accomplishments of 118 oncology patients, only three of the 11 brain tumor patients were found to have achieved academically anywhere near normal. The remainder were lagging markedly in academic development, with two being quite severely retarded. Even the three who did well experienced numerous learning problems, as well as social and emotional traumas. As in the Bamford study, in which 13 of 30 children experienced significant emotional problems, the brain tumor patients at DCH were subjected to peer ridicule and other forms of social rejection, which culminated for most in depression and withdrawal into a quite isolated life-style. The psychological costs for these individuals are thus very high and call into question whether survival under such circumstances is really worth the tremendous cost. Surely an evaluation of the true success of therapy for brain tumor patients must take into account the overwhelming detrimental effects on the child's mental processes.

While the location of the neoplasm in the brain has the most severe direct effect on the mental functioning of the pediatric oncology patient, ill effects of therapy are also seen. Because these effects are much more subtle, they are only now being recognized as substantial barriers to the child's attainment of psychological normalcy. Of greatest concern in this regard are the effects on the intellect of prophylactic irradiation of the central nervous system in leukemia patients. While early studies suggest the absence of harmful effects (Verzosa et al. 1976, Soni et al. 1975), more recent investigations have begun to recognize the detrimental consequences of the therapy, especially for younger patients (Eiser and Lansdown 1977). Children irradiated shortly after diagnosis have been found to have the greatest degree of alteration, with diminishment in performance IQ, as well as abstract and short-term memory ability. Mathematical skills are especially impaired (Eiser 1978). While the full extent of this impairment is not yet known, it appears that a substantial proportion of patients so treated are adversely affected. That such therapy greatly affects the child's ability to learn is shown by the fact teachers in the DCH study reported three quarters of patients who had received CNS irradiation experienced a decrease in the ability to retain knowledge, compared to only one fifth who had such difficulties in the nonirradiated group. These findings are, thus, not just psychological testing curiosities, but meaningful indicators of the ability of these children to intellectually advance. Perhaps equally significant, they highlight the importance of the lack of special teaching for these children, which is due to failure to recognize their problem.

Even subtler, direct effects on the child's mental capabilities result from the general nature of the systemic illnesses and their therapies. Fatigue was found in the DCH study to be an important factor lessening concentration, diminishing academic interest, and impeding learning. Less directly, this side effect, along with malaise and nausea, contributed to excessive absenteeism from school, which in turn interfered with the educational process. Further indirect effects will be discussed subsequently.

It must be recognized that the malignant disease and its treatment have very real effects on the child's ability to function on a normal mental level. An understanding of these consequences is important not only to facilitate efforts to assist the patient past the barriers, but also to measure the value of therapy against its effects on the subsequent quality of life.

INDIRECT EFFECTS ON THE CHILD'S PSYCHOLOGICAL STATE

The direct effects may damage the patient's intellectual abilities the most severely, but only a relatively few oncology patients are afflicted by a CNS tumor. All children with malignant disease, however, are subjected to the very complicated and encompassing social and emotional factors that accompany these maladies. The problems of negative peer reaction and isolation for patients with brain tumors have already been described, but they also exist for patients with leukemia-lymphoma and solid tumors. The total milieu surrounding patients with cancer has an effect on their psychological functioning.

The Patient's Reaction to the Illness

While the patient's immediate reaction to the illness can be considered temporary, in the evaluation of long-term psychological costs, it has an important influence on the patient's development of coping mechanisms and personality characteristics. Spinetta (1977) found that children are indeed attuned to the seriousness of their illness, and their awareness results in a substantial degree of anxiety. However, previous forms of anxiety described by Morrissey (1963), including death anxiety in older patients, mutilation fears in the middle group, and separation anxiety in the very young, were regarded by Spinetta (1974) as functions of the manner in which children were studied. Goggin et al. (1976) used projective testing to study pediatric oncology patients and found that the younger boys tended to be more anxious than girls, but with age the latter's anxiety levels increased. Further, they found that this anxiety contributed to the fact that strong emotional stimulation and interpersonal relationships were more traumatic and disruptive for children with malignant diseases, even though their responsiveness to emotional stimuli did not diminish.

While the testing by Goggin and co-workers suggested that the patients had good ego strength and object relations, alterations in personality characteristics seem to be common. The parents of half of the patients in the DCH study perceived permanent alterations in personality after the diagnosis. Heightened anger, depression, and introversion were the most commonly mentioned changes. Hoffman and Futterman (1971) also noted the tendency of children with cancer to be more passive, depressed, and isolated, as well as excessively dependent on their parents.

Patient Isolation

What is especially worrisome is the possibility of an isolated life-style's becoming a permanent mode of behavior for childhood oncology patients. Two thirds of the children in the DCH study were found to be substantially isolated, and this was as true for long-term survivors as for those ill 4 years or less. The words "loner" and "introverted" were commonly encountered in teachers' descriptions of the patients. In some cases the withdrawal from others was quite severe. The isolation was manifested by a decrease in number of best friends, loss of other close acquaintances, and diminished participation in extracurricular activities and interactions with the community. Children also tended to participate less in classroom activities and, because of somatic impediments of the illness, frequently were not so physically active, thus losing opportunities to interact with others.

The causes of the child's isolation are numerous, with the withdrawal being self-imposed as well as initiated by others. Fear of or actual ridicule because of physical changes, such as hair loss, can prompt the patient to avoid others. Inability to keep up in school because of fatigue and other previously mentioned effects of the disease or treatment may also lead to avoidance of school and thus lessen contacts with others. Kaplan et al. (1974) have pointed out that school personnel tend to isolate these children to avoid the emotional trauma associated with dealing with such children.

This resultant separation from others is detrimental to the child's development on all levels. Social and emotional growth are most obviously affected, but academic and physical development can also be delayed if the child avoids school and physical activity. This leads to a substantial diminishment in the patient's overall level of functioning and psychological well-being.

Reactions of Others to the Patient

Another factor affecting interaction with others is the general uncertainty about the diseases known as cancer. Van Eys (1977) has pointed out that the tendency of others to regard the child's illness as invariably fatal leads to "psychological euthanasia," leaving a "dead mind in a live body." The mystique surrounding cancer does indeed lead to preconceived notions of how the individual should be treated. Denial of employment because of the potential employer's fear the patient cannot perform is common, as are decreased academic expectations on the part of teachers. While hard to document, the latter phenomenon appears quite prevalent and can severely damage the child's intellectual development and sense of well-being.

Parents also tend to alter their attitudes toward their child because of the trauma of the illness and the threat of death. Dependence on the parents is fostered by the necessities of medical care, and this poses a threat to developing independence particularly for the adolescent. Extremes of separation anxiety and mother-child symbiosis are seen in school phobia, which, as Lansky et al. (1975) noted, occurs at a much higher rate than normal in oncology patients. The attendant regression and isolation would seem to be as important as overdependence in interfering with personality integration and psychological well-being in these instances.

The reactions of others also play a part in the home, the primary source of the patient's emotional support. Preexisting problems can be exacerbated by the illness and render the family unable to provide such backing. Separation of the parents and the family's financial distress or poor coping with the illness can undermine the provision of support to the patient. This lack of support can further tax the child's ability to adjust and lead to poor coping mechanisms.

Long-Term Effects on Patient Personality

O'Malley (1977) found, in a long-term follow-up study, that patients' psychological alterations and difficulties persist. In standard psychiatric interviews, he noted that only half of 72 patients had no psychiatric symptoms and 14% were quite impaired. Anxiety and depression were most prominent, and one fifth of the patients had diminished self-concepts. At least 30% had lost friends and thus seemed to be involved to some degree in the isolated life-style described earlier.

While further study is necessary to evaluate the extent and persistence of such problems, it is evident that some patients suffer altered life-styles because of their illness and its sequelae. The subjective nature of personality changes makes it difficult to ascertain the true damage done to the child's ability to perform in society. However, if the performance level is substantially below that otherwise expected, remedial efforts are called for to eliminate, if possible, obstacles to normal development created by the illness.

THE PSYCHOLOGICAL COSTS INDUCED BY IMPAIRED EDUCATIONAL DEVELOPMENT

Many problems the child encounters are impediments to education, as well as to nonacademic development. Fatigue, social isolation, depression, and poor family support interfere with the child's schooling, but two of the greatest hindrances in this regard are the previously mentioned decreased teacher expectations and excessive student absenteeism. The former appears related to the educator's lack of knowledge about how to relate to a child with cancer. As a consequence, preconceived concepts prevail and requirements are frequently reduced in the expectation the patient will die fairly soon. The consequences of such attitudes can be devastating, as children idle away their time in school, are allowed to be truant with no questions raised, and generally are not required to perform at the level at which they are capable. In the extreme, resultant disinterest in school may lead to dropping out. The child who survives the illness is thus left unprepared for future life because survival was not anticipated. Cured of the physical ailment, such patients are beset with a whole new spectrum of social and sometimes emotional difficulties because of the reaction of others to their disease. While not all children are affected to this degree, most have at least one teacher who expects less of them, and for some the consequences are quite severe. The very existence of this behavior among teachers calls into question the validity of using school records to evaluate such children's academic performance.

Another side effect of the illness is a substantial increase in the amount of classtime missed by the child. The DCH study showed that three quarters of the patients missed more than a month of school per year in the first 3 years after the diagnosis. Furthermore, at least a quarter of the patients were habitually truant and many others were suspected of having multiple unwarranted absences. While medical care and its attendant side effects necessitate some absences, the social factors previously elucidated contribute heavily to unjustified absenteeism. School phobia has already been noted as the most severe form of nonattendance and in this study characterized 14% of the patients.

A child who is not in school cannot be expected to perform at the level of other children the same age. The social variables contributing to absenteeism combine with the effects of nonattendance to further impede the child's intellectual, social, and emotional development. The resulting poor self-image, in turn, deters the child from interacting with others and reinforces the desire to avoid school. Deteriorating learning abilities due to absenteeism, physical effects of the illness, and falling behind in schoolwork are other reasons for disliking school and thus attempting truancy. The end result is a substandard educational experience for the patient, which may lead to underachievement in employment and other life activities. This, in turn, reinforces the patient's feelings of inadequacy and poor self-concept. While the dropout rate among patients in the DCH study was not above the norm, it is important to note that some patients did drop out because of their illness. Truly, for them, the psychological cost of being cured of cancer was quite high.

THE PSYCHOLOGICAL COST OF CURE TO ADOLESCENTS

Even though the disease process creates vicissitudes for all children with cancer, adolescents seem particularly vulnerable. For all patients, the dynamic processes of growth, physical, social, emotional, and intellectual, must continue throughout the course of the illness and its therapy. For the adolescent, however, the process requires the initiation of independence, development of a good self-concept and ego strength, planning for the future, and perfection of interpersonal relationships. All these growth skills are impeded by the illness and the hardships it inflicts. As Holton (1971) has pointed out, these hardships lead to loss of self-esteem and creation of a sense of inferiority.

It is notable that all those dropping out of school in the DCH study were teen-agers, as were half of those who had school phobia. Lansky and co-workers (1975) found the same percentage of adolescents exhibiting this syndrome, which is usually regarded as most common in early elementary school children. Physical changes also appeared to be especially traumatic for these individuals, especially hair loss in teen-age girls. For two this problem led to school phobia.

While intervention may help adolescents through the difficult periods, they clearly suffer emotional traumas that can affect their future lives. Their concern about peer interaction and tendency to withdraw make teen-agers especially vulnerable to developing an isolated behavior pattern that could persist into later life.

SUMMARY

One is left with the impression that children with cancer are faced with multiple threats to their psychological well-being, including physical alterations in their mental ability and the influence of complex, interwoven social and emotional variables. The more direct the effect on the central nervous system, the greater the apparent interference in intellectual functioning. Those with brain tumors are thus the most severely impaired, while certain types of therapy brought to bear on the brain, such as irradiation, seem to have lesser, but still significant, effects.

For all patients, the intricate combination of social and emotional factors surrounding the illnesses known as cancer pose real obstacles to normal development and integration into society. Diminished expectations by others, particularly teachers, handicap the child's efforts to attain the level of excellence that would otherwise be expected.

Isolation is a substantial problem that may leave the patient relatively unsupported in dealing with stresses of the illness and predisposed to a lifelong pattern of decreased interaction with others. Further long-term effects are unclear, but it appears that anxiety and depression persist for many of these patients.

It is clear that rather substantial psychological costs must be paid by the young person who is cured of cancer. What is not clear is how long such impediments will persist and whether some may be altered by changes in therapy or intervention into social and emotional problems. Future efforts in treating childhood cancer must include attempts to ameliorate the insults to mental status that are now recognized. A truly cured patient must be capable of achieving near previously expected levels of intellectual development. The simple survival of a human organism is not sufficient. If that person is psychologically handicapped, we have accomplished only the elimination of the disease, not the cure of the child.

ACKNOWLEDGMENTS

The author gratefully acknowledges the assistance of Bernard Spilka, Ph.D., Georgia M. Zwartjes, M.Ed., Dorothy R. Heideman, M.Ed., and Katherine A. Cilli, B.S., in conducting the research undertaken at The Children's Hospital, Denver.

The investigation was supported by grant CA-19581, awarded by the National Cancer Institute, Department of Health, Education and Welfare.

REFERENCES

Bamford, F. N., P. Morris-Jones, D. Pearson, G. G. Riberio, S. M. Shalet, and C. G. Beardwell. 1976. Residual disabilities in children treated for intracranial space occupying lesions. Cancer 37:1149–1151.

Bloom, H. J., E. N. Wallace, and J. M. Henk. 1969. The treatment and prognosis of medulloblastoma in children—A study of 82 verified cases. Am. J. Roentgenol. 105:43–62.

Eiser, C. 1978. Intellectual abilities among survivors of childhood leukaemia as a function of CNS irradiation. Arch. Dis. Child. 53:391–395.

Eiser, C., and R. Lansdown. 1977. Retrospective study of intellectual development in children treated for acute lymphoblastic leukaemia. Arch. Dis. Child. 52:525–529.

Goggin, E. L., S. B. Lansky, and K. Hassanein. 1976. Psychological reactions of children with malignancies. J. Am. Acad. Child. Psych. 15:314–325.

Hoffman, I., and E. H. Futterman. 1971. Coping with waiting. Compr. Psychiatry 12:67–81.

Holton, C. P. 1971. Psychological aspects of the management of adolescents with malignancy. Med. Coll. Va. Q. 7:112–119.

Kaplan, D. M., A. Smith, and R. Grobstein. 1974. School management of the seriously ill child. J. Sch. Health 44:250–254.

Lansky, S. B., J. T. Lowman, T. Vats, and J. Gyulay. 1975. School phobia in children with malignant neoplasms. Am. J. Dis. Child. 129:42–46.

Morrissey, J. R. 1963. Children's adaptation to fatal illness. Soc. Work 8:81–88.

O'Malley, J. E. 1977. Long-term follow-up of survivors of childhood cancer: Psychiatric sequelae. Presented at the American Psychological Association 85th Annual Convention, San Francisco, August 28, 1977.

Soni, S. S., G. W. Morten, S. E. Pitner, D. A. Duenas, and M. Powazek. 1975. Effects of central nervous system irradiation on neuropsychologic functioning of children with acute lymphocytic leukemia. N. Engl. J. Med. 293:113–118.

Spinetta, J. J. 1974. The dying child's awareness of death. Psychol. Bull. 81:256–260.

Spinetta, J. J. 1977. Adjustment in children with cancer. J. Pediatr. Psych. 2:49–51.

van Eys, J. 1977. The outlook for the child with cancer. J. Sch. Health 47:165–169.

Verzosa, M. S., R. J. A. Aur, J. V. Simone, H. O. Hustu, and D. P. Pinkel. 1976. Five years after central nervous system irradiation of children with leukemia. Int. J. Radiat. Oncol. Biol. Phys. 1:209–215.

Status of the Curability of Childhood Cancers,
edited by J. van Eys and M. P. Sullivan.
Raven Press, New York © 1980.

Population Studies of Incidence, Survival, and Follow-up

G. J. Draper

*Childhood Cancer Research Group, Department of Paediatrics, University of Oxford,
Oxford, England*

In this paper we shall discuss incidence, survival, and follow-up in childhood cancer from a population viewpoint. Estimates of incidence and survival rates are now available from several sources and it is possible to combine these data to obtain a general picture of the magnitude of the problem of treating and following up children with cancer.

INCIDENCE

We shall consider a hypothetical center serving a population of 1 million children under age 15; in Britain or the United States this would correspond to a total population of about 3–4 million. Table 1 shows for each of the main diagnostic groups the approximate number of cases that would be expected to occur in 1 year in such a population; this is based mainly on data from the United States (Young and Miller 1975), Britain (Draper et al. 1980), and the

Table 1. *Estimated Annual Numbers of Cases of Neoplasms in 1 Million Children Below Age 15, North American and European Populations*

Diagnosis	No. Cases
Leukemia	37
Hodgkin's disease	5
Non-Hodgkin's lymphomas	7
Neuroblastoma	9
Wilms' tumor	8
Retinoblastoma	3
Brain tumors (including nonmalignant)	23
Osteosarcoma	3
Ewing's tumor	2
Rhabdomyosarcoma	4
Others	13
Total	114

285

Manchester Children's Tumour Registry (quoted in Draper et al. 1980). Slightly less than half of the cases would occur in children in the age range 0–4 years, and a quarter or rather more in each of the age ranges 5–9 and 10–14 years.

For different types of tumor there are wide differences in the ages at which cases most frequently occur. Examples of age distributions for the British data already referred to have been reported by Draper and co-workers (1980). These age distributions are based on data from cancer registries throughout Britain and the diagnoses were not subjected to specialist review. However, at least for most groups, they give a good indication of the true age distribution. The histograms for the three main categories of embryonic tumors, neuroblastoma, Wilms' tumor, and retinoblastoma, are similar, with peaks in early life. Hodgkin's disease and bone tumors show the opposite pattern. Lymphoid and myeloid leukemia differ in their age distributions; the lymphoid peak at around age 3 or 4 has been discussed by Miller (1977).

Data from the United States, Britain, other European countries, and Israel show a considerable degree of similarity in the total incidence of childhood cancer and even in the incidence for individual diagnostic types. It has been suggested that the incidence of Wilms' tumor is remarkably constant between different countries (Innis 1972). This seems to be true for some other diagnostic groups, as well, though the evidence does not come from a very wide range of countries. However, for some diagnostic groups there are striking differences in incidence between different races or areas. Examples include the rarity of Ewing's tumor in black populations in both Africa and the United States and the difference in the proportions of lymphoid and myeloid types of leukemia between Japan and Africa, on the one hand, and the United States and Britain, on the other. It has also been suggested that the incidence of retinoblastoma is greater in underdeveloped countries than in developed ones, though this could be attributable to ascertainment bias, in that patients may be referred to specialized centers even though they live outside the notional catchment area.

For reviews of some of these and other points, see Davies (1976) and Miller (1977).

Very little can be said about factors affecting incidence, since little is known about etiologic factors in childhood cancer. Many epidemiologists agree that obstetric radiography can cause childhood cancer; Bithell and Stewart (1975) present a comprehensive analysis of one set of data that support this. However, with modern X-ray equipment the numbers of cases so caused will be very small indeed. Virus infections during pregnancy have also been suggested as possible causative agents, but even if this suggestion is correct, the number of cases attributable to this cause is unknown and seems likely to remain so. Transplacental carcinogenesis has been widely discussed, but the only well-documented and epidemiologically important finding is the association between diethylstilbestrol given to pregnant women and adenocarcinoma of the vagina and cervix among daughters of these women (Herbst et al. 1977); the great majority of these tumors occur in adolescents and young adults, rather than in children.

Genetic factors are of great interest in relation to childhood cancer, and a variety of interesting associations have been reported. Around 30–40% of cases of retinoblastoma appear to be genetically determined. However, in general, no quantitative estimates are available concerning the importance of the genetic element in childhood cancer.

SURVIVAL RATES AND FOLLOW-UP

The resources needed for the medical care of children with cancer depend not only on disease incidence, but also on the number of children surviving and the length of time treatment continues. Table 2 shows, for major diagnostic categories, the proportions of patients who might reasonably be expected to survive with modern methods of treatment. These figures are based on data from a variety of sources and derived from estimates made independently by J. Pritchard and the present author. They are presented only as a very rough guide; any such estimates are subject to considerable error since they reflect experience at a limited number of centers and involve a considerable degree of extrapolation and guesswork.

More than 50% of all childhood cancer patients can now be expected to survive at least 3 years, and many will be long-term survivors. Thus, at any one time in a population of 1 million children, there might be expected to be more than 200 surviving patients who were treated within the preceding 3 years

Table 2. *Predicted 3-Year Survival Rates for Patients with Various Forms of Cancer, Assuming Results from Specialized Centers Can Be Attained**

Diagnosis	Survival Rate (%)
Lymphoid leukemia	60
Myeloid leukemia	25
Hodgkin's disease	90
Non-Hodgkin's lymphomas	50
Neuroblastoma	25
Wilms' tumor	75
Retinoblastoma	90
Brain tumors (including nonmalignant)	45
Osteosarcoma	40
Ewing's tumor	50
Rhabdomyosarcoma	50
Other malignant neoplasms	50
All types	50+

* There is, of course, a considerable element of extrapolation and sheer guesswork in making these estimates. I am indebted to Dr. J. Pritchard for the use of his estimated figures, which differ slightly from those given here.

and many more on long-term follow-up; the number of long-term survivors would increase by about 60 per year. Allowing for the fact that some patients are treated with chemotherapy for 2 years or even longer, it can be very roughly calculated that in this population around 130 patients might actually be on therapy, and hence under regular medical care, at any one time, though many of these would be between courses of chemotherapy, rather than receiving treatment.

Survival curves for children treated in Britain for various diseases have been presented by Draper et al. (1980). The rates are based on data from cancer registries throughout Britain for 1962–70, and may to some extent underestimate the true rates even for this period because of the way cancer registry data are collected. These and other data suggest that for some tumors, such as retinoblastoma, Wilms' tumor, and neuroblastoma, 3-year survival is almost equivalent to long-term cure, whereas for others, particularly brain tumors, this is not true. These data relate to the period before modern chemotherapy; not only the proportion of survivors but also the shape of the survival curve may change with current methods of treatment. In particular, the proportions of late deaths among survivors may change, but information on this will take some time to become available since recently treated children have necessarily not been followed up for long periods.

Occurrence of Late Deaths

An idea of the number of late deaths can be obtained by examining the portions of survival curves for periods beyond, say, 3 or 5 years after treatment. Another, exactly equivalent, way of looking at this problem is to calculate death rates directly for various intervals after diagnosis from the numbers of patients still alive and the numbers of deaths occurring during those intervals. Table 3 gives such rates for 2-year periods after 3 years' survival, again for patients treated in Britain during 1962–70. Because of the method of follow-up, deaths occurring later than 1975 or after age 20 have been omitted, but the general picture is unlikely to be much affected by these omissions.

Two quite different patterns emerge from Table 3 (or, equivalently, from the survival curves). For neuroblastoma and retinoblastoma (and also for Wilms' tumor, not shown here) death rates are very low after 3 years' survival. Remembering again that these data relate largely to the period before modern methods of treatment, it is clear that for some diagnostic groups there is little risk of death following successful survival to 3 years after diagnosis. It is important, however, to sound a warning about extrapolating these results to recently treated patients. Although a greater proportion of patients are now successfully treated, in some cases the effect of treatment may be to postpone rather than to prevent tumor recurrence or metastases. If this is true, there could be a higher proportion of late deaths than is observed in the data presented here.

There is, for the period considered, another type of pattern, exemplified in

Table 3. Annual Death Rates Among 3-Year Survivors at Various Intervals from Diagnosis*

Diagnosis	3–4 Years		5–6 Years		7–8 Years		9–10 Years	
	No. Deaths	Rate (%)	No. Deaths	Rate (%)	No. Deaths	Rate (%)	No. Deaths	Rate (%)
Hodgkin's disease	40	8.6	19	7.1	4	4.0	0	0.0
Neuroblastoma	7	2.1	1	0.4	0	0.0	0	0.0
Retinoblastoma	1	0.2	2	0.4	2	0.5	1	0.4
Ependymoma	9	8.0	5	6.0	1	2.5	2	14.4

* Cases diagnosed in Britain between 1962 and 1970. Death rates for patients below 20 years of age dying before 1976.

Table 3 by Hodgkin's disease and ependymoma, of a continuing high death rate. This pattern is found also with some other types of tumor, in particular some bone and brain tumors. The current 3-year survival rate for Hodgkin's disease is much higher than that reported here; it is obviously important to determine whether today's 3-year survivors are effectively cured or at an appreciable risk of late death, following the pattern of earlier years.

The occurrence of late deaths among childhood cancer survivors has also been studied by Li et al. (1978), who reported on two independent series of 1,807 and 425 children who survived at least 5 years after diagnosis. The results of that study are generally similar to those given here.

Hospital Admissions

We have carried out a special study to estimate the numbers of hospital admissions and days spent in the hospital by a group of long-term survivors, including both admissions related to the neoplasm and admissions for other causes.

Using cancer registry data, we identified 313 3-year survivors diagnosed in Scotland between 1962 and 1970. Records relating to these children were matched with data on hospital admissions throughout Scotland for the period from 1968 to 1974 using computer record linkage methods. The same procedure was carried out for a control group of 552 children who did not have cancer. As a result of this record linkage, we identified 364 admissions among the cancer patients; of these, 263 were classified as tumor related and 101 as apparently unrelated to the tumor. For the controls, 226 admissions were identified. These results must, of course, be treated with some caution since mistakes could have occurred in the record linkage procedures and hospital admissions outside Scotland are not covered.

Numbers of admissions and rates per 100 patients per year for tumor-related causes are presented in Table 4. The most notable feature of this table is the continuing high admission rate for patients with leukemia, lymphomas (mainly Hodgkin's disease), and brain and bone tumors. This high rate was due in part to repeated admissions for a few patients. This was particularly true, for instance, for the group classified as "other," in which a few retinoblastoma patients were frequently admitted, mainly, we think, for examinations of the unaffected eye. Similarly, a few patients with Hodgkin's disease were admitted on several occasions, one of them 18 times in less than 2 years.

Admission rates for causes apparently unrelated to the neoplasm are presented in Table 5, together with control data. The object of this analysis was to determine whether there was a high general level of morbidity among the survivors. It appears, at least as judged by hospital admissions, that this was not so. The rates for all cancer patients taken together are very similar to those for controls, and, indeed, for the youngest patients they appear to be somewhat lower, though this difference may be only an artifact or a chance result. Among individual

Table 4. Hospital Admissions for Tumor-Related Causes for 313 3-Year Survivors at Various Intervals from Diagnosis (Preliminary Results)

Diagnosis	3–4 Years		5–6 Years		7–12 Years	
	No. Admissions	Rate per 100 Persons per Year	No. Admissions	Rate per 100 Persons per Year	No. Admissicns	Rate per 100 Persons per Year
Leukemia	17	147	0	0	—*	—
Lymphoma	17	35	33	72	3	5
Neuroblastoma	3	9	3	8	0	0
Wilms' tumor	6	17	1	4	2	6
Brain tumor (including nonmalignant)	48	34	24	19	10	6
Malignant bone tumor	12	70	3	20	0	0
Other	35	18	32	17	14	6
Total	138	29	96	22	29	5

* No patients at risk.

Table 5. Hospital Admissions for Causes Not Directly Tumor-Related Among 313 3-Year Survivors and 552 Controls by Age (Preliminary Results)

Diagnosis	3–8 Years		9–14 Years		15+ Years	
	No. Admissions	Rate per 100 Persons per Year	No. Admissions	Rate per 100 Persons per Year	No. Admissions	Rate per 100 Persons per Year
Leukemia	2	9.6	0	0.0	0	0.0
Lymphoma	1	2.8	5	6.5	3	2.6
Neuroblastoma	8	9.1	1	3.0	1	12.7
Wilms' tumor	9	10.5	1	2.2	0	0.0
Brain tumor (including nonmalignant)	4	3.0	19	7.5	18	8.0
Malignant bone tumor	0	0.0	0	0.0	0	0.0
Other	12	4.0	11	3.9	6	2.5
All cancer patients	36	5.4	37	5.1	28	4.4
Controls	97	8.6	80	5.8	49	4.5

Table 6. *Second Primary Malignant Neoplasms in 410 Childhood Cancer Patients**

Years Since Diagnosis of First Tumor	No. Second Malignant Tumors	Rate Per 1,000 Person-Years	Cumulative Incidence (%)
5–9	4	2.3	1.2
10–14	4	3.6	3.0
15–19	6	14.0	10.0
20–24	1	5.1	12.5 (S.E. = 4%)

* Adapted from Li et al. (1975).

tumor types, only the rates for brain tumors appear particularly high, and examination of individual case records might reveal that some of these admissions were in fact directly related to the tumor.

Second Malignant Neoplasms

One long-term hazard for cancer survivors that has been much discussed is the occurrence of second primary tumors, but the only estimate of *incidence rates* of second malignant neoplasms among children with cancer appears to be that given by Li et al. (1975), and updated by Li (1977), on 410 5-year survivors treated at the Sidney Farber Cancer Institute, Boston. Most of the second malignant primaries observed appeared to be radiation induced. It was estimated that in the 20 years after 5-year survival, i.e., in the period 5 to 25 years after diagnosis, childhood cancer patients had a 12% chance of developing a second malignant tumor (Table 6). Only a small number of patients were actually followed for a long period, so the true incidence of second primary tumors may be considerably different from the figure given. Li gives the standard error of the estimate as 4%, which means that the true risk might well be as low as 8% or even 4% or as high as 16% or even 20% for patients treated in the same way. Moreover, the rate will depend on the doses of radiation and presumably the amounts and types of chemotherapy used, as well as the proportions of different types of tumor included in the series. Thus, for another series completely different figures might be obtained. No corresponding data appear to be available from other countries.

ACKNOWLEDGMENTS

I am very grateful to many colleagues in the Childhood Cancer Research Group who carried out much of the work on which this paper is based and helped in preparing the manuscript. The Childhood Cancer Research Group is supported by the Department of Health and Social Security, the Scottish Home and Health Department, and the Leukaemia Research Fund. In the collection of the data much help was given by the staff of cancer registries and hospitals, and I am very grateful for this. The data on which Tables 4 and 5 are based were provided by the Information Services Division of the Common Services Agency, the Scottish Health Service, and I thank Dr. M. A. Heasman, Dr. I. Kemp, Dr. J. Clarke, and their colleagues for all their help.

REFERENCES

Bithell, J. F., and A. Stewart. 1975. Pre-natal irradiation and childhood malignancy: A review of British data from the Oxford survey. Br. J. Cancer 31:271–278.

Davies, J. N. P. 1976. Some variations in childhood cancers throughout the world. Recent Results Cancer Res. 13:28–58.

Draper, G. J., J. M. Birch, J. F. Bithell, L. M. Kinnier Wilson, I. Leck, H. B. Marsden, P. H. Morris Jones, C. A. Stiller, and R. Swindell. 1980. Childhood Cancer in Britain, 1953–1975. Her Majesty's Stationery Office, London, on behalf of The Office of Population Censuses and Surveys, London (in press).

Herbst, A. L., P. Cole, T. Colton, S. T. Robboy, and R. E. Scully. 1977. Age-incidence and risk of diethylstilbestrol-related clear cell adenocarcinoma of the vagina and cervix. Am. J. Obstet. Gynecol. 128:43–50.

Innis, M. D. 1972. Nephroblastoma: Possible index cancer of childhood. Med. J. Aust. 1:18–20.

Li, F. P. 1977. Second malignant tumors after cancer in childhood. Cancer 40:1899–1902.

Li, F. P., J. R. Cassady, and N. Jaffe. 1975. Risk of second tumors in survivors of childhood cancer. Cancer 35:1230–1235.

Li, F. P., M. H. Myers, H. W. Heise, and N. Jaffe. 1978. The course of five-year survivors of cancer in childhood. J. Pediatr. 93:185–187.

Miller, R. W. 1977. Ethnic differences in cancer occurrence: Genetic and environmental influences with particular reference to neuroblastoma, *in* Progress in Cancer Research and Therapy, vol. 3, Genetics of Human Cancer, J. J. Mulvihill, R. W. Miller, and J. F. Fraumeni, eds. Raven Press, New York, pp. 1–14.

Young, J. L., and R. W. Miller. 1975. Incidence of malignant tumors in U.S. children. J. Pediatr. 86:254–258.

Status of the Curability of Childhood Cancers,
edited by J. van Eys and M. P. Sullivan.
Raven Press, New York © 1980.

Genetics and the Child Cured of Cancer

Alfred G. Knudson, Jr., M.D., Ph.D.

*The Institute for Cancer Research, The Fox Chase Cancer Center,
Philadelphia, Pennsylvania*

The greatly improved survival of children with cancer is raising questions only faintly heard a decade ago. Chief among these questions, of course, is, What are the deleterious effects of the treatment and should our therapies be modified to avoid them? But we also see that some subsequent problems in cured children are attributable to genetic differences acting alone or in concert with our well-intentioned therapy. These differences sometimes place other family members at increased risk of the same cancer, and this risk may be greatest for offspring of the cured patient. Offspring may also be at risk of a genetic defect caused by the therapeutic agents that made cure possible. I wish to discuss these two types of genetic features of the child cured of cancer.

GENETIC TRANSMISSION OF CHILDHOOD CANCER

Cancers of children—and, indeed, of adults, too—occur in both hereditary and nonhereditary forms. This is a relatively new idea. It was formerly taught that some cancers, e.g., retinoblastoma and neurofibrosarcoma, occurred in genetically predisposed children, while most occurred by chance in normal children. Now we know that retinoblastoma and neurofibrosarcoma can strike children who are evidently not genetically predisposed, and that Wilms' tumor, neuroblastoma, brain tumors, bone sarcoma, leukemia, and lymphoma sometimes develop in children at genetic risk. Most of our understanding of these phenomena derives from the study of relatives of cured patients.

Retinoblastoma

It is no surprise that retinoblastoma has been the richest source of genetic information, for its high rate of cure has been of long duration. The study of survivors has revealed that bilaterally affected persons carry a dominant "retinoblastoma gene" that is transmitted to half of their offspring, who in turn are most often afflicted bilaterally. On the other hand, a minority of patients with unilateral disease transmit such a dominant gene. It is estimated that about 40% of retinoblastoma cases are associated with the dominant gene and that 60% occur in children who are genetically normal (Knudson 1978).

In one small group of retinoblastoma cases, genetic abnormality can be seen microscopically. In these cases somatic cells, including lymphocytes and fibroblasts, reveal a deletion in the long arm of one chromosome 13, a defect designated by the term 13q⁻. The deletions vary from case to case, but band 13q14 is affected in all cases. In fact, a new technique introduced by Yunis and Ramsay (1978) has shown that retinoblastoma can result from deletion of a particular part of the 14 band. However, most hereditary cases do not show a deletion at this site, suggesting the genetic change is usually too subtle to be seen. This would, of course, be true for very small deletions or point mutations. Nevertheless, the deletion cases and these other cases are so similar clinically that we can presume that both groups result from some genetic change at a retinoblastoma locus (Knudson 1978).

We can make reasonable estimates of risk of retinoblastoma for a patient's offspring. The offspring of patients with bilateral disease are at an approximately 50% risk of this tumor, and in that 50% the tumor will most often be bilateral. If patients with deletions are fertile, they also transmit a 50% risk. About 10% of patients with unilateral disease transmit a risk of 50%, but unfortunately we do not yet know how to identify the subgroup that transmits the risk.

Wilms' Tumor

For many years some patients with Wilms' tumor have been cured, and the proportion has increased with the advent of chemotherapy. More and more familial cases are also being reported. These familial cases are much more often bilateral than is true for Wilms' tumor generally, and it may be that bilateral cases are always the result of genetic predisposition. On the basis of such considerations, Knudson and Strong (1972a) estimated that 38% of Wilms' tumor cases might be prezygotically determined. This estimate was based on an incidence of 8% bilaterality, which is probably too high. If the incidence of bilateral tumors is 4–5%, the genetic form may have an incidence of 15–20%. Most genetic cases are attributable to a new germinal mutation; the patients do not have a family history of the disease. The familial cases show a genetic pattern that is compatible with dominant inheritance.

There is an unusually high coincidence of Wilms' tumor with aniridia. Of further interest is the fact that patients with both diseases have the sporadic form of aniridia, whereas most patients with aniridia have inherited it from an affected parent. As suggested by Knudson and Strong (1972a), patients with aniridia and Wilms' tumor have a chromosomal deletion in every cell. The various deletions are all in the short arm of chromosome 11 (Riccardi et al. 1978, Francke et al. 1978, Bader et al. 1979) and evidently include closely linked loci for aniridia and Wilms' tumor. It is not known how often such deletions occur without the development of Wilms' tumor, but they have been observed in a pair of identical twins, both of whom had aniridia but only one of whom had the tumor (Maurer et al. 1979), so penetrance is not complete.

Generally, hereditary cases of Wilms' tumor do not show such a deletion. It is not known, of course, whether these hereditary cases involve submicroscopic change such as point mutation at the same or some other site. In any event, Wilms' tumor and retinoblastoma are the only tumors in humans for which a tumor gene site has been identified.

Estimation of the risk of Wilms' tumor among the offspring of patients cannot be performed as for retinoblastoma. Knudson and Strong (1972a) estimated that approximately 60% of gene carriers develop the tumor. If this were true, then 30% of the offspring of those with known hereditary disease (including those with chromosomal deletions) or with bilateral disease should be affected, since 50% would be expected to carry the mutant gene or deletion. Most cases of Wilms' tumor are unilateral and it is for patients with unilateral disease that there is the greatest uncertainty. If 10–15% of these patients have the genetic form and are combined with those with bilateral disease to give a total of 15–20% genetic cases, then 5–8% of the offspring of patients with unilateral disease should be gene carriers and 3–5% should develop tumor. So far there are not sufficient data to test whether this is true. Li et al. (1979) have gathered reproductive data on 12 patients with Wilms' tumor, all unilateral, and found that none of the 7 offspring are affected, whereas almost one might have been expected to be. In any case, the risk of tumor is estimated to be no more than 5% for the offspring of patients with unilateral disease.

Neuroblastoma

Familial cases of neuroblastoma have also been observed. Sometimes one family member may have neuroblastoma and another ganglioneuroma, so these two tumors seem closely related. They may even occur in the same patient. The pedigrees of neuroblastoma patients are consistent with dominant inheritance (Knudson and Strong 1972b), the isolated sib pairs being compatible with gonadal mosaicism of a parent. In one remarkable family, one parent of several affected children was found to have a ganglioneuroma (Chatten and Voorhess 1967, Gerson et al. 1974). The percentage of all cases that are genetic has been estimated at 22% (Knudson and Strong 1972b), based on the analysis of multiple primary tumors in familial and nonfamilial cases.

Chromosomal localization has not yet been accomplished for a neuroblastoma gene. In one fascinating report (Pegelow et al. 1975), an affected child had two chromosomal abnormalities ($21p^-q^-$ and atypical 11) in his lymphocytes; one of these was found in one parent and one in the other. Each parent had had a child with neuroblastoma by a previous marriage. On the other hand, Brodeur et al. (1977) have analyzed several tumors in children whose lymphocytes were normal on the assumption that the same chromosomal aberration might be found, regardless of whether it arose germinally or somatically. A significant fraction of tumors were found to show a deletion of the short arm of chromosome 1, distal to band 31. The finding of such a deletion in all somatic cells in a case of neuroblastoma would add great weight to the argument that the deleted segment contained a neuroblastoma gene site.

As with Wilms' tumor, risk estimates for the offspring of neuroblastoma survivors are not possible yet, but they should not be very different from those for Wilms' tumor survivors if the calculations of Knudson and Strong (1972b) are correct.

Other Solid Tumors

There are numerous familial cases of brain tumors, and again the pattern of inheritance is consistent with mendelian dominance (Knudson and Meadows 1978). Within a family the histologic type may vary, although there is rarely an overlap between gliomas and medulloblastoma. Supporting the view that some brain tumors are genetic in origin are the observations that two well-known dominantly inherited conditions, von Recklinghausen's disease and the nevoid basal cell carcinoma syndrome, are accompanied by a significant incidence of brain tumors, nearly always glioma in the former and medulloblastoma in the latter. There has been no chromosomal localization of brain tumor genes.

Familial sarcomas are also well known. Familial rhabdomyosarcoma has been noted in connection with dominantly inherited breast cancer (Li and Fraumeni 1969a,b). The affected pedigrees seem to be a portion of the pedigrees of a broader syndrome that embraces not only breast cancer, but other sarcomas and brain tumors, as well (Lynch et al. 1978, Blattner et al. 1979). Neurofibrosarcomas may be either genetic or nongenetic in origin. Chabalko et al. (1974) have shown that approximately half of all cases in children are associated with von Recklinghausen's disease. Osteosarcoma is occasionally familial and has been found in a small fraction of patients with genetic retinoblastoma independently of radiation, indicating that the retinoblastoma gene imposes a small risk, perhaps 5% or so, of osteosarcoma in addition to a greater than 90% risk of retinoblastoma (Abramson et al. 1976).

Familial cases of germinal and teratoid tumors have been reported in both children and adults, suggesting that dominant genes exist for these neoplasms, too (Knudson 1977). The inheritance patterns suggest the existence of separate genes for testicular and ovarian tumors. For familial testicular tumors there is little specificity, as teratomas, embryonal carcinomas, choriocarcinomas, and seminomas have been reported in males of different ages in various combinations. Among ovarian tumors, granulosa cell tumors seem separable, but there is overlap between dysgerminomas and dermoid cysts. Nongonadal teratoid tumors have also been reported in families; the usual forms have been presacral teratomas and frontal endodermal sinus tumors.

Risk estimates for the offspring of survivors of these tumors will not be possible until more genetic information is available. However, judging from the low frequency of multiple tumors and familial cases, it seems likely that the risks are no worse than for Wilms' tumor and neuroblastoma.

von Recklinghausen's Disease

von Recklinghausen's disease has been associated with so many different tumors of childhood that it must be discussed separately. The development of neurofibrosarcomas is well known and has been alluded to already. Gliomas, especially of the optic chiasm, constitute another major type of tumor. Pheochromocytomas occur in some adults with von Recklinghausen's disease, but neuroblastomas and ganglioneuromas have been found only rarely. Especially interesting is the relationship between neuroblastoma IV-S and neurofibromatosis. Bolande and Towler (1970) have observed the differentiation of cutaneous neuroblastomas into lesions indistinguishable from neurofibromas.

All of the above tumors are of neural or neural crest origin and develop in cells whose differentiation is somehow impaired by the neurofibromatosis mutation. The site of action of the affected gene seems to be different from those of the genes associated with the specific tumors. Recently, however, there have been reports of unexpectedly high frequencies of associations with Wilms' tumor (Stay and Vawter 1977), rhabdomyosarcoma (McKeen et al. 1978), and leukemia (Bader and Miller 1978). The mechanism of action of the neurofibromatosis mutation in such cases is especially puzzling.

Leukemia and Lymphoma

Although some pedigrees show dominant transmission of leukemia and lymphoma, the phenomenon is rare (Knudson 1977). As more patients are cured and survive to adulthood, we shall learn whether some patients had disease attributable to new germinal mutations by surveying the incidence of leukemia and lymphoma in their offspring.

There are also rare cases of leukemia and lymphoma in subjects with well-recognized recessively inherited conditions, especially Fanconi's anemia, Bloom's syndrome, ataxia-telangiectasia, and Wiskott-Aldrich syndrome. These conditions are all very rare and readily diagnosed, so they should not present great difficulty in genetic counseling. Of great interest are the mechanisms by which leukemogenesis occurs in these genetic states.

GENETIC EFFECTS OF TREATMENT

The agents of therapy for childhood cancer include some potent carcinogens and mutagens, such as ionizing radiation and alkylating agents. More is known about the carcinogenic and mutagenic effects of X irradiation than of any other agent. With reference to second tumors, it should be noted that patients who develop second tumors in response to irradiation may be genetically predisposed to tumors. Thus, the development of osteosarcoma in an irradiated orbit in a patient with bilateral retinoblastoma may be attributable to both genetic and environmental factors.

What we are especially concerned with here is the possibility that some therapeutic agent may produce a germinal mutation in the ovary or testis of the treated child and that this mutation will later manifest itself as a genetic disorder in the cured child's offspring. We do not have enough experience to be able to predict risk, but some general estimates can be offered.

Phenotypic Effects of Mutation

Gross chromosomal aberrations can produce any of a wide spectrum of congenital defects, including the classical trisomic and deletion syndromes. The same is true of dominant gene mutations, including such distinctive phenotypes as those for achondroplasia and osteogenesis imperfecta. Any specific abnormality would be rare; we are concerned with the total probability that *some* defect will occur.

Of course, many mutations will result in no visible abnormality, a subtle abnormality, or an abnormality that will appear only in some individuals who have the mutation. Thus, if the mutation affects susceptibility to an acquired disease, it could easily escape recognition. Then there are recessive mutations that are apparent only in those rare individuals who incidentally inherit the same mutation from both parents. X-linked recessive mutations, such as that for hemophilia, would be manifest only in the male offspring of treated females. A female offspring inheriting such a mutation could, of course, later produce a male child who would manifest the mutation.

The Role of the Patient's Sex

The genetic effect of exposure to a mutagen is a function of the sex and age of the exposed subject because germ cells exist at different developmental stages in the two sexes between birth and puberty and sensitivity to mutagenesis is stage dependent. Oogonial mitoses are completed in fetal life, so the cells in the ovary are in the oocyte stage during childhood. On the other hand, male germ cells are in the spermatogonial stage during childhood. The oocyte is much less vulnerable to point mutation than is the spermatogonium, but its long residence in the dictyotene state of meiosis renders it susceptible to chromosomal nondisjunction. Mutagens in the female are therefore not expected to increase readily the incidence of single-gene mutations and structural rearrangements in the offspring, but are expected to increase the incidence of nondisjunction, thus leading to increased numbers of offspring with chromosomal aneuploidy. By contrast, among the offspring of treated males, the frequency of single-gene mutations and structural rearrangements should be elevated and the incidence of aneuploidy affected little or not at all.

The Background Frequency of Mutational Events

The effects of mutagens are measured above a background of spontaneous mutations, and it cannot be specified that·a defect in a particular offspring has been induced by treatment administered to the parent; the role of a mutagen is defined statistically. The background rates of interest here are those for newly arising genetic conditions, not for conditions that are inherited from affected parents. Dominant conditions that are clinically apparent have been estimated to occur at a rate of at most 1% of births, with 20% of these, or two per 1,000, resulting from new mutations (BEIR Report III, in press). These spontaneous dominant mutations occur in the germ cells of the male parent postnatally and in the germ cells of the female parent prenatally. It is thought that dominant mutations are derived nearly equally from male and female parents. Therefore, if the frequency of new cases of all dominant conditions is two per 1,000, we can deduce that the background mutation rate for dominants is approximately one per 1,000 in both male and female germ cells. Similarly, chromosomal rearrangements are estimated to occur at a rate of approximately two per 1,000 (Friedrich and Nielsen 1973). These are the two classes of events that would be expected to be induced with much greater frequency in the offspring of males exposed to mutagens in childhood than in the offspring of females so exposed because the exposure in females occurs after the main period during which mutations take place.

Aneuploid states of clinical significance occur at a rate of approximately three per 1,000 births (Lewis 1975, Friedrich and Nielsen 1973). Autosomal trisomies and the triplo-X condition occur at rates of 1.4 per 1,000 births and 0.9 per 1,000 female births, respectively, and all result from maternal nondisjunction. We can presume that the incidence of these defects increases among the offspring of females treated with mutagens. The XYY and XO conditions occur at rates of 1.2 and 0.2 per 1,000 males and females, respectively, and virtually all result from paternal nondisjunction. These incidences should not be increased among the offspring of treated females or males. Klinefelter's syndrome (XXY) occurs at a rate of about 1.3 per 1,000 male births. An estimated 0.8 cases per 1,000 births develop as a result of nondisjunction in females; this incidence should be increased in the offspring of treated females. On the other hand, the 0.5 cases per 1,000 births that develop after nondisjunction in males should not be increased among the offspring of treated males.

Dose-Response Relationships

Virtually nothing is known regarding the relationship of genetic effect to dose of chemical mutagen in man, and even for irradiation much controversy surrounds quantitative estimates. Nevertheless, there are two tentative conclusions, based in large part upon investigations in mice. One is that the general nature of the dose-response curve is quadratic, with the linear term being of greater importance for single-gene mutations and both terms for chromosomal rearrangements (Lewis 1975). The second is that a useful quantitative indicator of genetic effect is the doubling dose, or that dose of mutagen that will double the background frequency of the mutant germ cell under consideration. Thus, if the background rate of new dominant gene mutations is one per 1,000 germ cells, a doubling dose would add one more new mutation per 1,000 germ cells. For different kinds of radiation the biological effectiveness varies, so a more appropriate unit is the rem. For X rays, the value in rad is approximately the same as that in rem. Although the doubling dose is not accurately known, the range of estimates has been from 35 to 200 rem (Lewis 1975). If we assume a low doubling dose of 35 rem in male parents only, the frequency of newborns affected by new dominant mutations would be two per 1,000 at a background level of radiation, three per 1,000 with 35 rem, four per 1,000 with 70 rem, and so on.

For chromosomal aberrations of the structural type, the dose-response relationship is more complex. If the dose of X irradiation is delivered in multiple small doses or a single dose at a low rate, the chromosomal effect will be nearly linear, as for gene mutations, but if it is delivered in a single large dose at a high rate, the quadratic expression applies. Thus, for a dose of 200 rem, Lewis (1975) estimates 2.2 new unbalanced translocations per 1,000 live births with the latter schedule to male parents in childhood, but 0.2 cases with the former schedule. Irradiation of the female parent in childhood is estimated to produce only a small fraction of this number of abnormalities.

There is more uncertainty about the induction of abnormalities of chromosome number as a function of dose. On the basis of mouse experiments it has been estimated that the rate of such abnormalities carries a doubling dose approximately the same as that for point mutations, except that when the male parent has been irradiated in childhood, the offspring are little affected. Lewis (1975) estimates that 200 rem delivered to the female gonad in childhood would impose an added risk of aneuploidy in the offspring of about 11 per 1,000 births.

It can be concluded, then, that for gonadal doses of 200 rem in childhood, the offspring may be at an added risk of genetic abnormality of 1% or so. In the offspring of irradiated males there will be primarily dominant mutations (approximately six induced per 1,000 births) and structural chromosomal aberrations (approximately two induced per 1,000 births). In the offspring of females there will be primarily chromosomal aneuploidy (approximately 11 induced per 1,000 births). At higher doses of gonadal irradiation a linear extrapolation applies for most of these, except for structural aberrations when irradiation is given in single doses at a high rate. At doses greater than 800–1,000 rem, however, sterility becomes very probable (Bender and Young 1978, Anonymous 1978, Shalet et al. 1978), so gonadal irradiation beyond those levels is of little practical significance for offspring. The highest level of irradiation likely to produce a genetic effect is, therefore, probably on the order of 1,000 rem. If the effect is linear, the added risk of defect would be imparted to about 5% of all births.

Risk Assessment

As these considerations make apparent, there are probably significant risks to the offspring of childhood cancer survivors treated with certain modalities.

The risks are as yet incompletely measured for chemicals (Bender and Young 1978). For ionizing radiation the risks are not great, but significantly above normal levels. Chromosomal abnormalities can be detected in utero and avoided, if desired, by selective abortion. Under those conditions, the chief undetectable defects would be those resulting from dominant mutations induced in the germ cells of the male parent.

These effects would not add greatly to our burden of congenital defects, given the fact that just one per 1,000 persons in the adult population will be a survivor of childhood cancer in the future (Meadows et al. 1980, see pages 263 to 275, this volume). Of course, these levels of risk would be disastrous for a population as a whole. But assuming that the kinds of induced genetic disorders that befall the offspring are no different from those afflicting newborn populations generally, we can place a limit upon the burden to society. It appears unlikely that the risk of new deleterious mutations will be increased more than tenfold for this population of children. So far we have only a small body of data on offspring of survivors, but these show no significant excess of congenital defects (Li et al. 1979, Li and Jaffe 1974, Holmes and Holmes 1975). Even if all survivors were normally fertile and their offspring were all at a tenfold increased risk, the burden of new mutations added to the general population would be 1% above that already observed. Thus, if μ were the total incidence of all new mutations in the general population, the incidence of extra mutations for this special population would be $\frac{1}{1,000} \cdot 10 \cdot \mu$, or 0.01μ. To the extent that infertility, lower risk, and selective abortion operated, the incidence would be lower.

I have not discussed the risks to still later generations because there are too many variables to evaluate. It is important to note, however, that many of these mutations may be transmitted. The incidence of disorders would therefore rise from both new mutations affecting each generation of offspring and mutations transmitted from previous generations.

CONCLUSIONS

The offspring of survivors of childhood cancer are at increased risk of genetic disorder for two reasons: they may inherit the genes that caused the parents' cancers and so be at risk of the total effects of those genes, and they may acquire new genetic abnormalities, genic or chromosomal, induced in the parental germ cells by therapeutic agents. The first of these risks will fall heavily upon a subpopulation of children whose parents had the genetic form of a particular cancer; the second will apply to all offspring of survivors whose treatment included carcinogenic agents, but will probably be small. Inheritance of cancer genes therefore seems to be the principal risk. Recent progress suggests that we shall be better able to identify which parents are at risk of the first type of disorder and, in some instances, which of their offspring are, too. The second type of disorder can be found only in the offspring. The problems with their detection are the same as those for detecting dominant conditions and chromosomal aberrations generally. We conclude, then, that the offspring of survivors of childhood cancer constitute a high-risk group for genetic cancer and other genetic abnormalities and should be examined accordingly.

ACKNOWLEDGMENTS

This investigation was supported in part by U.S. Public Health Service Grant CA06927 from the National Cancer Institute, Department of Health, Education and Welfare, and by an appropriation from the Commonwealth of Pennsylvania.

REFERENCES

Abramson, D. H., R. M. Ellsworth, and L. E. Zimmerman. 1976. Nonocular cancer in retinoblastoma survivors. Trans. Am. Acad. Ophthalmol. Otolaryngol. 81:454–457.

Anonymous. 1978. Treatment of childhood cancer: Effects on the gonads (Editorial). Br. Med. J. 2:785–786.

Bader, J. L., F. P. Li, P. S. Gerald, S. L. Leikin, and J. G. Randolph. 1979. 11p chromosome deletion in four patients with aniridia and Wilms' tumor, *in* Proceedings of the 70th Annual Meeting of the American Association for Cancer Research, Abstract 850, p. 210.

Bader, J. L., and R. W. Miller. 1978. Neurofibromatosis and childhood leukemia. J. Pediatr. 92:925–929.

BEIR Report III. 1980. Effects on Population of Exposure to Low Levels of Ionizing Radiation. National Academy of Sciences, Washington, D.C., in press.

Bender, R. A., and R. C. Young. 1978. Effects of cancer treatment on individual and generational genetics. Semin. Oncol. 5:47–56.

Blattner, W. A., D. B. McGuire, J. J. Mulvihill, B. C. Lampkin, J. Hananian, and J. F. Fraumeni, Jr. 1979. Genealogy of cancer in a family. J.A.M.A. 241:259–261.

Bolande, R. P., and W. F. Towler. 1970. A possible relationship of neuroblastoma to von Recklinghausen's disease. Cancer 26:162–175.

Brodeur, G. M., G. S. Sekhon, and M. N. Goldstein. 1977. Chromosomal aberrations in human neuroblastomas. Cancer 40:2256–2263.

Chabalko, J. J., E. T. Creagen, and J. F. Fraumeni, Jr. 1974. Epidemiology of selected sarcomas in children. J. Natl. Cancer Inst. 53:675–679.

Chatten, J., and M. L. Voorhess. 1967. Familial neuroblastoma: Report of a kindred with multiple disorders, including neuroblastomas in four siblings. N. Engl. J. Med. 277:1230–1236.

Francke, U., V. M. Riccardi, H. M. Hittner, and W. Borges. 1978. Interstitial del(11p) as a cause of the aniridia-Wilms' tumor association: Band localization and a heritable basis. Am. J. Hum. Genet. 30:81A.

Friedrich, U., and J. Nielsen. 1973. Chromosome studies in 5,049 consecutive newborn children. Clin. Genet. 4:333–343.

Gerson, J. M., J. Chatten, and S. Eisman. 1974. Familial neuroblastoma—A follow up. N. Engl. J. Med. 290:1487.

Holmes, H. A., and F. F. Holmes. 1975. After ten years, what are the handicaps and life styles of children treated for cancer? An examination of the present status of 124 such survivors. Clin. Pediatr. 14:819–823.

Knudson, A. G. 1977. Genetics and etiology of human cancer. Adv. Hum. Genet. 8:1–66.

Knudson, A. G. 1978. Retinoblastoma: A prototypic hereditary neoplasm. Semin. Oncol. 5:57–60.

Knudson, A. G., and A. T. Meadows. 1978. Developmental genetics of neural tumors in man, *in* Cell Differentiation and Neoplasia (Proceedings of the 30th Annual Symposium on Fundamental Cancer Research), G. F. Saunders, ed. Raven Press, New York, pp. 83–92.

Knudson, A. G., and L. C. Strong. 1972a. Mutation and cancer: A model for Wilms' tumor of the kidney. J. Natl. Cancer Inst. 48:313–324.

Knudson, A. G., and L. C. Strong. 1972b. Mutation and cancer: Neuroblastoma and pheochromocytoma. Am. J. Hum. Genet. 24:514–532.

Lewis, E. B. 1975. Possible genetic consequences of irradiation of tumors in childhood. Radiology 114:147–153.

Li, F. P., W. Fine, N. Jaffe, G. E. Holmes, and F. F. Holmes. 1979. Offspring of patients treated for cancer in childhood. J. Natl. Cancer Inst. 62:1193–1197.

Li, F. P., and J. F. Fraumeni, Jr. 1969a. Soft-tissue sarcomas, breast cancer, and other neoplasms. A familial syndrome? Ann. Intern. Med. 71:747–752.

Li, F. P., and J. F. Fraumeni, Jr. 1969b. Rhabdomyosarcoma in children: Epidemiologic study and identification of a familial cancer syndrome. J. Natl. Cancer Inst. 43:1365–1373.

Li, F. P., and N. Jaffe. 1974. Progeny of childhood-cancer survivors. Lancet 2:707–709.

Lynch, H. T., G. M. Mulcahy, R. E. Harris, H. A. Guirgis, and J. F. Lynch. 1978. Genetic and pathologic findings in a kindred with hereditary sarcoma, breast cancer, brain tumors, leukemia, lung, laryngeal, and adrenal cortical carcinoma. Cancer 41:2055–2064.

Maurer, H. S., T. W. Pendergrass, W. Borges, and G. R. Honig. 1979. The role of genetic factors in the etiology of Wilms' tumor. Cancer 43:205–208.

McKeen, E. A., J. Bodurtha, A. T. Meadows, E. C. Douglass, and J. J. Mulvihill. 1978. Rhabdomyosarcoma complicating multiple neurofibromatosis. J. Pediatr. 93:992–993.

Meadows, A. T., N. L. Krejmas, and J. B. Belasco for the Late Effects Study Group. 1980. The medical cost of cure: Sequelae in survivors of childhood cancer, in Status of the Curability of Childhood Cancers, J. van Eys and M. P. Sullivan, eds. Raven Press, New York, pp. 263–275.

Pegelow, C. H., A. J. Ebbin, D. Powers, and J. W. Towner. 1975. Familial neuroblastoma. J. Pediatr. 87:763–765.

Riccardi, V. M., E. Sujansky, A. C. Smith, and U. Francke. 1978. Chromosomal imbalance in the aniridia–Wilms' tumor association: 11p interstitial deletion. Pediatrics 61:604–610.

Shalet, S. M., C. G. Beardwell, P. H. Morris Jones, and D. Pearson. 1978. Treatment of childhood cancer: Effects on gonads. Br. Med. J. 2:1290–1296.

Stay, E. J., and G. Vawter. 1977. The relationship between nephroblastoma and neurofibromatosis (von Recklinghausen's disease). Cancer 39:2550–2555.

Yunis, J. J., and N. Ramsay. 1978. Retinoblastoma and subband deletion of chromosome 13. Am. J. Dis. Child. 132:161–163.

Status of the Curability of Childhood Cancers,
edited by J. van Eys and M. P. Sullivan.
Raven Press, New York © 1980.

Prevention—The Ultimate Solution

Robert W. Miller

Clinical Epidemiology Branch, National Cancer Institute, Bethesda, Maryland

Children are not just little people with respect to carcinogenesis or other matters. They have special susceptibilities and special exposures, and even cancers with the longest latent periods can arise well within a child's expected life-span. Carcinogens may be encountered not only in the uterine environment, but also in breast milk. We now know that carcinogens may be found in schools, playgrounds, and homes.

PHYSICAL AGENTS

Ionizing Radiation

The carcinogenic effects of X-ray exposure during childhood or in utero have apparently been markedly diminished by the adoption of more stringent protective measures in the use of radiological procedures, particularly fluoroscopy, since 1956. In that year, potential hazards from medical X rays were cited in reports by the National Academy of Sciences (NAS) (1956) and the (British) Medical Research Council (MRC) (1956). As a result, unnecessary fluoroscopy and radiotherapy for benign disorders have been progressively reduced. Children under 5 years of age experienced about 1000 fewer deaths from leukemia in 1960 through 1966 than expected on the basis of rates for the previous decade (Miller 1969). This reduction, which was not attributable to improved therapy, may have been due in part at least to a decrease in heavy exposures to X rays after the NAS and MRC reports.

Cancer of the thyroid in adults has been widely induced by radiation administered to the thymus gland in infancy to reduce enlargement or to prevent status thymicolymphaticus (Lambert 1978), once thought to be a cause of sudden infant deaths. The frequency of thyroid cancers should be substantially lower in persons born since 1960 than it was in those born in the half-century before, when thymic irradiation was common. Such a decrease in rates is the ultimate proof of the cause of a disease; when the suspected agent is removed or blocked, the effect no longer occurs.

Ultraviolet Radiation

Overexposures of children to sunlight are presumably cumulative in effect, and may produce skin cancer many years later. Skin cancers are rare in children unless they have a genetic disorder, such as xeroderma pigmentosum, that makes them especially susceptible to the carcinogenic effects of ultraviolet light. Protecting these genetically handicapped children from such exposures has clearly prevented the occurrence of skin neoplasia (Lynch et al. 1977). Children, especially those with fair complexions, should be advised against overexposure, a measure that would reduce the frequency of skin cancer in adults in the future. One need not stay out of the sun to avoid ultraviolet light since noncarcinogenic sunscreen ointments are effective.

Asbestos

Asbestos has not caused cancer during childhood because the latent period has been too long. The discovery that asbestos could induce mesothelioma was made in South Africa when a cluster of cases was observed not primarily among asbestos workers, but among people of various occupations who had grown up near the open-pit mines (Wagner et al. 1960). Selikoff's group has reported on four children of asbestos workers who developed mesothelioma in middle age, apparently because of childhood exposure to dust on their fathers' workclothes (Anderson et al. 1976). A dramatic example of this hazard has been reported by Li et al. (1978): cancer of the lung developed in a man 60 years of age who was a cigarette smoker and who had worked as a pipe-insulator in a shipyard for 25 years, and mesothelioma developed in his wife at age 50 and his daughter at age 34. The father had often worn his dust-laden workclothes home. Chisolm (1978) has referred to this sort of contamination as "fouling one's own nest."

The carcinogenicity of asbestos is related to its physical properties, the length and diameter of the fibers. Rats exposed to glass fibers especially manufactured to duplicate the dimensions of carcinogenic forms of asbestos develop tumors (Stanton et al. 1977). Among asbestos workers, the frequency of bronchogenic carcinoma is greatly potentiated by cigarette smoking; the risk is about 90 times greater in such persons than in people who don't smoke or work with asbestos, and about nine times greater than in people who smoke but are not exposed to asbestos.

An unknown number of schoolrooms with asbestos-board walls or asbestos-sprayed ceilings are exposing children to floating fibers (Sawyer 1977). The Yale University School of Art and Architecture had an incredible misadventure with asbestos-sprayed ceilings, which caused heavy pollution as they frayed over time. The offending material had to be wetted down and carefully removed at substantial expense. A determination of the extent of such hazards in schoolrooms is needed, and the question arises: will childhood exposure to asbestos potentiate lung cancer occurrence if the exposed person takes up cigarette smoking as a teen-ager or adult? If childhood exposure to asbestos has been widespread for the last 20 years, and if pulmonary cancer is potentiated by later cigarette smoking, an upturn in lung cancer rates among people in their thirties may soon be upon us. Research is needed to determine the amount and source of asbestos fibers lodged in the lungs of children who die accidentally, and to determine if cigarette smoking has the same potentiating carcinogenic effect when it occurs simultaneously with asbestos exposure as when it occurs sequentially. A study might be made of asbestos-exposed shipyard workers of World War II who took up smoking later, if enough can be found for a proper evaluation. Methods for prevention are obvious but difficult to implement: rid the child's environment of asbestos and persuade the child not to smoke.

CHEMICALS

Intrauterine Exposures

The incidence of clear cell adenocarcinoma of the cervix or vagina, usually rare in young women, is 0.14–1.4 per 1000 women under 30 years of age whose mothers were treated with diethylstilbestrol (DES) at some time during the first 17 weeks of pregnancy (Herbst et al. 1977). This transplacental chemical carcinogen, the first discovered in humans, does not follow the pattern of carcinogens in animal models. In animals, carcinogenic effects appear when exposures occur late in pregnancy, after organogenesis (Rice 1973). In humans, the effect of exposure early in pregnancy is presumably related to the minor developmental anomalies seen in a high proportion of DES-exposed daughters (Robboy et al. 1977). In males, hypospermia and anomalies of the genitalia have been reported, but no cancers so far (Bibbo et al. 1977). Later effects are still unknown, but there is one unconfirmed report of abnormal outcomes of pregnancy in a small number of DES-exposed daughters, possibly related to the abnormal shape of the uterus, as revealed by X-ray film studies (Kaufman et al. 1977).

Any carcinogen that crosses the placenta may be carcinogenic in the offspring. One such agent is diphenylhydantoin (DPH), which is used to treat epilepsy. DPH can cause a lymphoma-like disease, which sometimes disappears if administration is stopped (Hoover and Fraumeni 1975). When taken by a pregnant woman, DPH occasionally causes malformations in the child: hypoplasia of the bones in the midface, which gives the infant a cute appearance, and, more readily apparent, hypoplasia or aplasia of the fingernails or toenails (Hanson and Smith 1975). DPH might be expected to induce lymphoma in some of these children, but instead, neuroblastoma has been reported in three such children (Pendergrass and Hanson 1976, Sherman and Roizen 1976, Seeler et al. 1979). DPH is the second human transplacental chemical carcinogen to be discovered.

As yet, no evidence has been presented for other transplacental chemical carcinogens, but the effects of such carcinogens may occur in middle or even late life, when the intrauterine exposure can no longer be traced, or the high rate of cancer may be masked because the cancer is of a common type and the additional cases due to prenatal influence are not recognizable. What sorts of chemicals now enter the fetus through the placenta? Dowty and co-workers (1976) have identified more than 100 volatile organic chemicals in umbilical-cord blood, including benzene, styrene, plastics, and food additives.

Pollution of the environment (and the fetus) is dramatically illustrated by a public health advisory issued by the Michigan State Department of Public Health on September 12, 1978, which lists some waterways within the state so polluted with various industrial wastes and contaminants that the fish cannot be eaten, and others, including the Great Lakes, that are less polluted, so the fish caught there can be eaten once a week. One wonders what other state health departments issue such advisories.

Breast Feeding

There is no evidence that carcinogens in breast milk cause human cancer, but in theory they could. Some pollutants are stored in fat and can best be excreted in the fat of breast milk, including polychlorinated biphenyls (PCBs), polybrominated biphenyls (PBBs), and DDT. No change in breast feeding practice is recommended because at present there is no known danger from the levels of these substances in human breast milk (American Academy of Pediatrics 1978). If the mother has been subjected to unusual occupational exposure or has ingested large quantities of food known to be contaminated, such as sport fish from waters polluted by PCBs, breast milk can be analyzed to help determine if breast feeding should be continued.

Drugs

Drugs used to treat several serious ailments are known to be carcinogenic within a few years of administration. Immunosuppressant therapy for renal transplantation can induce lymphoma or hepatobiliary tract tumors in children within a few months of initiation of treatment (Hoover 1977). Anabolic androgenic steroids given for aplastic anemia, particularly the Fanconi type, may induce tumors of the liver (Meadows et al. 1974). Apparently the underlying disease predisposes the patient to the carcinogenic effects of the drug. Chemotherapy for other types of cancer may induce leukemia (Reimer et al. 1977). Some cancer-inducing drugs are used for serious but nonfatal illnesses, and one must weigh the benefits against the risks more carefully in these cases than in those involving potentially fatal neoplasms. As more is learned about alternative means of treatment and about the doses or patient characteristics that increase the risk of second primary tumors, adjustments in therapy may be possible to eliminate or reduce the risk of such tumors.

Habits

The carcinogenic effects of cigarette smoking exceed by far those of all other known environmental agents. The example set by the parents or other household members markedly affects the probability that a child will become a cigarette-smoker. The etiologist in this instance can define the cause, but is a novice at suggesting means of persuading children not to smoke.

Life-Style and Diet

Among the 96 counties in the United States with average populations of 300,000 or more between 1950 and 1969, San Francisco ranked 11th in male mortality from cancer (all types) and Denver ranked 91st (Miller and McKay, unpublished observation). These two counties are highly urban areas coextensive with the cities. Why the difference in cancer rates? Some say life-style is the reason—all the environmental influences that affect people in one place more than the other, including smoking, drinking, diet, water supplies, automobile emissions, medical care, occupation, and neighborhood factories. The difference in mortality rates between San Francisco and Denver is substantial; identifying the causes seems formidable.

Unidentifiable seeds of cancer can obviously be sown early in life, as indicated by the retention of old-country cancer rates by migrants but not their children (Haenszel 1975), and by the substantially lower rates among Seventh-Day Adventists than the general population (Phillips 1975), apparently related to their dietary habits.

A word of caution about diet: if parents are too restrictive, the child may be adversely affected psychologically or even physically. Substantial reduction of fats in the diet can lead to chronic nonspecific diarrhea, and can be cured by giving the child a glass of milk (Cohen et al. 1979). Too little vitamin B_{12} in the breast milk of a vegetarian caused her infant to develop severe megaloblastic anemia, metabolic disorders, and coma (Higginbottom et al. 1978). The disorders were treated with vitamin B_{12}, which could have prevented them had it been given to the mother during pregnancy and lactation.

VIRUSES

Much attention has been focused in the past on time-space clusters of childhood leukemia as evidence for a viral etiology of the disease, but the disease was never shown to be horizontally transmitted in a fashion that would suggest infectious origins (Caldwell and Heath 1976). Two new reports, however, indicate that, under special circumstances at least, Epstein-Barr virus (EBV) is oncogenic: in Burkitt's lymphoma in Africa (de-Thé et al. 1978) and in X-linked lymphoproliferative disorders described by Purtilo and associates (1977). The latter report describes several families in which brothers were afflicted with lymphoma-like diseases, agammaglobulinemia and fatal infectious mononucleosis, which are different manifestations of B-lymphocyte disease. These are instances of interactions between a virus and genetic susceptibility for which no animal models are as yet known. A vaccine may prevent these diseases in high-risk groups.

Carcinoma of the uterine cervix has epidemiologic characteristics that strongly suggest it is due to a transmissible agent, and it has been described as a venereal disease (Kessler 1976). With initiation of sexual activity and contact with multiple partners now occurring early in life, the origins of this neoplasm can sometimes be traced into the pediatric age-range. Prevention depends on psychosocial research and application.

GENETIC INFLUENCES

There is a common misunderstanding that genetic influences refer only to heredity, when in fact somatic cell genetics is very much involved in the origins of the vast majority of cancers. When reference is made to initiation and promotion as steps in the carcinogenic process, it should be noted that initiation is virtually synonymous with mutation in a body cell at any time during the life-span. An extended consideration of this subject was presented earlier in this conference (Knudson 1980, see pages 295–305, this volume), as well as in the volume *Genetics of Human Cancer* (Mulvihill et al. 1977). Of particular interest is the dramatic interaction between cancer-predisposing genetic disorders and radiant energy.

When children with ataxia-telangiectasia (AT), an autosomal recessive disease accompanied by a marked predisposition to lymphoma (Kersey et al. 1973), were treated with conventional doses of radiotherapy, they sometimes suffered severe acute radiation reactions (Cunliffe et al. 1975). Exposure of their skin fibroblasts in culture to various doses of X rays revealed an inverse relationship between survival and dose (Taylor et al. 1976) and a DNA-repair defect (Paterson et al. 1976). At least two complementation groups and one variant have been identified. The defect in AT is thus an X-ray analog of the DNA repair defect after ultraviolet-light damage in xeroderma pigmentosum (XP), which apparently predisposes its bearers to skin cancer.

Cells from patients with these two diseases are being evaluated for use as screening devices for chemical mutagens and carcinogens. Chemicals do not cause DNA-repair defects in XP, but certain carcinogens increase the frequency of sister-chromatid exchanges (SCE) (Wolff et al. 1977). A recent report from Sweden indicates that studies of SCE in the newborn may reveal much about maternal exposures during pregnancy to such chemicals as benzene (Funes-Cravioto et al. 1977).

CONCLUSIONS

We need to know not only what causes cancer, but also who is most or least susceptible and why. Important clues to the biology of cancer can come from the study of relatively rare "spontaneous" cancers in children genetically predisposed to neoplasia. These rare diseases may represent human models of carcinogenesis for which no corresponding animal models are yet known. Studies of such patients may lead to fresh concepts for prevention, early detection, and treatment.

REFERENCES

American Academy of Pediatrics, Committee on Environmental Hazards. 1978. PCBs in breast milk. Pediatrics 62:407.

Anderson, H. A., R. Lilis, S. M. Daum, A. S. Fischbein, and I. J. Selikoff. 1976. Household-contact asbestos: Neoplastic risk. Ann. N.Y. Acad. Sci. 271:311–323.

Bibbo, M., W. B. Gill, F. Azizi, R. Blough, V. S. Fang, R. L. Rosenfield, G. F. B. Schumacher, K. Sleeper, M. G. Sonek, and G. L. Wied. 1977. Follow-up study of male and female offspring of DES-exposed mothers. Obstet. Gynecol. 49:1–8.

Caldwell, G. G., and C. W. Heath, Jr. 1976. Case clustering in cancer. South. Med. J. 69:1598–1602.

Chisolm, J. J., Jr. 1978. Fouling one's own nest. Pediatrics 62:614–617.

Cohen, S. A., K. M. Hendricks, E. J. Eastham, R. K. Mathis, and W. A. Walker. 1979. Chronic nonspecific diarrhea: A complication of dietary fat restriction. Am. J. Dis. Child. 133:490–492.

Cunliffe, P. N., J. R. Mann, A. H. Cameron, K. D. Roberts, and H. W. C. Ward. 1975. Radiosensitivity in ataxia-telangiectasia. Br. J. Radiol. 48:374–376.

de-Thé, G., A. Geser, N. E. Day, P. M. Tukei, E. H. Williams, D. P. Beri, P. G. Smith, A. G. Dean, G. W. Bornkamm, P. Feorino, and W. Henle. 1978. Epidemiological evidence for causal relationship between Epstein-Barr virus and Burkitt's lymphoma from Ugandan prospective study. Nature 274:756–761.

Dowty, B. J., J. L. Laseter, and J. Storer. 1976. The transplacental migration and accumulation in blood of volatile organic constituents. Pediatr. Res. 10:696–701.

Funes-Cravioto, F., C. Zapata-Gayon, B. Kolmodin-Hedman, B. Lambert, J. Lindsten, E. Norberg, M. Nordenskjold, R. Olin, and A. Swensson. 1977. Chromosome aberrations and sister-chromatid exchange in workers in chemical laboratories and a rotoprinting factory and in children of women laboratory workers. Lancet 2:322–325.

Haenszel, W. 1975. Migrant studies, *in* Persons at High Risk of Cancer: An Approach to Cancer Etiology and Control, J. F. Fraumeni, Jr., ed. Academic Press, New York, pp. 361–371.

Hanson, J. W., and D. W. Smith. 1975. The fetal hydantoin syndrome. J. Pediatr. 87:285–290.

Herbst, A. L., P. Cole, T. Colton, S. J. Robboy, and R. E. Scully. 1977. Age-incidence and risk of diethylstilbestrol-related clear cell adenocarcinoma of the vagina and cervix. Am. J. Obstet. Gynecol. 128:43–50.

Higginbottom, M. C., L. Sweetman, and W. L. Nyhan. 1978. A syndrome of methylmalonic aciduria, homocystinuria, megaloblastic anemia and neurologic abnormalities in a vitamin B_{12}-deficient breast-fed infant of a strict vegetarian. N. Engl. J. Med. 299:317–323.

Hoover, R. 1977. Effects of drugs—Immunosuppression, *in* Origins of Human Cancer. A. Incidence of Cancer in Humans (Cold Spring Harbor Conferences on Cell Proliferation, Vol. 4), H. H. Hiatt, J. D. Watson, and J. A. Winsten, eds. Cold Spring Harbor Laboratory, Cold Spring Harbor, New York, pp. 369–379.

Hoover, R., and J. F. Fraumeni, Jr. 1975. Drugs, *in* Persons at High Risk of Cancer: An Approach to Cancer Etiology and Control, J. F. Fraumeni, Jr., ed. Academic Press, New York, pp. 185–198.

Kaufman, R. H., G. L. Binder, P. M. Gray, Jr., and E. Adam. 1977. Upper genital tract changes associated with exposure in utero to diethylstilbestrol. Am. J. Obstet. Gynecol. 128:51–59.

Kersey, J. H., B. D. Spector, and R. A. Good. 1973. Primary immunodeficiency diseases and cancer: The Immunodeficiency-Cancer Registry. Int. J. Cancer 12:333–347.

Kessler, I. I. 1976. Human cervical cancer as a venereal disease. Cancer Res. 36:783–791.

Knudson, A. G., Jr. 1980. Genetics and the child cured of cancer, *in* Status of the Curability of Childhood Cancers, J. van Eys and M. P. Sullivan, eds. Raven Press, New York, pp. 295–305.

Lambert, E. C. 1978. Errors in concepts, *in* Modern Medical Mistakes. Indiana University Press, Bloomington, Indiana, pp. 15–49.

Li, F. P., J. Lokich, J. Lapey, W. B. Neptune, and E. W. Wilkins, Jr. 1978. Familial mesothelioma after intense asbestos exposure at home. J.A.M.A. 240:467.

Lynch, H. T., B. C. Frichot III, and J. F. Lynch. 1977. Cancer control in xeroderma pigmentosum. Arch. Dermatol. 113:193–195.

Meadows, A. T., J. L. Naiman, and M. Valdes-Dapena. 1974. Hepatoma associated with androgen therapy for aplastic anemia. J. Pediatr. 84:109–110.

Medical Research Council. 1956. Hazards to Man of Nuclear and Allied Radiations. Her Majesty's Stationery Office, London, 128 pp.

Miller, R. W. 1969. Decline in U.S. childhood leukaemia mortality. Lancet 2:1189–1190.

Mulvihill, J. J., R. W. Miller, and J. F. Fraumeni, Jr., eds. 1977. Genetics of Human Cancer. Raven Press, New York, 519 pp.

National Academy of Sciences. 1956. The Biological Effects of Atomic Radiation: Summary Reports from a Study. National Academy of Sciences–National Research Council, Washington, D.C., 108 pp.

Paterson, M. C., B. P. Smith, P. H. M. Lohman, A. K. Anderson, and L. Fishman. 1976. Defective excision repair of γ-ray-damaged DNA in human (ataxia telangiectasia) fibroblasts. Nature 260:444–447.

Pendergrass, T. W., and J. W. Hanson. 1976. Fetal hydantoin syndrome and neuroblastoma. Lancet 2:150.

Phillips, R. L. 1975. Role of life-style and dietary habits in risk of cancer among Seventh-Day Adventists. Cancer Res. 35:3513–3522.

Purtilo, D. T., D. DeFlorio, Jr., L. M. Hutt, J. Bhawan, J. P. S. Yang, R. Otto, and W. Edwards. 1977. Variable phenotypic expression of an X-linked recessive lymphoproliferative syndrome. N. Engl. J. Med. 297:1077–1081.

Reimer, R. R., R. Hoover, J. F. Fraumeni, Jr., and R. C. Young. 1977. Acute leukemia after alkylating-agent therapy of ovarian cancer. N. Engl. J. Med. 297:177–181.

Rice, J. M. 1973. An overview of transplacental chemical carconogenesis. Teratology 8:113–126.

Robboy, S. J., R. E. Scully, W. R. Welch, and A. L. Herbst. 1977. Intrauterine diethylstilbestrol exposure and its consequences: Pathologic characteristics of vaginal adenosis, clear cell adenocarcinoma, and related lesions. Arch. Pathol. Lab. Med. 101:1–5.

Sawyer, R. N. 1977. Asbestos exposure in a Yale building: Analysis and resolution. Environ. Res. 13:146–169.

Seeler, R. A., J. N. Israel, J. E. Royal, C. I. Kaye, S. Rao, and M. Abulaban. 1979. Ganglioneuroblastoma and fetal hydantoin-alcohol syndromes. Pediatrics 63:524–527.

Sherman, S., and N. Roizen. 1976. Fetal hydantoin syndrome and neuroblastoma. Lancet 2:517.

Stanton, M. F., M. Layard, A. Tegeris, E. Miller, M. May, and E. Kent. 1977. Carcinogenicity of fibrous glass: Pleural response in the rat in relation to fiber dimension. J. Natl. Cancer Inst. 58:587–603.

Taylor, A. M. R., J. A. Metcalfe, J. M. Oxford, and D. G. Harnden. 1976. Is chromatid-type damage in ataxia telangiectasia after irradiation at G_0 a consequence of defective repair? Nature 260:441–443.

Wagner, J. C., C. A. Sleggs, and P. Marchand. 1960. Diffuse pleural mesothelioma and asbestos exposure in the North Western Cape Province. Br. J. Ind. Med. 17:260–271.

Wolff, S., B. Rodin, and J. E. Cleaver. 1977. Sister chromatid exchanges induced by mutagenic carcinogens in normal and xeroderma pigmentosum cells. Nature 265:347–349.

Status of the Curability of Childhood Cancers,
edited by J. van Eys and M. P. Sullivan.
Raven Press, New York © 1980.

A Veteran's Extrapolation—1979

John R. Hartmann, M.D., and F. Leonard Johnson, M.D.

Division of Hematology/Oncology of The Children's Orthopedic Hospital and Medical Center and The Fred Hutchinson Cancer Research Center, Seattle, Washington

"In most series the mortality rate in malignant disease exceeds 80%, with death usually occurring within one year after the diagnosis has been established. In many instances the tumor is incurable from its inception. . . .

"The achievements in diagnosis and therapy have been many and inspiring during the past decade. . . . However, the sum total is indeed small and only surface depth with what lies ahead" (Michael 1964).

Since Wardrop (1809) published the first series of descriptions of malignant tumors in children, the unique spectrum of childhood malignant diseases has been well defined, a fact that has had a major effect on the therapy and prognosis of childhood cancer. The tumors of childhood, involving most commonly the hematopoietic system, kidney, and soft tissue, are usually of mesodermal origin, in contrast to the common adult carcinomas, which are ectodermal or endodermal in origin (Sutow 1977).

Up until 30 years ago, the only progress that had been made in pediatric oncology was this definition of the unique types of tumors affecting children, for aside from surgical removal of a completely localized neoplasm, no specific therapy was available and cure was rare. Farber's introduction of aminopterin into the therapy of acute lymphoblastic leukemia (Farber et al. 1948) was the first step of many that would eventually result in over 50% of children with cancer being offered the possibility of cure (Pinkel et al. 1972) and a step that would lay to rest Dargeon's complaint that "childhood cancer has been a conspicuous example of the traditional inertia attending any seemingly insoluble human problem" (1960). Our therapeutic progress has been slow, and largely empirical, but nevertheless, when one compares the situation in 1964, when the textbooks said childhood leukemia was incurable (Michael 1964), to the present, when most children with acute lymphoblastic leukemia are able to discontinue therapy without ever having relapsed (Simone et al. 1975), there is no doubt that significant progress has been made.

Farber's first step was followed by at least eight subsequent steps along the path to our present situation:

1. The development of individual cytotoxic agents, many, such as 6-mercapto-purine, based on the principle of antimetabolic processes (Elion et al. 1952), and others, such as vincristine, found by serendipity (Johnson 1968);

2. The definition, derived from clinical studies in late-stage metastatic solid tumors and leukemia, of an effective role for a particular drug in a particular malignant disease, e.g., actinomycin D in Wilms' tumor (Farber et al. 1960), prednisone and vincristine in acute lymphoblastic leukemia (Harris 1979);

3. The recognition and understanding of the most effective way in which to use chemotherapeutic agents, especially in a localized malignant tumor, such as Wilms' tumor, namely, as an adjuvant to localized therapy with radiotherapy and surgery (Wolff et al. 1968);

4. The recognition in acute lymphoblastic leukemia that certain drugs are most effectively used in induction (vincristine and prednisone) and others in maintenance (methotrexate and 6-mercaptopurine), and that some sites, such as the central nervous system, require aggressive adjuvant therapy early in the course of treatment (Pinkel et al. 1972);

5. The development of more effective supportive care, with blood component therapy and broad-spectrum antibiotics permitting more aggressive chemothera-peutic protocols, such as the LSA_2-L_2 protocol for non-Hodgkin's lymphoma, to be successfully used (Wollner et al. 1975);

6. The development of centers designed to study and treat cancer in childhood and cooperation between centers both within and beyond specific cancer groups;

7. The recognition of and attempts to deal with the tremendous psychosocial effects of the diagnosis of childhood cancer on a family (Lansky et al. 1978); and

8. Finally, and perhaps most important, the development of the attitude that cancer in a child need not be fatal and, based on that premise, the development of curative therapeutic regimens with the resources available.

An idea of current progress can be gauged from our experiences at The Children's Orthopedic Hospital and Medical Center in Seattle with 283 children who presented consecutively with cancer between January 1, 1972, and December 31, 1974, all of whom have been followed at least 3½ years (Table 1). Forty-nine percent of these children are still alive, including 45% who have never had a recurrence of their tumor. Impressive therapeutic gains have been made in acute lymphoblastic leukemia, Hodgkin's disease, Wilms' tumor, rhabdomyo-sarcoma, and bone tumors. With the introduction of a more aggressive approach to non-Hodgkin's lymphoma (Woolner et al. 1975), the overall survival rate of patients with this once rapidly progressing malignant disease has increased to over 50%.

These steps, however, have taken us only a short way along the path to eventual understanding and cure, or ideally prevention, of childhood cancer. In acute nonlymphoblastic leukemia, neuroblastoma, and brain tumors, consis-tently effective therapy has yet to be devised. In addition, the long-term effects

Table 1. *Status of Patients Presenting Between 1/1/72 and 12/31/74*

Diagnosis	No. Patients	No. Alive, NED (%)	No. Dead, with Cancer (%)	No. Alive, with Disease (%)
Acute lymphocytic leukemia	87	44 (50.6)	37 (42.5)	6 (6.9)
Acute nonlymphocytic leukemia	25	1 (4.0)	24 (96.0)	
Brain tumors	37	17 (45.9)	15 (40.5)	5 (13.6)
Hodgkin's disease	13	12 (92.3)	1 (7.7)	
Non-Hodgkin's lymphoma	19	7 (36.8)	12 (63.2)	
Wilms' tumor	14	11 (78.6)	3 (21.4)	
Neuroblastoma	23	7 (30.4)	16 (69.6)	
Rhabdomyosarcoma	10	7 (70.0)	3 (30.0)	
Ewing's sarcoma	3	1 (33.3)	1 (33.3)	1 (33.3)
Osteogenic sarcoma	7	4 (57.1)	3 (42.9)	
Histiocytosis	12	9 (75.0)	3 (25.0)	
Retinoblastoma	2	1 (50.0)	1 (50.0)	
Other sarcomas	14	4 (28.6)	10 (71.4)	
Other carcinomas	7	3 (42.9)	3 (42.9)	1 (14.3)
Misc. others	10	6 (60.0)	4 (40.0)	

of current radiotherapy and chemotherapy regimens remain to be precisely defined and may present a significant dilemma for oncologists in the next several decades.

We must continue to evaluate and, if possible, modify therapy, the delayed complications of which may lead to growth retardation, intellectual impairment, abnormalities of the cardiovascular, hepatic, endocrine, exocrine, nervous, reproductive, and respiratory systems, and possibly even the development of secondary cancers in 8–16% of patients (Harris 1979, Li et al. 1975, Meadows and D'Angio 1974, Meadows et al. 1977).

It would seem that we have now reached a plateau in the therapy of pediatric cancer. Our most recent advances appear to be descriptive rather than therapeutic, as we try to learn more about the unique pathophysiology of the cancer cell. We have seen advances in our understanding of tumor cell kinetics, but cannot use this understanding reproducibly and consistently in the treatment of pediatric cancer. We have seen better definition of prognostic groups in leukemia, but are unable to devise therapy that will improve the poorer prognosis of children in certain of these categories. We have recognized morphological and enzyme markers of cancer cells, such as the L_1–L_2–L_3 morphology (Bennett et al. 1976) and terminal deoxynucleotidyl transferase (TdT) associated with leukemic lymphoblasts (McCaffrey et al. 1973), but are as yet unable to use this information to improve the outlook for childhood cancer. With solid malignant tumors such as Wilms' tumor, we now understand why certain children, despite having localized disease at diagnosis, do extremely poorly. Having recognized that a particular histological picture of anaplasia or sarcoma augers an especially poor prognosis, however, we are still unable to devise effective therapy to help these children (Beckwith and Palmer 1978).

In certain malignant diseases, such as non-Hodgkin's lymphoma, it is clear that a more aggressive cytotoxic approach has been therapeutically beneficial. In acute nonlymphoblastic leukemia or relapsed acute lymphoblastic leukemia, approaches using high-dose cyclophosphamide and total body irradiation followed by marrow transplantation from a suitably matched donor may improve the prognosis of these patients (Thomas et al. 1975). There is, however, a major problem associated with this more aggressive approach, in that it leads us away from therapy based on a precise knowledge of the biochemistry and physiology of the tumor cell or mechanisms aimed at promoting the body's own immunologic defenses in helping to eradicate a cancer.

The ultimate pathway to our goal of curing or preventing cancer must come from basic research into the biochemistry, pathophysiology, and immunology of the tumor cell. In the meantime, we can be encouraged by the tremendous progress that has been made in treating childhood cancer and that has been discussed in this symposium—encouraged but not complacent, for we must still work largely in the darkness of empiricism as we strive to make pediatric oncology centers as obsolete as tuberculosis sanitariums.

ACKNOWLEDGMENTS

This work was partially supported by grants CA-10382, CA-15704, and CA-18039 from the National Cancer Institute. Dr. Johnson is the recipient of A.C.S. Junior Faculty Clinical Fellowship 401.

REFERENCES

Beckwith, J. B., and N. S. Palmer. 1978. Histopathology and prognosis of Wilms' tumor. Cancer 41:1937–1948.
Bennett, J. M., D. Catovsky, M. T. Daniel, G. Flandrin, D. A. G. Galton, H. R. Gralnick, and C. Sultan. 1976. Proposals for classification of the acute leukemias. Br. J. Haematol. 33:451–458.
Dargeon, H. W. 1960. Tumors of Childhood: A Clinical Treatise. Paul B. Hoebner, Inc., New York, 476 pp.
Elion, G. B., E. Burgi, and G. H. Hitchings. 1952. Studies on condensed pyrimidine systems. IX. The synthesis of some 6-substituted purines. J. Am. Chem. Soc. 74:411–414.
Farber, S., G. D'Angio, A. Evans, and A. Mitus. 1960. Clinical studies of actinomycin D with special reference to Wilms' tumor in children. Ann. N.Y. Acad. Sci. 39:421–424.
Farber, S., L. K. Diamond, R. D. Mercer, R. S. Sylvester, and J. A. Wolff. 1948. Temporary remission in acute leukemia in children produced by folic acid antagonist 4-aminopteroyl-glutamic acid (aminopterin). N. Engl. J. Med. 238:787–793.
Harris, C. C. 1979. A delayed complication of cancer therapy—Cancer. Guest editorial. J. Natl. Cancer Inst. 63:275–277.
Johnson, I. S. 1968. Historical background of vinca alkaloid research and areas of future interest. Cancer Chemother. Rep. 52:455–461.
Lansky, S. B., N. U. Cairns, R. Hessanein, J. Wehr, and J. T. Lowman. 1978. Childhood cancer: Parental discord and divorce. Pediatrics 62:184–188.
Li, F. P., J. R. Cassady, and N. Jaffe. 1975. Risk of second tumors in survivors of childhood cancer. Cancer 35:1230–1235.
McCaffrey, R., D. F. Smoler, and D. Baltimore. 1973. Terminal deoxynucleotidyl transferase in a case of childhood acute lymphoblastic leukemia. Proc. Natl. Acad. Sci. U.S.A. 70:521–525.

Meadows, A. T., and G. J. D'Angio. 1974. Late effects of cancer treatment: Methods and techniques for detection. Semin. Oncol. 1:87–90.

Meadows, A. T., G. J. D'Angio, V. Miké, A. Banfi, C. Harris, R. Jenkins, and A. Schwartz. 1977. Pattern of second neoplasms in children. Cancer 40:1903–1911.

Michael, P. 1964. Tumors in Infancy and Childhood. J. P. Lippincott Co., Philadelphia, 461 pp.

Pinkel, D., J. Simone, H. D. Huston, and R. J. A. Aur. 1972. Nine years' experience with "total therapy" of childhood acute lymphocytic leukemia. Pediatrics 50:246–251.

Simone, J. V., M. S. Verzosa, and J. A. Rudy. 1975. Initial features and prognosis in 363 children with acute lymphoblastic leukemia. Cancer 36:2099–2108.

Sutow, W. W. 1977. General aspects of childhood cancer, *in* Clinical Pediatric Oncology, W. W. Sutow, T. J. Vietti, and D. J. Fernbach, eds. 2nd ed. C. V. Mosby Company, St. Louis, pp. 1–15.

Thomas, E. D., R. Storb, R. A. Clift, A. Fefer, F. L. Johnson, P. E. Nieman, K. G. Lerner, H. Glucksberg, and C. D. Buckner. 1975. Bone marrow transplantation. N. Engl. J. Med. 292:832–843, 895–902.

Wardrop, J. 1809. Observations on Fungus Haematodes. A. Constable, Edinburgh, 205 pp.

Wolff, J. A., W. Krivit, W. A. Newton, and G. J. D'Angio. 1968. Single versus multiple dose dactinomycin therapy of Wilms' tumor. N. Engl. J. Med. 279:290–294.

Wollner, N., J. H. Burchenal, P. H. Lieberman, P. R. Exelby, G. J. D'Angio, and M. L. Murphy. 1975. Non-Hodgkin's lymphoma in children. Med. Pediatr. Oncol. 1:235–263.

Author Index*

See also List of Contributors, pp. xiii–xv.

Subject Index

577246

3 1378 00577 2465